DONALD M. GOLDBERG

Principles of
Speech Audiometry

Principles of Speech Audiometry is a volume in the **PERSPECTIVES IN AUDIOLOGY SERIES**—Lyle L. Lloyd, Ph.D., series editor. Other volumes in the series include:

Published:

Forensic Audiology edited by Mark B. Kramer, Ph.D., and Joan Armbruster, M.S.

Aging and the Perception of Speech by Moe Bergman, Ed.D.

Communicating with Deaf People: A Resource Manual for Teachers and Students of American Sign Language by Harry W. Hoemann, Ph.D.

Language Development and Intervention with the Hearing Impaired by Richard R. Kretschmer, Jr., Ed.D., and Laura W. Kretschmer, Ed.D.

Noise and Audiology edited by David M. Lipscomb, Ph.D.

The Sounds of Speech Communication: A Primer of Acoustic Phonetics and Speech Perception by J. M. Pickett, Ph.D.

Hearing Assessment edited by William F. Rintelmann, Ph.D.

Auditory Management of Hearing-Impaired Children: Principles and Prerequisites for Intervention edited by Mark Ross, Ph.D., and Thomas G. Giolas, Ph.D.

Introduction to Aural Rehabilitation edited by Ronald L. Schow, Ph.D., and Michael A. Nerbonne, Ph.D.

Acoustical Factors Affecting Hearing Aid Performance edited by Gerald A. Studebaker, Ph.D., and Irving Hochberg, Ph.D.

American Sign Language and Sign Systems by Ronnie Bring Wilbur, Ph.D.

In Preparation:

Acoustic Amplification: A Unified Treatment by Harry Levitt, Ph.D.

Speech of the Hearing Impaired: Research, Training, and Personnel Preparation edited by Irving Hochberg, Ph.D., Harry Levitt, Ph.D., and Mary Joe Osberger, Ph.D.

Publisher's Note

Perspectives in Audiology is a carefully planned series of clinically oriented and basic science textbooks. The series is enriched by contributions from leading specialists in audiology and allied disciplines. Because technical language and terminology in these disciplines are constantly being refined and sometimes vary, this series has been edited as far as possible for consistency of style in conformity with current majority usage as set forth by the American Speech-Language-Hearing Association, the *Publication Manual of the American Psychological Association,* and the University of Chicago's *A Manual of Style.* University Park Press and the series editors and authors welcome readers' comments about individual volumes in the series or the series concept as a whole in the interest of making **Perspectives in Audiology** as useful as possible to students, teachers, clinicians, and scientists.

A Volume in the Perspectives in Audiology Series

PRINCIPLES OF SPEECH AUDIOMETRY

Edited by

Dan F. Konkle, Ph.D.
Division of Hearing and Speech Sciences
Vanderbilt University School of Medicine, and
Bill Wilkerson Hearing and Speech Center
Nashville, Tennesee

and

William F. Rintelmann, Ph.D.
Department of Audiology
Wayne State University School of Medicine
Detroit, Michigan

University Park Press

Baltimore

UNIVERSITY PARK PRESS
International Publishers in Science, Medicine, and Education
300 North Charles Street
Baltimore, Maryland 21201

Copyright © 1983 by University Park Press

Typeset by Maryland Composition Company
Manufactured in the United States of America by The Maple Press Company

All rights, including that of translation into other languages, reserved. Photomechanical reproduction (photocopy, microcopy) of this book or parts thereof without special permission of the publisher is prohibited.

Chapter 10 is the work of the United States government and thus is not under copyright.

Library of Congress Cataloging in Publication Data
Main entry under title:

Principles of speech audiometry.

(Perspectives in audiology series)
Includes indexes.
1. Audiometry, Speech.   I. Konkle, Dan F.
II. Rintelmann, William F.   III. Series.
RF294.5.S6P74   1983   617.8′0754   82-13612
ISBN 0-8391-1767-1

CONTENTS

Contributors / vii
Preface to *Perspectives in Audiology* / ix
Preface / xi

CHAPTER 1 **Introduction to Speech Audiometry**
Dan F. Konkle, Ph.D. and William F. Rintelmann, Ph.D. / 1

CHAPTER 2 **Historical Foundations of Speech Audiometry**
S. Richard Silverman, Ph.D. / 11

CHAPTER 3 **Acoustics and Perception of Speech**
Thomas H. Townsend, Ph.D. / 25

CHAPTER 4 **Calibration Measurements for Speech Audiometers**
Dan F. Konkle, Ph.D. and Thomas H. Townsend, Ph.D. / 55

CHAPTER 5 **Measurements of Auditory Thresholds for Speech Stimuli**
Richard H. Wilson, Ph.D., and Robert H. Margolis, Ph.D. / 79

CHAPTER 6 **Clinical Assessment of Speech Recognition**
Fred H. Bess, Ph.D. / 127

CHAPTER 7 **Measures of Discomfort and Most Comfortable Loudness**
Donald D. Dirks, Ph.D., and Donald E. Morgan, Ph.D. / 203

CHAPTER 8 **Speech Stimuli for Assessment of Central Auditory Disorders**
William F. Rintelmann, Ph.D., and George E. Lynn, Ph.D. / 231

CHAPTER 9 **Masking in Speech Audiometry**
Dan F. Konkle, Ph.D., and Grant A. Berry, M.A. / 285

CHAPTER 10 **Speech Audiometry and Hearing Aid Assessment: A Reappraisal of an Old Philosophy**
Daniel M. Schwartz, Ph.D., and Brian E. Walden, Ph.D. / 321

CHAPTER 11 **Speech Recognition and Aural Rehabilitation**
Elmer Owens, Ph.D. / 353

CHAPTER 12 **Research Trends and Clinical Needs in Speech Audiometry**
Wayne O. Olsen, Ph.D. / 375

Author Index / 396
Subject Index / 407

CONTRIBUTORS

Grant A. Berry, M.A.
Clinical Coordinator
Speech and Hearing Center
Hospital of the University of
 Pennsylvania
3400 Spruce Street
Philadelphia, Pennsylvania

Fred H. Bess, Ph.D.
Professor and Director
Division of Hearing and Speech
 Sciences
Vanderbilt University School of
 Medicine
and
Director
Bill Wilkerson Hearing and Speech
 Center
1114 19th Avenue South
Nashville, Tennessee

Donald D. Dirks, Ph.D.
Professor
Division of Head and Neck Surgery
 (Audiology)
School of Medicine
University of California, Los
 Angeles
Los Angeles, California

Dan F. Konkle, Ph.D.
Assistant Professor
Division of Hearing and Speech
 Sciences
Vanderbilt University School of
 Medicine
and
Bill Wilkerson Hearing and Speech
 Center
1114 19th Avenue South
Nashville, Tennessee

George E. Lynn, Ph.D.
Professor, Department of Audiology
Associate, Department of Neurology
Wayne State University School of
 Medicine
University Health Center, 5E
4201 St. Antione
Detroit, Michigan

Robert H. Margolis, Ph.D.
Associate Professor
Communicative Disorders
Director, Hearing Clinic
Syracuse University
Syracuse, New York

Donald E. Morgan, Ph.D.
Associate Professor
Division of Head and Neck Surgery
 (Audiology)
and
Director of Audiology Clinic
School of Medicine
University of California, Los
 Angeles
Los Angeles, California

Wayne O. Olsen, Ph.D.
Professor
Department of Otorhinolaryngology
Mayo Clinic and Mayo Foundation
Rochester, Minnesota

Elmer Owens, Ph.D.
Professor, Audiology and Speech
Department of Otolaryngology
University of California, San
 Francisco
400 Parnassus
San Francisco, California

William F. Rintelmann, Ph.D.
Professor and Chairman
Department of Audiology
Wayne State University School of
 Medicine
University Health Center, 5E
4201 St. Antoine
Detroit, Michigan

Daniel M. Schwartz, Ph.D.
Director
Speech and Hearing Center
Hospital of the University of
 Pennsylvania
3400 Spruce Street
and
Associate Professor
Department of Otorhinolaryngology
 and Human Communication
University of Pennsylvania School
 of Medicine
Philadelphia, Pennsylvania

S. Richard Silverman, Ph.D.
Director Emeritus
Central Institute for the Deaf
and
Professor of Audiology, Emeritus
Washington University
St. Louis, Missouri

Thomas H. Townsend, Ph.D.
Appalachian Audiological
 Associates
40 Lunt Drive
Greenfield, Massachusetts

Brian E. Walden, Ph.D.
Supervisor of Research Section
Army Audiology and Speech Center
Walter Reed Army Medical Center
Washington, D.C.

Richard H. Wilson, Ph.D.
Audiology Section
Veterans Administration Medical
 Center
5901 East Seventh Street
Long Beach, California
and
Associate Clinical Professor
Division of Otolaryngology
University of California, Irvine
Irvine, California

PREFACE TO PERSPECTIVES IN AUDIOLOGY

Audiology is a young, vibrant, dynamic field. Its lineage can be traced to the fields of education, medicine, physics, and psychology in the nineteenth century and the emergence of speech pathology in the first half of this century. The term "audiology," meaning the science of hearing, was coined by Raymond Carhart in 1947. Since then, its definition has expanded to include its professional nature. Audiology is the profession that provides knowledge and service in the areas of human hearing and, more broadly, human communication and its disorders. Audiology is also a major area of study in the professional preparation of speech pathologists, speech and hearing scientists, and otologists.

Perspectives in Audiology is the first series of books designed to cover the major areas of study in audiology. The interdisciplinary nature of the field is reflected by the scope of the volumes in this series. The volumes (see p. ii) include both clinically oriented and basic science texts. The series consists of topic-specific textbooks designed to meet the needs of today's advanced level student and of focal references for practicing audiologists and specialists in many related fields.

The **Perspectives in Audiology** series offers several advantages not usually found in most texts, but purposely featured in this series to increase the practical value of the books for practitioners and researchers, as well as for students and teachers.

1. Every volume includes thorough discussion of relevant clinical and/or research papers on each topic.
2. Most volumes are organized in an educational format to serve as the main text or as one of the main texts for graduate and advanced undergraduate students in courses on audiology and/or other studies concerned with human communication and its disorders.
3. Unlike ordinary texts, **Perspectives in Audiology** volumes will retain their professional reference value as focal reference sources for practitioners and researchers in career work long after completion of their studies.
4. Each volume serves as a rich source of authoritative, up-to-date information and valuable reviews for specialists in many fields, such as administration, audiology, early childhood studies, linguistics, otology, psychology, pediatrics, public health, special education, speech pathology, and/or speech and hearing science.

Principles of Speech Audiometry, edited by Dan F. Konkle and William F. Rintelmann, is a major volume in the **Perspectives in Audiology Series** in that it covers one of the more significant single clinical topics in the field of audiology—the use of speech stimuli. The measurement of auditory abilities is a major facet of audiology. The broad topic of audiologic assessment was presented in an earlier series volume edited by Dr. Rintelmann entitled **Hearing Assessment**. The present volume on speech audiometry is a logical focus and refinement of that volume. The basic audiologic assessment protocol consists of a combination of pure tone and speech stimuli. Although various other stimuli may be used for specific procedures, such as those used to determine site of lesion and habilitative planning, speech stimuli play a critical role in a comprehensive audiologic assessment. **Principles of Speech Audiometry** is a comprehensive and integrated text on the use of speech stimuli. Although the primary intent of the book is to serve as a graduate level text, this volume reflects the thorough coverage of the various aspects of speech audiometry, making it a valuable professional reference for clinicians and researchers.

Lyle L. Lloyd, Ph.D.
Chairman and Professor of Special Education
Professor of Audiology and Speech Sciences
Purdue University

PREFACE

This book is intended primarily as a text for graduate level courses in speech audiometry. Thus, chapters are organized into content areas consistent with the editors' perceptions and experiences with the various topics typically taught in speech audiometry courses. The rationales, procedures, and strategies associated with commonly used speech threshold and suprathreshold evaluative techniques are presented as they relate to both auditory assessment and aural rehabilitative applications. Although the book is designed to provide coverage of traditional speech audiometric procedures and related areas, the focus of some chapters is neither traditional nor conventional in the treatment of the subject matter. Indeed, although the contributors to this book were charged with producing clinically oriented manuscripts, they also were encouraged to examine critically the applications of speech audiometry that have become accepted as routine clinical procedures by many audiologists. Hence, this book also should be of value to practicing audiologists, otologists, and researchers who have an interest in the principles of speech audiometry.

The text stresses the use of standardized speech stimuli presented through calibrated systems to assess parameters of auditory function. Further, while comparisons regarding the relative value of various speech audiologic measures are not stressed, an emphasis is placed upon selecting specific techniques to provide information consistent with the intended application of the test findings. Guidelines for the interpretation of test findings, however, generally are provided within the context of comparing the responses for an individual listener to findings established previously either for the same listener, or for a homogeneous group of listeners. In this respect, much of the text is based on the vast body of literature describing normal auditory function. Specific efforts have been directed toward reminding the reader that abnormal auditory function must be defined in terms of normal hearing behavior and that specific abnormalities are best classified based on a profile of audiometric data rather than the results of a single test procedure.

The book is divided into twelve chapters. The first three present general information designed to familiarize the reader with the process of speech audiometry. Chapter 1 is an overview of speech audiologic assessment, including a review of the rationale for using speech stimuli to assess hearing and a brief examination of the common assessment strategies and clinical applications used in speech audiometry. The second chapter provides the reader with an historical perspective of the development of speech audiometry during the 1940s and 1950s. Chapter 3 focuses on the acoustics and perception of speech and is intended to introduce the reader to the basic physical properties of speech stimuli and to the fundamental concepts associated with decoding, processing, and converting speech signals into meaningful linguistic units. These initial three chapters, especially Chapter 3, highlight specific basic concepts and are not intended to present an exhaustive coverage of the topic areas. Chapters 4 through 9 are devoted to strategies and procedures necessary for the clinical application of speech audiometry. Chapter 4 discusses audiometer calibration for both earphone and sound field presentations of speech stimuli. The fifth chapter focuses on threshold measurement procedures, Chapter 6 considers speech recognition assessment when stimuli are presented at suprathreshold intensity levels, and Chapter 7 discusses the reliability, validity, and applicaton of suprathreshold measurements for loudness discomfort and most comfortable listening levels. The 8th chapter considers the use of speech signals to assess central auditory dysfunction. Chapter 9 is devoted to the application of contralateral masking in speech audiometry. While these six chapters provide the basis for clinical audiologic assessment with speech stimuli, they also challenge the reader to examine critically the rationales that justify using various speech audiometric procedures. Chapters 10 and 11 examine the role of speech audiometry in the aural rehabilitation process. The first of these two chapters reviews the use of speech stimuli for evaluating and selecting amplification for individuals with hearing impairment. Chapter 11 provides a discussion of speech recognition measures as they relate to: 1) indicating a need for aural rehabilitation, and 2) evaluating improvement in communicative skills as a result of aural rehabilitative programs. The final chapter, 12, examines current research trends and suggests some future clinical directions in speech audiometry. The content of this chapter is directed toward clinical needs and focuses on several areas in which future research might result in improved clinical applications. Chapter 12, for the most part, requires a basic understanding of concepts, speech test materials, and procedures discussed in the preceding chapters. Hence, Chapter 12 is not intended for the beginning graduate student.

This book was completed as the result of the efforts of many individuals, and the editors would be remiss if these persons were not acknowledged. First, we wish to express our most sincere appreciation to the contributors both for their chapters, and also for their cooperation, understanding, and patience during the production of this text. Next, three universities permitted the editors to devote substantial time to this project. The initial planning of the book and the early stages of its production were accomplished while both editors were on the Faculty of the University of Pennsylvania School of Medicine. The book was completed through the generous support of Vanderbilt University School of Medicine (DFK) and Wayne State University School of Medicine (WFR). Our secretarial staffs at these three universities devoted many long hours to assist us in the production of the text. We hereby express our thanks to Deborah Wray, Barbara Coulson, Pat Himmelberg, Lillie Abner, and Andrea Phillips. Several of our colleagues reviewed and offered valuable criticisms and suggestions concerning various chapters of the text. In this regard we are indebted to Fred Bess, Gene Bratt, Larry Humes, Sabina Kurdziel, Ralph Ohde, Wayne Olsen, and Jay Sanders. We also wish to acknowledge Lyle L. Lloyd, the Series Editor, and Janet S. Hankin, from University Park Press, for the opportunity to produce this text. Finally, we are grateful for the patience, understanding and support of our families (Pam, Matt, and Fred Konkle and Anne Rintelmann) during this entire project.

Dan F. Konkle
William F. Rintelmann

In fond memory of Raymond Carhart, Ph.D.

An internationally respected pioneer in the field of Audiology who with keen foresight wrote three decades ago:

> ... speech audiometry supplies a tool which can significantly enhance the diagnosis of hearing losses and the planning of appropriate programs for managing hard of hearing patients. (Carhart, R. 1952. Basic principles of speech audiometry, p. 71. Acta Otolaryngol. 40:62–71).

Clearly, these words are equally as challenging today.

CHAPTER 1
INTRODUCTION TO SPEECH AUDIOMETRY

Dan F. Konkle and William F. Rintelmann

CONTENTS

RATIONALE	2
ASSESSMENT STRATEGIES AND CLINICAL APPLICATIONS	3
Types of Speech Stimuli	3
Types of Listener Responses	6
Procedures for Presenting Stimuli and Recording Responses	7
Applications of Speech Audiometric Data	8
SUGGESTIONS FOR INTEGRATING SUBSEQUENT INFORMATION	9
REFERENCES	9

Although the discipline of audiology encompasses a broad range of activities, most audiologists devote a substantial portion of their time and energy to the assessment of the integrity of the auditory system. This process is termed *audiometry* and literally means hearing measurement. In clinical settings, audiometry usually is performed by observing, recording, and interpreting a listener's responses to controlled acoustic stimuli. Although many different types of stimuli and response protocols can be used to assess hearing, the majority of procedures commonly used in clinical settings involve the employment of both pure tone and speech audiometric stimuli. Pure tone audiometry refers to audiometric procedures that use tonal signals to assess hearing, whereas speech audiometry denotes the array of techniques using speech stimuli to assess auditory function. The purpose of this book is to focus on basic principles and clinical applications of speech audiometry.

The reader should realize at the outset that the content of this book in no way implies that speech audiometric measures are more important to the assessment of auditory function than pure tone procedures. Rather, both pure tone and speech audiometry provide useful information for the assessment and management of hearing disorders. While subsequent chapters of this text provide detailed discussions of various facets of speech audiometry, such information is most useful to those readers who also have a basic understanding of pure tone audiometry. Interested readers are referred to Martin (1975), Green (1978), or Wilber (1979) for reviews of pure tone audiometry.

The intent of this introductory chapter is to provide a brief overview of the topic of speech audiometry. Specifically, this chapter concerns: 1) the rationale for using speech as a stimulus to assess hearing; 2) the assessment strategies and applications of test findings commonly used in speech audiometry; and 3) suggestions for integrating the information contained in other chapters.

Within this chapter, various terms are identified and defined as they relate to the application of speech audiometry. The reader should be aware that, although terms are used consistently throughout this book, some terms differ from those used in other treatments of the same topics. In such instances, an explanation is provided in support of using a particular term, and in most cases preference is given to accepted usage by related professional disciplines.

RATIONALE

As noted previously, the two most common stimuli used clinically to assess hearing are pure tones and speech. Each of these signals, when used with appropriate clinical procedures, can provide valuable information concerning the integrity of the auditory system. Pure tone measures, for example, permit the audiologist to assess auditory function at discrete frequencies within the range of audibility. Findings from pure tone testing can be used to quantify the severity and configuration of hearing loss, as well as to suggest the presumed anatomical site of lesion. Pure tones, however, are relatively nonmeaningful stimuli that seldom are important to everyday listening or communication. Thus, the results of pure tone tests are of limited use to the clinician in predicting communicative deficits that may be associated with hearing loss. Among the more common complaints expressed by individuals with hearing loss are "I can hear, but I can't understand" or "I have a difficult time understanding someone when other people are talking." Moreover, it is well recognized that two individuals with similar hearing loss patterns as measured by pure tone audiometry often report different complaints regarding communicative problems. Such factors as age at onset, site of lesion, psychosocial demands, motivation, and intelligence, among other parameters, interact in a complex manner with the hearing loss to contribute to communicative handicaps. Consequently, although pure tone audiometric techniques can provide important data to quantify hearing loss, alternative stimuli must be used to assess communicative skills.

Because speech is an auditory stimulus that is vital to everyday listening and fundamental to the communicative process, speech stimuli are used in audiologic evaluations to assess the ability to hear and understand spoken materials. Within this context, the results of speech audiometry contain a certain amount of "face validity" for assessing communicative function. The actual predictive accuracy (i.e., validity) of speech audiometric data to assist in estimating communicative ability, however, depends upon several important factors. These include variables associated with assessment strategies (i.e., the type of speech material used as stimuli, the response mode required from the listener, and the procedures used to present the stimuli and to record the listener's responses) and, most importantly, the intended application of the findings. These factors are critically important and demand serious consideration.

ASSESSMENT STRATEGIES AND CLINICAL APPLICATIONS

Types of Speech Stimuli

The speech material selected as stimuli for hearing assessment depends primarily upon the purpose of the evaluation. Whereas the general rationale for speech audiometry is to provide information about communicative abilities that cannot be derived from the pure tone audiogram, it is unrealistic to expect a given sample of speech to be representative of all forms of verbal communication. Thus, different types of speech materials are used in speech audiometry depending upon the purpose and nature of the test. The following discussion briefly considers five of the more commonly used forms of speech material and presents the basic advantages and limitations associated with each.

Syllables Syllables are used in speech audiometry to examine a listener's ability to recognize phonemic units of speech. Syllables are used rather than individual phonemes because it is difficult to produce a phoneme in isolation. The phoneme /b/, for example, typically is pronounced as "buh." Thus, consonant (C) phonemes usually are combined with a vowel (V) with the consonant either in the initial (CV) or final (VC) position, and less frequently as a vowel-consonant-vowel (VCV) or consonant-vowel-consonant (CVC) arrangement. Syllables may be either meaningful monosyllabic words or nonsense stimuli. The primary advantage of using nonsense stimuli, compared to meaningful words, is to avoid influences that the listener's vocabulary may have on the correct identification of phonemes. An example of a nonsense syllable test used in speech audiometry is that of Levitt and Resnick (1978) described in Chapter 6.

Monosyllabic Words One of the most popular types of speech materials used for hearing assessment is meaningful monosyllabic (one syllable) words. These stimuli are convenient for constructing audiologic tests because there are a large number of such words comprising a pool from which word lists may be developed based on various criteria. The so-called phonetically or phonemically balanced word lists that are comprised of phonetic or phonemic units in approximate proportion to their use in everyday conversation are examples of this type of test material. Other criteria that have been employed include the construction of word lists comprised of phonemes known to be difficult to identify by a particular hearing loss population, or lists that contain both easy and difficult words. Chapter 6 provides further discussion of these concepts. Another advantage associated with the large pool of monosyllabic words is that several equivalent alternative word lists can be developed based on the same criteria without having to repeat words several times. Thus, alternative word lists can be used to avoid the influence of learning effects upon audiometric tasks that require repeated measures.

Like syllables, meaningful monosyllabic words are usually of the CV, VC, or CVC variety. Unlike syllables, however, care must be taken so that the monosyllabic words selected as stimuli are within the vocabulary of the listener. The reader should also recognize that although monosyllables can be meaningful words that are indeed representative of speech, such words only are first order approximations of speech encountered in everyday communication, that is, conversations are not usually restricted to monosyllabic words spoken in isolation. Hence, audiometric findings based on monosyllabic materials must be viewed with caution when applied as an index of overall communicative function. In spite of this limitation, monosyllabic words have received widespread use for many speech audiometric purposes.

Spondaic Words Spondaic words constitute a subcategory of dissyllabic (two-syllable) words that are produced with equal stress on each syllable. Examples of spondaic words (spondees) include *baseball*, *cowboy*, *sidewalk*, and *toothbrush*. Spondees are used in speech audiometry primarily to measure various types of thresholds. The concept of speech threshold is given detailed consideration in Chapter 5 and will be defined for the present discussion simply as the minimum intensity of a stimulus necessary to evoke a predetermined type of auditory sensation. It is common clinical practice to obtain the threshold of intelligibility for speech by using spondaic words presented at different intensity levels until the listener is able to recognize correctly 50 percent of the items. Because the measure of interest in this test is the intensity level necessary for a 50 percent correct response, it is important that each spondee used as a stimulus item can be perceived at essentially the same intensity level. Spondaic words basically satisfy this criterion because they are two-syllable words that contain many acoustic cues, they are pronounced with equal stress on each syllable, and the listener must perceive both syllables in order to recognize the item correctly. The concept just discussed is typically referred to as homogeneity for intelligibility. This characteristic of spondaic words makes them appropriate stimuli for threshold measurements and accounts for their popular use in speech audiometric assessment. Thresholds that are derived from spondaic words, however, are not necessarily representative of everyday speech. This limitation should be recognized and care should be taken to avoid overgeneralizing spondee thresholds as "truly" indicative of everyday communicative ability.

Sentences The use of syllables and words to assess speech intelligibility has been criticized because such material fails to represent realistic stimuli encountered in most communicative situations. A unit of speech that contains greater face validity in this respect is the sentence. Various forms of sentence material have been developed for use in speech audiometry; but, because most sentence tests have proven to be too easy, this type of stimulus has not received wide clinical acceptance. This is unfortunate, because sentence stimuli offer many of the practical advantages associated with syllables and words and constitute a more realistic representation of everyday communication.

Connected Speech Connected speech is the most valid type of material in representing everyday communicative function. Use of this type of stimulus in speech audiometry, however, has been restricted to detection measures such as most comfortable or uncomfortable listening levels. It is difficult to devise listener response formats for connected speech that provide quantified information about intelligibility. It is equally difficult to control the physical parameters (i.e., intensity, frequency, and time) of connected speech so that changes in such parameters can be related to communicative function. Another common application of connected speech is its use as a competing message. When used as a competing message, connected speech is presented to the listener at the same time as the primary signal. Whereas the listener's task is to respond to the primary signal and ignore the competing stimulus, the presence of the connected discourse makes the listening task more difficult. At the same time, however, introduction of a competing message makes the listening condition more realistic in terms of certain everyday communication experiences.

The types of speech material just discussed were selected because they represent stimuli commonly used in speech audiometry. Although there are other materials that also could be used in hearing measurement, the reader should realize that the selection of speech stimuli requires careful consideration. In addition to the many practical considerations, the selection of speech materials should be based on the purpose of the measurement and the application of the test findings. The subsequent chapters of this book provide information necessary to understanding both the advantages and disadvantages related to the use of specific speech materials in various speech audiometric applications.

Types of Listener Responses

The majority of speech audiometric procedures used clinically require a simple recognition type response. Unfortunately, the nature of this type of response often is misunderstood, especially by persons who do not have knowledge of the various speech audiometric procedures. The reason for this is that the terms used to describe test procedures typically do not reflect either the type of speech stimulus or the type of response required of the listener. To illustrate, the traditional threshold measure obtained in most clinical settings is called the speech reception threshold (SRT). This measurement involves the presentation of spondaic words at various intensity levels until the listener is able to correctly identify fifty percent of the items. The term *speech reception threshold*, however, is misleading because the measurement does not represent a threshold for *speech*, but a threshold for spondaic words only. If other types of material were used it is probable that different intensity values would be obtained, each supposedly representing a speech threshold. Of equal concern is use of the term *reception* to denote the listening task. Indeed, the task of the listener is to recognize, not receive, the spondaic word. Thus, to avoid possible confusion, this task would best be described as a spondaic word recognition threshold. Another example of a poorly termed speech audiometric procedure that uses the recognition type response is the so-called *speech discrimination* test. This measurement commonly is obtained by presenting a list of syllables, meaningful monosyllables, or sentences at a constant suprathreshold intensity level and asking the listener to report what is heard after the presentation of each stimulus item. The task is scored by expressing the number of correctly identified items as a percentage of the total number of items presented. Again, it would be more meaningful and less confusing to describe this measure as a function of the type of stimulus material used, rather than the more general term *speech*. More importantly, however, this procedure does not represent a discrimination task. Discrimination entails distinguishing between two or more stimuli. Because the listener is required only to report what is heard based on the presentation of a single item, this clinical procedure should be classified as a recognition measure rather than a discrimination score.

Another category of listener response depends upon judgments made based on previously defined criteria. The listener, for example, may be asked to adjust the intensity of connected speech to a level considered suitable for 50 percent intelligibility, perceived to be most comfortable, or judged to be uncomfortable. These types of response modes are subjective in that they neither convey a correct or incorrect index nor imply a degree of acceptability. Probably the greatest drawback to this type of response is that it is difficult to establish the validity of such measurements because the listener depends upon internal criteria to make judgements.

Procedures for Presenting Stimuli and Recording Responses

Recall that the primary purpose of speech audiometry is to assess the integrity of the auditory system and often to attempt to make some judgement about communicative ability. Intelligent clinical decisions concerning hearing integrity, however, cannot be made unless the performance of normal-hearing persons on the same audiometric tasks also is known. Otherwise stated, one cannot define abnormal responses before defining the range of normal behavior. Furthermore, comparing the findings of an individual listener to normative data is appropriate only when the same stimuli and procedures are used to collect both sets of data. These concepts are stressed in subsequent chapters, and will not be amplified here.

Consider, also, that most of the procedures used for speech audiometry in clinical settings today are the same or similar to those employed during the 1940s and early 1950s. Although this probably reflects the foresight of those involved with the initial development and construction of speech audiometric materials and procedures, it also suggests a reluctance on the part of audiologists to alter such practices or adapt newer strategies. Continued use of many of these early procedures can no longer be justified in view of technologic advancements and research findings. To illustrate, Martin and Forbis (1978) conducted a survey of audiologic procedures used clinically by American audiologists. The findings from this survey, based on 319 usable questionnaires, revealed that more than 96 percent of all audiologists performed speech testing as part of audiologic assessment. The majority, however, preferred to present the speech stimuli to listeners using monitored live voice techniques rather than using recorded materials. This practice cannot be justified because there is a substantial body of research and clinical data to indicate that live voice presentations increase test-retest measurement variability to a substantial degree and thus reduce reliability (Brandy, 1966; Hirsh et al., 1952; Hood and Poole, 1980; Kruel et al., 1968; Penrod, 1979). It must be recognized that only the original utterance of the speech stimuli comprises the test material. Hence, unless the original material is recorded or stored in computer memory for reproduction, it is not possible to control within- or between-talker differences. A series of live voice presentations of the same material, either by the same or different talkers, therefore, constitutes exposing the listener to a series of different test stimuli. Under such circumstances, test findings are confounded and, hence, difficult to interpret. Thus, audiologists should avoid using live voice presentations during speech audiometry.

Other findings that emerged from the Martin and Forbis survey revealed that over 80 percent of the audiologists used speech materials that were developed before 1955. Over 85 percent of the audiologists presented word recognition materials at a single suprathreshold intensity level despite research data to suggest that such a practice seldom provides adequate information to make appropriate clinical decisions (Bess, 1982; Carhart, 1965; Dirks, 1978; Olsen and Matkin, 1979). More than one half of the audiologists surveyed did not familiarize listeners with spondaic words before obtaining recognition thresholds, even though nearly two decades ago Tillman and Jerger (1959) reported that such a practice increases response variability. It is hoped that the information contained in subsequent chapters of this book will convince readers to avoid many of these unjustified practices.

In addition to procedural effects on test results, the methods employed to record the listener's responses also will influence speech audiometric findings. The typical method of recording responses for both threshold and suprathreshold word recognition measures is to judge the listener's verbal response as simply correct or incorrect. A record is seldom kept of the errors made in response to stimuli, yet such a practice could provide valuable information for structuring aural rehabilitative programs. Also, the most frequently used response protocol requires that the listener verbally repeat what is heard, thereby also testing the ability of the examiner to correctly recognize what the listener actually said. More frequent use of "write down" types of responses could avoid the potential influence of examiner bias that may result from the verbal response. Both Chapters 6 and 11 provide more discussion of these topics.

Applications of Speech Audiometric Data

Clinical findings from speech audiometric tests are used to: 1) quantify the magnitude of hearing loss; 2) predict the potential site of auditory lesion; 3) estimate hearing handicap; 4) identify candidates for amplification and select and evaluate hearing aid systems; 5) structure rehabilitative programs; and 6) evaluate the success of medical, surgical, or rehabilitative interventions regarding the restoration of auditory function. The degree to which these various applications of speech audiometry are successfully achieved is considered in detail throughout the remaining chapters of this text. The clinical findings that guide these applications result from the assessment of various forms of auditory behavior including both threshold and suprathreshold recognition abilities, different types of loudness phenomena and subjective judgements of speech quality. Underlying the applications of speech audiometric data and assessment of auditory behavior is an array of procedures and materials, many of which may be used interchangeably to evaluate diverse auditory functions. This versatility in conjunction with the numerous clinical applications probably accounts for the popularity of speech audiometry. These same attributes, however, serve to stress the importance of having a complete and thorough understanding of the principles related to speech audiometry. Failure to understand adequately the strengths and, most importantly, the limitations of the variables (discussed throughout this text) concerning the application of speech audiometric data can result in gross misapplication of clinical findings. Conversely, careful and appropriate use of speech stimuli and measurement procedures can provide valuable audiologic information.

SUGGESTIONS FOR INTERGRATING SUBSEQUENT INFORMATION

As noted previously, speech audiometry is a versatile clinical tool because it has many applications. In order to obtain the most information from speech audiometric data, however, it is best to assess several aspects of auditory behavior so that a profile of results is available for interpretation. Consequently, the chapters of this book have been arranged in a sequence that relates more to the types of applications rather than to specific test procedures. It is recommended that the reader use this organization to integrate the information contained in this text. It would be most beneficial to progress through the book by reading each chapter in sequence, because much of the material in the latter chapters is based, in part, on concepts explained in the first several chapters.

Finally, the reader should be aware that the charge to the contributors of this book was to provide a clinical treatment. In many cases, space restrictions have required contributors to confine their discussions to those areas considered to be of greatest clinical relevance. Regardless of the depth of treatment, however, references are provided throughout the book to assist the reader who wishes to pursue specific topics further.

REFERENCES

Bess, F. 1982. Basic hearing measurement. In N. Lass, L. McReynolds, J. Northern, and D. Yoder (eds.), Speech, Language, and Hearing. W. B. Saunders Company, Philadelphia.

Brandy, W. T. 1966. Reliability of voice tests of speech discrimination. J. Speech Hear. Res. 9:461–465.

Carhart, R. 1965. Problems in the measurement of speech discrimination. Arch. Otolaryngol. 82:253–260.

Dirks, D. 1978. Effects of hearing impairment of the auditory system. In E. Caterette and M. Friedman (eds.), Handbook of Perception, Volume IV: Hearing, pp. 567–608. Academic Press, Inc., New York.

Green, D. 1978. Pure tone air-conduction testing. In J. Katz (ed.), Handbook of Clinical Audiology, pp. 98–109. 2nd Ed. Williams & Wilkins Company, Baltimore.

Hirsh, I., H. Davis, S. Silverman, E. Reynolds, E. Eldert, and R. Benson. 1952. Development of materials for speech audiometry. J. Speech Hear. Disord. 17:321–337.

Hood, J., and J. Poole. 1980. Influence of the speaker and other factors affecting speech intelligibility. Audiology 19:434–455.

Kruel, E., J. Nixon, K. Kryter, D. Bell, J. Lang, and E. Schubert. 1968. A proposed clinical test of speech discrimination. J. Speech Hear. Disord. 11:536–552.

Levitt, H., and S. Resnick. 1978. Speech reception by the hearing impaired: Methods of testing and the development of new tests. Scand. Audiol. 6 (Suppl.):107–130.

Martin, F. 1975. Introduction to Audiology. Prentice-Hall, Inc., Englewood Cliffs, N.J.

Martin, F., and N. Forbis. 1978. The present status of audiometric practice: A follow-up study. Asha 20:531–541.

Olsen, W., and N. Matkin. 1979. Speech audiometry. In W. Rintelmann (ed.), Hearing Assessment, pp. 133–206. University Park Press, Baltimore.

Penrod, J. 1979. Talker effects on word-discrimination scores of adults with sensorineural hearing impairment. J. Speech Hear. Disord. 44:340–349.

Tillman, T., and J. Jerger. 1959. Some factors affecting the spondee threshold in normal-hearing subjects. J. Speech Hear. Res. 2:141–146.

Wilber, L. 1979. Pure tone audiometry: Air and bone conduction. In W. Rintelmann (ed.), Hearing Assessment, pp. 20–50. University Park Press, Baltimore.

CHAPTER 2

HISTORICAL FOUNDATIONS OF SPEECH AUDIOMETRY

S. Richard Silverman

CONTENTS

EARLY USES OF SPEECH AS TEST MATERIAL 11
IMPACT OF WORLD WAR II 14
INCREASE IN CLINICAL APPLICATIONS 18
REFERENCES 24

EARLY USES OF SPEECH AS TEST MATERIAL

Although this chapter deals with the early modern era of the development of speech audiometry, roughly the 1940s and 1950s, it is interesting to note that speech was used as test material for an audiologic purpose as long as two centuries ago. The specific application then and in the nineteenth century was on the evaluation of what, in current terminology, we would call auditory training. According to Urbantschitsch (1895), Ernaud in 1761, Pereire in 1767, and Itard in 1805, among others, all attempted to document the value of concentrated and sustained auditory stimulation by pre- and post-training responses of severely and profoundly hearing-impaired children to syllables, words, and sentences. In his classic monograph on auditory training, Urbantschitsch (1895) included detailed speech recognition data on 60 subjects. Of course, lack of modern instrumentation precluded precise quantification of testing conditions and of results, but the important historical point is that speech was considered to have significant face validity in evaluating a procedure much as it is done today, for example, in evaluating the effects of surgery or of an instrument, a hearing aid. Audiology does indeed have a prehistory.

Modern speech audiometry and its application to various aspects of current audiologic practice developed originally in the context of testing communication systems during World War II. To the extent that the middle and inner ear function as a physical acoustic system, there is no logical break from the testing of communication systems. Fletcher and Steinberg (1929) and their associates at the Bell Telephone Laboratories (BTL) laid the groundwork for the subsequent wartime activity as their ideas for using speech as test material was applied to assess the efficiency of speech transmission of any kind. They were especially interested in measuring not only the performance of elements or components of a system but also in determining the amount of distortion, such as selective filtering, that could be tolerated without undue degrading of speech transmission. In other words, how *little* information can be transmitted without jeopardizing accurate reception of the message?

In developing tests for these purposes, the people at BTL were guided by two fundamental criteria for choice of speech material. The material had to be representative of English speech and it also had to be suitable for making tests the results of which could be properly quantified. The test framers recognized that these two criteria were frequently in conflict and that compromises were called for. The compromise consisted of the construction of two general classes of tests. One concerned with analysis of accuracy of reception of fundamental units of speech, vowels, consonants, syllables, and, occasionally, words, was called an articulation test. The other employed sentences as test items and was called an intelligibility test.

Much of what is currently subsumed under the rubric *speech audiometry* was what Fletcher and his group referred to as *articulation testing*. As is elaborated elsewhere in this book, the articulation function is a basic concept involved in articulation testing and essentially it expresses the relation between percentage of speech units (syllables, words, sentences) heard correctly and the intensity of the speech at the ear of the listener.

Articulation test items were generally of the consonant-vowel (CV) type: wi, key word: wi(th) or the consonant-vowel-consonant (CVC) type: shol, key word shoal. Many lists of 50 words were compiled, with each word list characterized by what was determined to be adequate sampling. These were written on cards; and the tester read them to a listener, who then wrote his responses. The data were then plotted as an articulation function an example of which is given in Figure 2-1. It was soon apparent that subjects required a good deal of training to participate in the CV and CVC type tests. An alternate procedure was developed using simple word lists wherein only the vowel or only the consonant was varied (for example bat-bet-bait, etc. and sigh-shy-thigh). For the purposes of the laboratory, however, the syllabic lists were preferable because they sampled more sounds with fewer items and hence used less time to get the information that was being sought. When a large amount of time was not a crucial factor as in the case of testing the untrained hearing-impaired individual, the word lists were to be preferred.

Nevertheless, importance was also attached to intelligibility tests as defined by Fletcher (1929). He stated that ". . . the intelligibility of a system transmitting speech is defined as the percent of ideas ex-

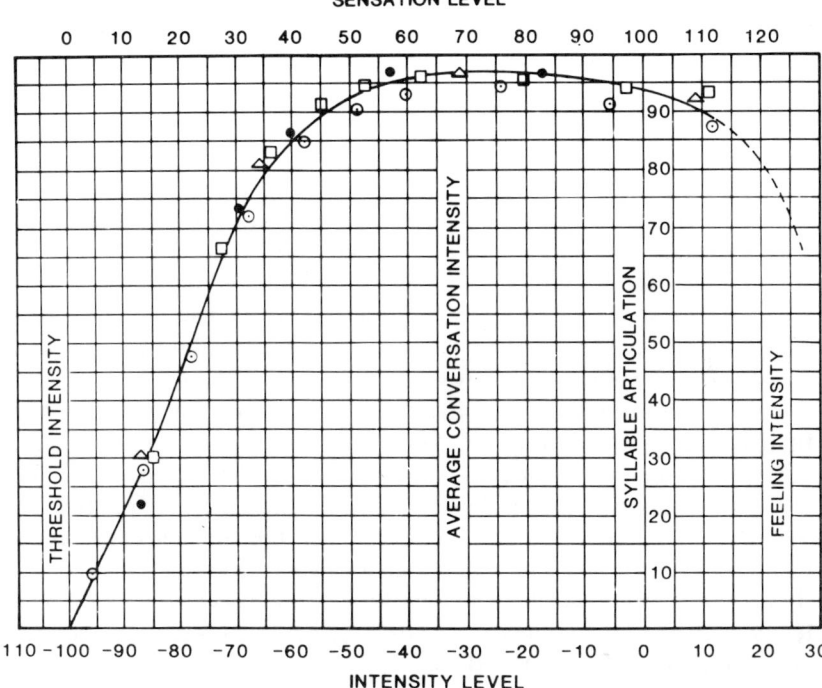

Figure 2-1. Articulation versus intensity of received speech. (Adapted from Fletcher, 1929)

pressed in the form of simple test sentences, which, after transmission, are correctly understood by a number of observers'' (p. 264). He suggested that "it is probable that the intelligibility is more directly related to the thing which it is desired to measure than is articulation" (p. 264). Forty-nine lists of 50 simple interrogative and imperative sentences each were compiled. The idea was to test observers' "acuteness of perception" that required hearing and understanding of key "thought" words related to many subjects of common public interest (for example, How large is the sun compared with the earth? or Explain why a corked bottle floats). The nagging problems, especially in a clinical context, of sentence intelligibility testing that in a sense still persist were evident in these early tests. Among them were difficulties of scoring, linguistic and cultural sophistication of subjects, optimum response mode, syntactic and semantic sampling, equivalence of lists, and others referred to later in this chapter and elsewhere in this book.

The next obvious step for the BTL group was to determine experimentally the relation between syllable articulation and intelligibility tests. The general approach was to relate recognition of test items to distortion. In general it was found that test sentences are useful for testing systems in which distortions are large, but are of little value for testing ordinary transmission systems with lesser distortion (Fletcher, 1929). This finding appears to be currently pertinent to the tough problem of valid evaluation of hearing aids.

At about the same time Fletcher (1929) described speech audiometry for screening school children for hearing loss. The test material was recorded pairs of digits, *one* through *nine* omitting the bisyllable *seven*, presented to multiple headphones in descending steps of 3 dB. Given the message set, this was essentially a vowel discrimination test. The children wrote their responses on a form prepared for the purpose. The test in its latest version was officially called the 4C test but was popularly referred to as the fading numbers test. The 4C test was fundamentally not too different from the conversation and whispered voice test. The end point of this latter test was the distance at which a listener could just repeat digits spoken by the examiner related to a "standard" distance, much as is done with the Snellen chart in the testing of vision. The conversational voice presumably sampled low frequency hearing and the whispered voice the high frequencies. This test was used in examining the hearing of potential inductees into the armed forces in World War II.

Experience with the application of the 4C test sounds a note of caution for those of us who resort to the numbers game in emphasizing the seriousness of all manner of human ailments. Out of a survey in New York City came a spectacular statistic that figured rather prominently in an advertising controversy many years later, claiming "3,000,000 hard-of-hearing children in the United States." The total was estimated by applying to the U.S. population of children the percentage that failed the 4C screening test. No one seemed to know or care that the percentage of failures was built into the scoring system. It was the percentage that fell outside the two-standard deviations limit of the scores of the group. But perhaps this bit of statistical legerdemain actually helped the cause of hearing conservation in children.

IMPACT OF WORLD WAR II

The need and the potential usefulness of speech audiometry came to the fore in the context of the World War II military "aural rehabilitation" programs developed to serve personnel whose hearing was impaired for whatever reason. An estimated 15,000 servicemen received help for their hearing impairments in these military centers established specifically for their needs. These services were available at Deshon (Butler, Pennsylvania), Borden (Chickasha, Oklahoma), and Hoff (Santa Barbara, California) General Hospitals for the Army and at the United States Naval Hospital (Philadelphia, Pennsylvania). These centers merit our citation because many of their personnel were stimulated in the post-war period to pursue productive professional and academic careers in some aspect of the emerging field of audiology. Among them were Moe Bergman, Raymond Carhart, Louis DiCarlo, Leo Doerfler, Grant Fairbanks, William Hardy, Miriam Hardy, Ira Hirsh, and Herbert Koepp-Baker. Associated with them in an advisory, consultative, or collaborative capacity were a substantial number of the workers at the Psycho-Acoustic Laboratories (PAL) at Harvard University including Hallowell Davis, James Egan, Clarence Hudgins, Clifford Morgan, Gordon Peterson, Douglas Ross and S. S. Stevens. Leo Beranek, at Harvard's Cruft Laboratory, was also involved, as were Rudolph Nichols at the Bell Telephone Laboratories and this writer at Central Institute for the Deaf (CID).

As prominent as any activity in the military rehabilitation programs was the provision of a hearing aid to the hearing-impaired serviceman. This required some measure of the relative effectiveness of instruments from among a number that were available. Needed was a test that involved presentation of material in the "free field" to the microphone of a body-worn aid, the results of which could be compared with unaided responses of a listener. Speech was chosen as the input signal because of high face validity and because it was not as sensitive to the acoustic conditions in the test room as were pure tones. It was decided to develop a test that would determine the threshold for speech and the threshold shift in the aided ear would determine the improvement in sensitivity of the listener.

The concept of the threshold, as it is derived from speech audiometry, requires some clarification. Three thresholds can be distinguished: 1) the threshold of detectability, defined as the point at which the listener is just able to detect speech sounds about half the time and is not able ordinarily to identify any of the sounds themselves; 2) the threshold of perceptibility, defined as the point at which the listener begins to perceive some words but can barely follow the gist of connected speech; and 3) the threshold of intelligibility, defined as the point at which the listener understands half the material presented to him and can presumably follow without perceptible effort the gist of connected speech. In the clinical context, the threshold of intelligibility turned out to be most frequently used.

In constructing a test to determine the threshold of intelligibility, Hudgins et al. (1947) suggested that the test items should meet the following criteria: 1) familiarity, the vocabulary should be within the intellectual ken of the listener; 2) phonetic dissimilarity, fine discriminations (cowboy-plowboy) should not be necessary, because no useful purpose is served by them in threshold tests; 3) normal sampling of English speech sounds, not essential for threshold testing, but a reasonable sampling is desirable; and 4) homogeneity with respect to basic audibility, the ease with which test words are understood should be as equivalent as possible so that small numbers of items can be scrambled and the articulation function will rise steeply over a narrow range of intensity.

A test which meets these criteria was developed by Hudgins and associates at the PAL. It consisted of lists of dissyllabic words of the spondee stress pattern, that is, such words as *earthquake*, *hardware*, in which both syllables are generally accented equally. The level at which the subject repeats half the words correctly is the threshold of hearing. From the standpoint of hearing impairment, the hearing loss was defined as the number of decibels more required by the impaired ear to hear the equivalent number of words. Early in its history this test was referred to as Psycho-Acoustic Laboratory Test Number 9 because it was the ninth of a series using speech as the test material. The stimulus words can be presented by recordings or by live voice. The modification of the recorded version which is widely used clinically is discussed later in this chapter. Obviously, live voice presentation requires a well trained talker.

Like the Bell Laboratory group before them, the PAL workers constructed a sentence intelligibility test (Number 12). Aware of the information and vocabulary load placed on listeners by the Bell sentences, the PAL group used sentences that were all questions, were much simpler, and could be answered by a single word (for example, What number comes before 10? What day comes before Sunday?; Hudgins et al., 1947). These sentences have been recorded in groups of four at successively lower intensities and are thus useful in obtaining a threshold for speech. The level thus obtained is about 4 dB above the threshold measured by the spondaic words. Its difficulty of scoring and its high correlation with the spondee test designed to obtain the same end point has resulted in very little, if any, clinical use.

Another speech test (not using the concept of the articulation function) was described by Falconer and Davis (1947). In this test the subject listens to a sample of recorded connected discourse and manipulates the attenuator until he is just able to get the gist of what is being said. His hearing loss is the number of decibels more that his ear requires than the normal ear to reach his threshold of intelligibility for connected discourse. This test had the advantage of economy of time and high face validity. The end point, on the other hand, was relatively not very definitive. Dr. Davis dubbed the material of the test *cold running speech*. However, Thurlow et al. (1948) found that hearing losses for speech determined by a variety of the types of tests described correlated so closely with one another that only one of them need be used in any clinical routine.

As is stressed elsewhere in this book, not only is it important to determine the faintest speech an ear can hear, measured by threshold tests, but it is of clinical significance to know how the ear hears speech at any intensity, particularly that above threshold. Clinicians are familiar with the patient who says, "I hear but I can't understand; I can hear better if you speak clearly rather than loudly." This patient's problem is not delineated by the threshold test. Granted that a sound must be audible before it can be distinguished from the other sounds, the fact that it is audible does not necessarily guarantee that it can be recognized accurately. The ability to distinguish one sound from another when both are audible is called discrimination as distinguished from sensitivity, which refers to the faintest sound that the ear can hear. In addition to sensitivity, a high degree of discrimination is needed to distinguish *sin* from *thin* and *pit* from *pith*.

In constructing a test to measure the power of discrimination (or, clinically, the discrimination loss) Egan (1948) suggested consideration of these points: 1) phonetic balance (PB), reasonable proportional representation in the test lists of the sounds that occur in everyday speech insures that the test measures what it sets out to measure, that is, how the ear copes with the task of discriminating speech that it is likely to have to discriminate in routine oral communication; 2) types of test items, words appear to be preferable to nonsense syllables, which may require recording by phonetic symbols and to sentences that may afford contextual clues; and 3) difficulty and reliability of test lists, the test items must be selected so that the distribution of item difficulty in each list will create a sensitive measuring instrument. In other words, those items which, under conditions of the tests, are always recorded correctly or are always missed should be eliminated from the test lists. Of course, for both sensitivity tests and discrimination tests many equivalent lists should be available to cut down the learning factor when more than one test is necessary.

Egan (1948) and his associates at the PAL constructed a test that consists of 20 equivalent phonetically balanced lists of 50 words each. It is worth noting that what constitutes phonetic balance in samples of the English language is an open question. Egan's referent for phonetic balance was the work of Godfrey Dewey (1923), who made an extensive study of the frequency of occurrence of words, syllables, and fundamental vowel and consonant sounds in written material from

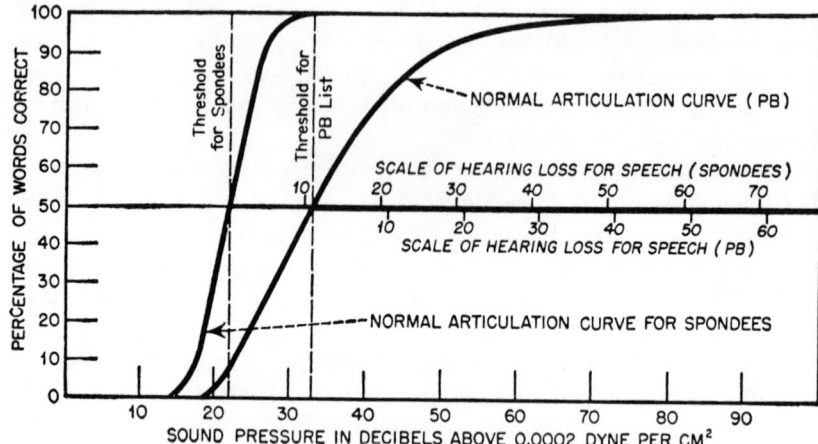

Figure 2-2. Relation of spondee and PB tests. (Adapted from Davis, 1947)

various conventional sources. However, French, Carter, and Koenig's (1930) analysis of telephone conversation differed considerably from the Dewey data. Nevertheless, the Egan lists became the material of choice for clinical purposes, probably because they appeared quite early in the post-war clinical literature.

A comparison of the shapes of the spondee test and phonetically balanced curves taken from Davis (1947) is shown in Figure 2-2. Notice that the spondee curve rises steeply because the words are almost equally audible and intelligible, whereas the phonetically balanced curve rises more gradually because the words represent the broad range of difficulty encountered in everyday speech.

INCREASE IN CLINICAL APPLICATIONS

An early and legitimate application of speech audiometry to a clinical problem was in the selection of patients suitable for the fenestration operation (Walsh and Silverman, 1946). This surgery involved fenestration of the horizontal semicircular canal in cases of otosclerosis. Speech material presented at high intensity levels conventionally about 30 to 40 dB above threshold served to assess the so-called "cochlear reserve" that might be used successfully if more efficient conduction could be provided. In this context the distinction was made between sensitivity (measured by spondaic words) and discrimination, independent of sensitivity, measured as the maximum score on a list of phonetically balanced words delivered to the ear at an appropriate level above threshold ("PB Max"). It was recognized that complete loss of sensitivity for high frequencies might reduce the discrimination score. The application to evaluation of surgery is shown in Figure 2-3, displaying the articulation functions of an ear before and after the fenestration operation related to the curve for the normal ear (Silverman et al., 1948).

Another clinical application appeared at this time. Certain disorders of the sensorineural class lead to much greater impairment of discrimination than can be explained on the basis of selective loss of sensitivity. This condition has often been wrongly termed *recruitment* and the distinction has not always been clear between sense organ dysfunction and a selective loss of sensitivity for high frequencies which may be based on an anatomical loss of high-frequency sensory units. At this time, too, speech audiometry as applied in the Doerfler-Stewart Test (1946) was employed to address the difficult problems of feigned and psychogenic hearing loss. This test depends on the interference by noise with the understanding of speech. Speech and noise levels given to the same ear are systematically varied, making it difficult for the feigning listener to retain a constant ratio of noise to speech.

A second and independent use of speech audiometry was the assessment of the social adequacy of hearing. This is based on the concept of hearing and understanding everyday speech, that is, simple speech in context, although the actual tests were usually done with lists of monosyllabic words. As we have seen, speech audiometry has been used to evaluate the results of surgery and other therapy and also the effectiveness of hearing aids. It has been made, in principle, the basis of medico-legal systems of determining compensation for industrial hearing loss although, ironically enough, the pure tone audiometer is the instrument of choice for making the actual measurements and the presumed hearing level for speech is obtained by averaging the hearing levels for certain selected audiometric frequencies.

Davis (1948) elaborated the notion of the social adequacy index suggested by Walsh and Silverman (1946) and brought various tests into quantitative relation. This is shown in Figure 2-4. He also presented a table for the rapid calculation of the social adequacy index.

The growing popularity of speech audiometry suggested a need for standardization in order to accomplish useful exchange of clinical findings. This led to the development by Hirsh et al. (1952), at Central Institute for the Deaf, of recorded tests W-1 and 2 and W-22, which were refinements of the spondee and PB tests, respectively.

Tests W-1 and W-2 were modifications of PAL Test No. 9 designed to measure threshold for speech by reducing the number of items in six different scramblings to 36, selecting those that ranked high in familiarity and were equal in intelligibility when spoken at the same

20 Silverman

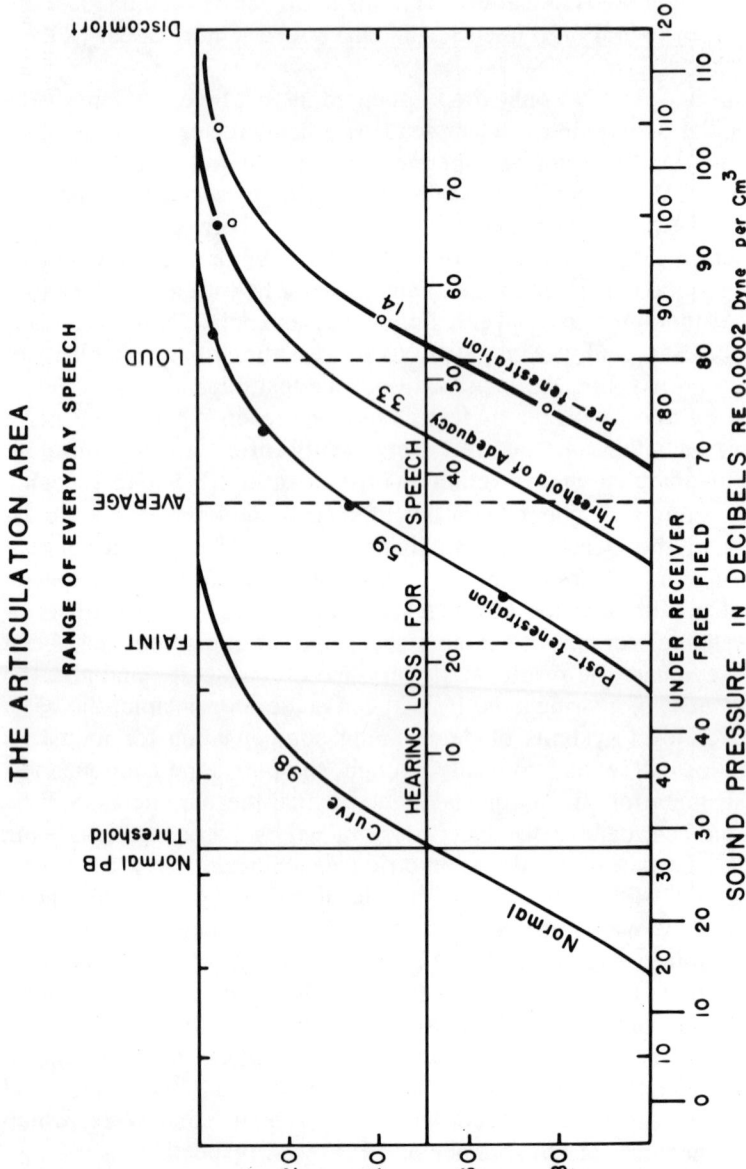

Figure 2-3. Graph showing change in articulation in fenestrated ear. (Adapted from Silverman et al., 1948)

Historical Foundations 21

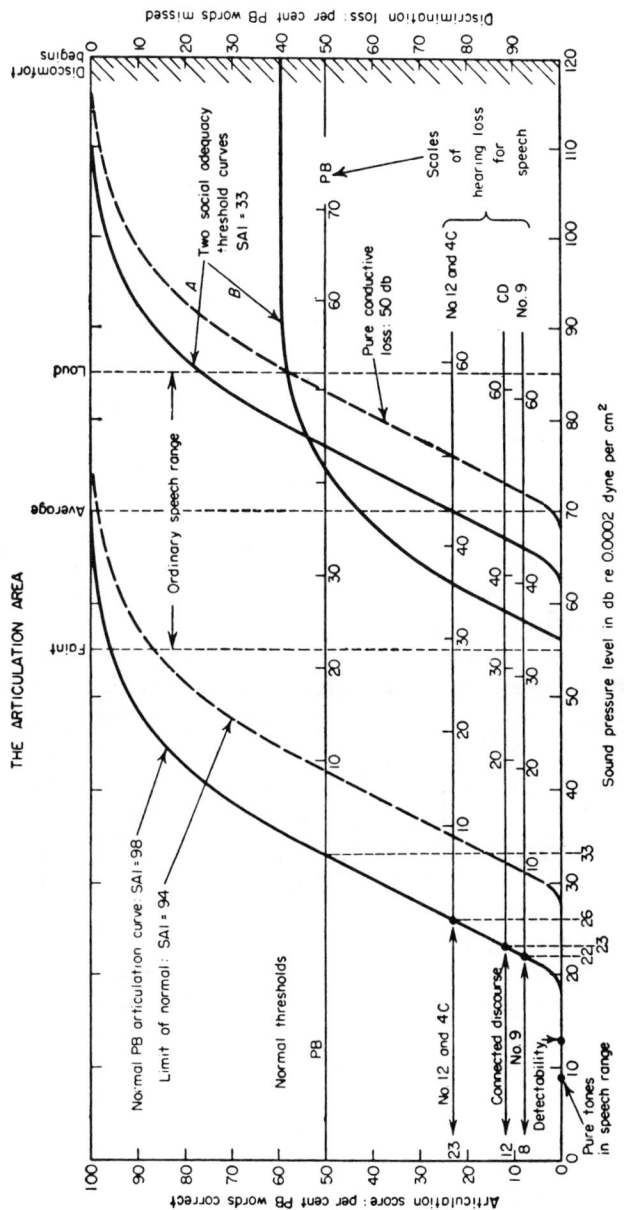

Figure 2-4. The articulation area. These curves are based on the phonetically balanced word lists of the Psycho-Acoustic Laboratory, as recorded at the Central Institute for the Deaf, as of January 1948. The other thresholds are for recorded tests used with the same apparatus: No. 9 (spondee words) and No. 12 (sentences), Psycho-Acoustic Laboratory, Harvard; 4C (pairs of one-digit numbers), Western Electric Company, and connected discourses (thresholds of intelligibility and detectability), newscast by Fulton Lewis Jr., Central Institute for the Deaf. The social adequacy index is the average percentage of phonetically balanced words that would be correctly understood by the patient at the three speech levels indicated by the dotted lines. (Adapted from Davis, 1948)

intensity into a volume unit (VU) meter. In test W-1 all of the spondaic words are recorded at the same intensity with a carrier phrase recorded at a level 10 dB higher. A 1000-Hz calibration tone is also recorded at this level. In W-2 the intensity of the words descends systematically by 3 dB for each successive group of three words. With this form of test it is necessary only to count the number of words repeated correctly. Each word correct lowers the threshold level by 1 dB.

CID Auditory Test W-22 is a modification of Egan's phonetically balanced word lists. It consists of a set of recordings of such lists that represent a more restricted and simpler vocabulary than the original PAL lists. In general, the CID modifications of the original PAL tests have accomplished improved item selection, more accurate specification of recording characteristics, and greater flexibility, resulting in a sufficient degree of uniformity that has contributed substantially to useful and frequent communication among investigators and clinicians of speech threshold and discrimination data.

After the introduction of CID test W-22, informal reports to Silverman and Hirsh (1955) raised questions about the power of the test to distinguish between conductive and nonconductive hearing losses. There seemed to be a difference between W-22 and previously recorded versions of the PB lists, especially the Rush Hughes recordings. Tests of patients showed that this was, in fact, so. Silverman and Hirsh (1955) urged caution in the use of the tests. They suggested that in the measurement of discrimination loss for *diagnosis* it is not speech as the basis of communication that is important but what is significant is speech as a *particular kind of auditory stimulus* whose properties they were not able to specify. On the other hand, for assessment for hearing disability it is the practical feature of speech communication that is the basic factor for choice of material for a test that ultimately must be validated in the field. To accomplish this the Armed Forces National Research Committee on Hearing and Bio-Acoustics (CHABA) in 1958 appointed a working group (Chairman, Grant Fairbanks) to formulate a set of criteria for a representative sample of everyday speech, with the one a priori assumption that the sample item should be the sentence. The CID Everyday Sentence Test, developed in 1959, was the result of this activity (Davis and Silverman, 1978).

Clinical experience with simpler forms of speech audiometry suggested a variety of other uses described in this book which are currently applied. It was recognized that speech is a series of complex acoustic signals that are part of an established code, namely, language. Speech carries meaning. The ability or the failure of individuals to deal with such signals may be used to separate clinical cases into categories. For example, low PB Max discrimination scores for monosyllabic words may separate sense-organ from conductive impairment. Almost all of the modifications of speech audiometry, however, represent some deliberate distortion of speech signal to make more difficult the necessary interpolations or the resynthesis of partial or disjointed patterns, or perhaps the performance of the usual tasks at unusually high speed. Favorite varieties of distortion have been: 1) selective filtering; 2) frequency transposition; 3) binaural separation of acoustic information, such as giving high frequencies to one ear and low frequencies to the other, or giving alternate temporal segments of the message to opposite ears; or 4) temporal distortions, such as differences in phase relation or speed of presentation. A variant of passive filtering is the introduction of masking noise, either steady or intermittent. In general, the deficits that are revealed by such modifications of speech audiometry are neurologic rather than otologic deficits but they represent an important advance in the field of neuro-otology. The functions that are tested are essentially functions of perception and belong among the "high" mental processes. Clinical application of such materials include the assessment of central auditory lesions and are discussed in Chapter 8.

Speech audiometry has also been applied to the analysis of normal speech from the linguistic point of view and has led to study in detail of the phonetic and phonemic structure of English speech in general and of word lists that might be used as laboratory tools for the study of communication by speech. A number of such lists have been prepared, and certain ways of using them may be suitable for clinical use as well (Davis and Silverman, 1978).

The rapidly accumulating clinical experience with speech audiometry suggested the need for critical investigation of assumptions and variables associated with its application. Among these were variations in equipment, live voice versus recorded speech, equivalence of lists, correlation with pure tone tests, some of which still exist, and, among other speech materials, listener indoctrination and message set, listener familiarity with syntactic structure and vocabulary, "normal" thresholds, reduction of number of items in the interest of saving time, and redundancy and sequential probabilities of occurrence of linguistic units. The important studies addressed to these problems are cited elsewhere in this book.

The foregoing brief account of the early history of speech audiometry emphasizes, at least implicitly, that its foundation required the participation in its development of disciplined workers from a variety of academic and professional fields. Prominent among them were acoustics, electrical engineering, experimental phonetics, linguistics, otology, physiology, psychology, and statistics. Thoughtful consideration of how speech audiometry grew out of the convergence of many pertinent disciplines addressed to a particular problem may be productive as audiology seeks to define itself and to delineate its role in the current and future professional scene.

REFERENCES

Davis, H. 1947. Tests of hearing. In Davis, H. (ed.), Hearing and Deafness: A guide for laymen, pp. 125–160. Murray Hill Books, Inc., New York.

Davis, H. 1948. The articulation area and the social adequacy index for hearing. Laryngoscope 58:761–778.

Davis, H., and S. R. Silverman. 1978. Appendix: Tests of hearing. In Davis, H., and S. R. Silverman (eds.), Hearing and Deafness, pp. 525–538. 4th Ed. Holt, Rinehart and Winston, New York.

Dewey, G. 1923. Relative Frequency of English Speech Sounds. Harvard University Press, Cambridge, Mass.

Doerfler, L. G., and K. Stewart. 1946. Malingering and psychogenic deafness. J. Speech Disord. 13:181–186.

Egan, J. P. 1948. Articulation testing methods. Laryngoscope 58:955–991.

Falconer, G. A., and H. Davis. 1947. The intelligibility of connected discourse as a test for the "Threshold of Speech." Laryngoscope 57:581–595.

Fletcher, H. 1929. Speech and Hearing. D. Van Nostrand Company, New York.

Fletcher, H., and J. C. Steinberg. 1929. Articulation Testing Methods. Bell Syst. Tech. J. 8:806–854.

French, N. R., C. W. Carter, and W. Koenig 1930. The words and sounds of telephone conversations. Bell Syst. Tech. J. 9:290–324.

Hirsh, I. J., H. Davis, S. R. Silverman, E. G. Reynolds, E. Eldert, and R. W. Benson. 1952. Development of materials for speech audiometry. J. Speech Hear. Disord. 17:321–337.

Hudgins, C. V., J. E. Hawkins, J. E. Karlin, and S. S. Stevens. 1947. The development of recorded auditory tests for measuring hearing loss for speech. Laryngoscope 40:57–89.

Silverman, S. R., and I. J. Hirsh. 1955. Problems related to the use of speech in clinical audiometry. Ann. Otol. Rhinol. and Laryngol. 64:1234–1245.

Silverman, S. R., W. R. Thurlow, T. E. Walsh, and H. Davis. 1948. Improvement in the social adequacy of hearing following the fenestration operation. Laryngoscope 58:607–631.

Thurlow, W. R., S. R. Silverman, H. Davis, and T. E. Walsh. 1948. A statistical study of auditory tests in relation to the fenestration operation. Laryngoscope 58:43–66.

Urbantschitsch, V. 1895. Über Hörübingen bei Taubstumheit und bei Ertaubung im Späteren Lebensalter. (Auditory Training for Deafmutism and for Deafness Acquired in Later Life). Urban and Schwarzenberg, Vienna.

Walsh, T. E., and S. R. Silverman. 1946. Diagnosis and evaluation of fenestration. Laryngoscope 56:536–555.

CHAPTER 3

ACOUSTICS AND PERCEPTION OF SPEECH

Thomas H. Townsend

CONTENTS

COMPOSITION OF SPEECH SOUNDS	26
ANALYSIS OF SPEECH	27
Waveform	27
Spectrum	29
Spectrogram	31
PRODUCTION OF SPEECH SOUNDS	33
Vowels	33
Consonants	36
Continuous Speech	38
DIMENSIONS OF SPEECH	38
COMMENTS ON PERCEPTION AND EARLY RESEARCH	40
Frequency	40
Intensity	41
Time	42
LEVELS OF PROCESSING	42
SPEECH MODE	43
Categorical Perception	43
The Syllable	44
DECODING ACOUSTIC PATTERNS	45
Implementation of Perception	45
Invariance and Segmentation	46
Feature Detectors	47
MODELS OF PERCEPTION	49
REFERENCES	50

Material on the acoustics and perception of speech in a book on speech audiometry may seem to have no more in common than the word "speech." Yet audiologists must continually remind themselves that both of their most basic functions, measurement of hearing and (re)habilitation of the hearing impaired, demand an intimate knowledge of the perceptual processes that decode the acoustic patterns commonly referred to as speech. Likewise, these events cannot be comprehended fully until one understands something about the acoustic architecture of speech utterances. Hence, the purpose of this chapter is to provide an overview of current concepts of speech production and perception. It is assumed that the reader has had some exposure to basic courses in audiology, such as phonetics, speech and hearing

---

This chapter was written while the author was Professor and Chairman of Audiology, Central Michigan University, Mt. Pleasant, Michigan.

science, and anatomy. Comprehensive treatment of the topics of this chapter would require a separate text—or two! Thus, references will be cited generously.

In particular, as the audiologist becomes more involved with the selection, evaluation, and fitting of hearing aids, the necessity for a thorough mastery of speech perception becomes paramount. Because hearing aid technology is becoming increasingly sophisticated, the audiologist's success as the primary professional in the management of personal amplification devices will depend greatly on the ability to utilize the current state of the science of perception in conjunction with the interpretation of hearing aid specifications.

This chapter begins by reviewing the acoustic parameters of speech signals and how they are generated and represented. Next, specific frequency-intensity-time patterns of phonemes are described. The first topic in the section on perception covers the effects of distortions of the acoustic signal. Then, basic terminology is discussed, such as speech mode, categorical perception, invariance, and feature detectors. Finally, the status of models of speech perception is presented.

It is the hope of the author that the material contained in this chapter will ignite sufficient curiosity that the reader will refer to other sources for more thorough compendiums on these subjects. The most up-to-date state of knowledge for each topic presented is reflected in the literature. Two excellent sources for the topics at hand are the *Journal of the Acoustical Society of America* and *Perception and Psychophysics*.

COMPOSITION OF SPEECH SOUNDS

Speech sounds are made up of both periodic and aperiodic components. Periodic waves result from vibration of the vocal folds in the larynx and are complex rather than sinusoidal. By definition, a complex, periodic sound results when the vibrational pattern is repetitious, but the pattern is not simple harmonic motion. It can be proven mathematically and demonstrated electronically that these complex waves are composed of at least two and, frequently, several pure tones that are harmonically related. The lowest frequency in a complex waveform is the fundamental (f_0); and the higher frequencies, or harmonics, are integer multiples of f_0. The distinguishing perceptual feature of periodic sound is that of tonality.

A speech sound that is aperiodic has a random vibrational pattern, that is, it theoretically never repeats itself. Aperiodic sounds are produced when air is forced through a narrow aperture causing turbulence and, hence, random movement. The consequence is a sound consisting of continuous frequencies, usually extending over a wide range. In contrast to periodic sound, aperiodic sound has no tonality although certainly the attribute of a pitch sometimes may be assigned to aperiodic speech sounds.

ANALYSIS OF SPEECH

Because of the invisible nature of acoustic patterns in air, they can be difficult to conceptualize; accordingly, several means of representing them exist. It is important to emphasize that any sound can be described by specifying three attributes: frequency, intensity, and time. Time must be further delineated into duration and phase; the latter describes the time relationship between two different sounds. Unfortunately, because we live basically in a two-dimensional world, it is difficult to represent graphically these three characteristics of sound simultaneously. Indeed, such a depiction would be highly desirable; however, the conventional means of portrayal consist of the waveform, the spectrum, and the spectrogram.

Waveform

One way of displaying sound patterns is by means of the waveform, which depicts intensity as a function of time. In engineering terminology this also is referred to as the time domain. The instrument most frequently used to examine waveforms is the oscilloscope. Figure 3-1 shows both a periodic (Figure 3-1A) and an aperiodic (Figure 3-1B) waveform represented on an oscilloscope. The intensity of both waves and the period (T) of the wave in Figure 3-1A can be determined by means of the calibrated vertical and horizontal scales. The period is the amount of time required for one complete vibration. From this the fundamental frequency can be calculated using the reciprocal relation, that is $f_0 = 1/T$. Also, by enlarging the time scale, it would be feasible to represent more than one speech sound, and determine the intensities and durations of each.

From the waveform it is furthermore possible to envision the actual vibrational pattern that yielded the sound displayed. Recall that sound creates longitudinal wave motion. Each element in the elastic medium (usually air when considering speech) vibrates back and forth about its rest position, and this movement can be retrieved from the waveform. The *vertical* displacement on the oscilloscope is proportional to the longitudinal motion of the actual vibrating components of the sound wave. To view the exact replication of the vibrational event, it is necessary only to stop the time sweep across the oscilloscope so that the dot (trace) then moves up and down on the screen about a fixed point just as an air particle would vibrate back and forth. The movement

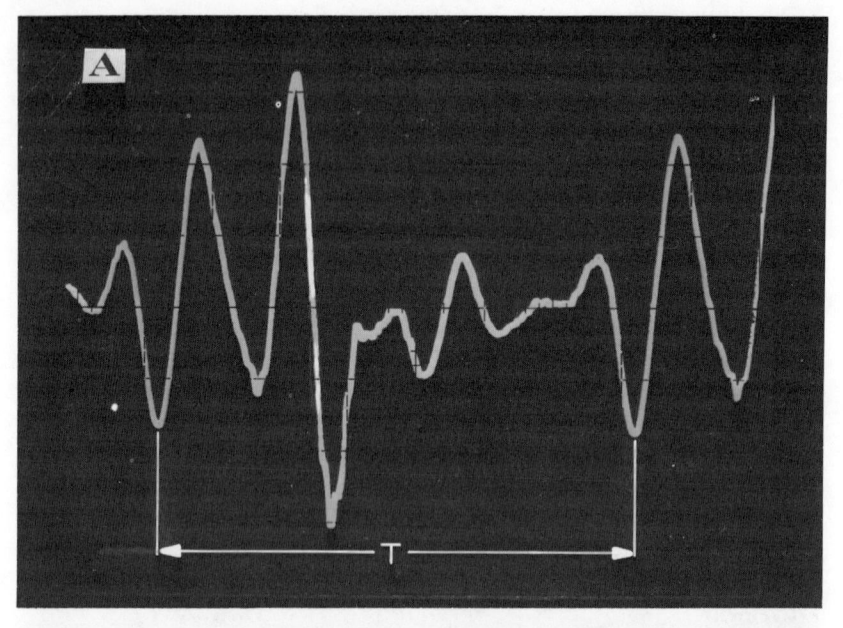

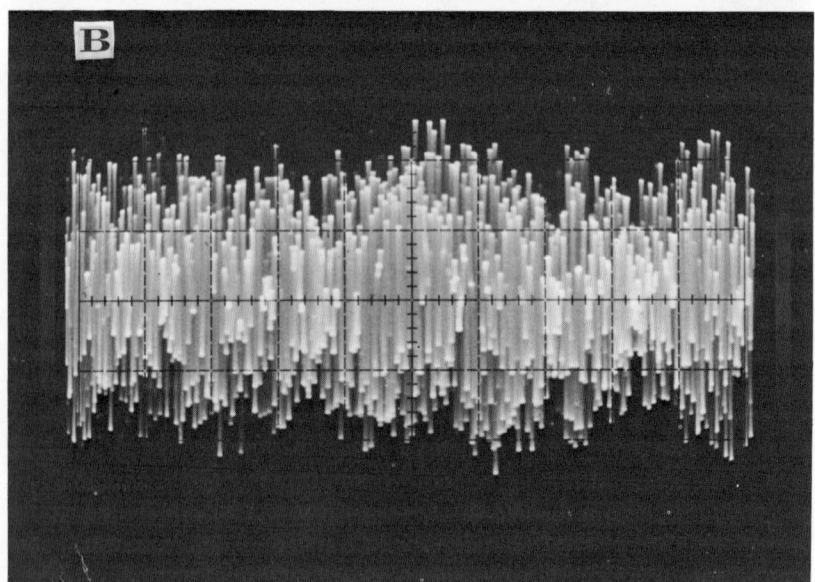

Figure 3-1. Two speech sounds represented as waveforms. The top portion of the figure (A) reveals a periodic sound, whereas the bottom portion (B) represents an aperiodic sound.

of any audible sound (i.e., ≥ 20 Hz), however, will move too rapidly on the oscilloscope to follow with the eye; therefore, stretching the pattern horizontally (across a known time scale) yields the opportunity for precise examination of the vibration.

Figure 3-1B represents an oscilloscopic pattern for an aperiodic sound. It is important to note that it is impossible to extract any frequency information from this trace. Hence, the inability to obtain frequency data for aperiodic sounds is the principal limitation of the waveform: frequency content can be realized only for periodic waves; and, if it is a complex sound, only f_0 can be calculated.

Spectrum

Another way of viewing a speech signal is by means of the spectrum, which reveals intensity on the ordinate and frequency along the abscissa. In Figure 3-2A, a periodic sound is seen to have many harmonically related frequency components of varying intensity. Each vertical line represents a discrete frequency, that is, a pure tone. Conversely, the aperiodic sound displayed in Figure 3-2B, because it is composed of a continuous spread of frequencies, yields a continuous spectrum. Frequently, it is convenient to show the overall shape of the spectrum by drawing a line connecting the top of the individual frequency components (Figure 3-2A) or across the continuous energy of the aperiodic sound (Figure 3-2B). Such a representation is known as the envelope, and when shown alone *without* the individual harmonics, it allows a convenient summary of the changes in intensity across frequency. These displays are more specifically termed the amplitude spectra to distinguish them from a related representation known as the phase spectrum, which reveals the phase relationship among the various frequencies. In general, the ear is not sensitive to phase differences, so the phase spectrum is frequently omitted. That is to say, the ear generally will perceive a complex sound in the same way, regardless of the relative phases of the different components.

Note that when the spectrum is used, exact intensity information is available for each frequency component, but there is no representation of time. Because time is not displayed, this mode is also referred to as the frequency domain. The obvious limitation is that the time attribute is absent, so there is no means to determine the duration of the sound or the changes in the frequency-intensity image over time.

A spectrum can be derived in two ways. The first is to write the mathematical equation of a waveform, and then calculate the frequency segments and their intensities. This method, Fourier analysis, is cumbersome to accomplish by hand; but a computer program first described in the mid 1960s (Cooley and Tukey, 1965) called the fast Fourier transform (FFT), does it with facility. A second means of obtaining

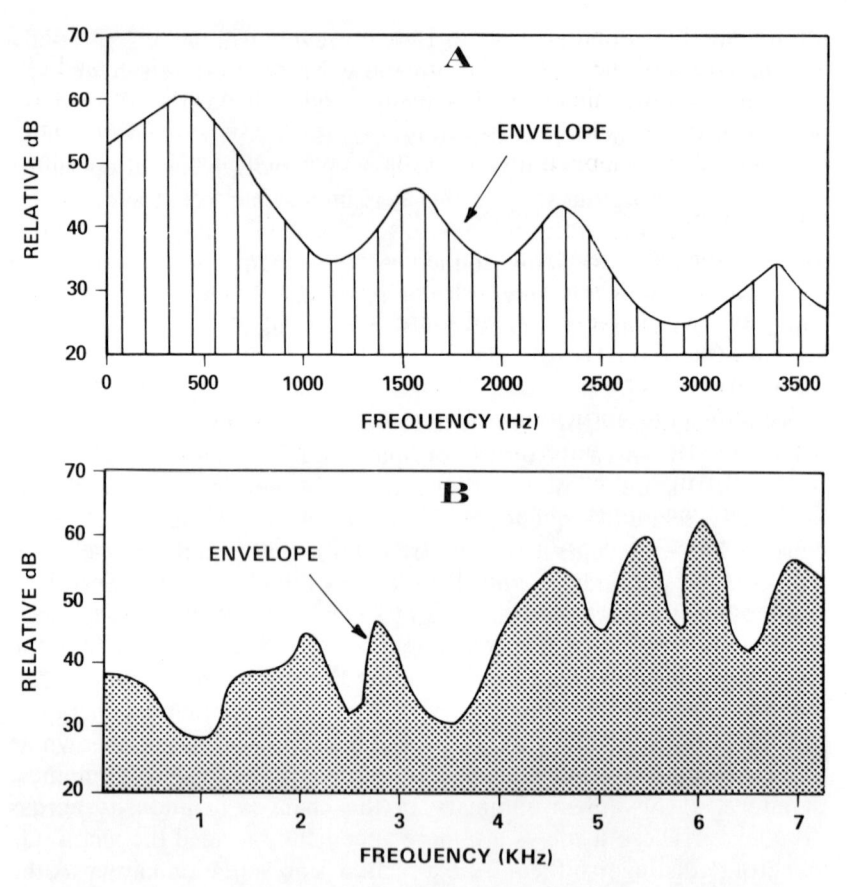

Figure 3-2. Two speech sounds represented as (amplitude) spectra. The top portion of the figure (A) shows a periodic sound, and the bottom portion (B) depicts an aperiodic sound.

the spectrum can be realized in the laboratory using filters, but not always to the same degree of accuracy as with the FFT. Generally, the narrower the band-pass of the filter available, the better the resolution. The trade off, however, is that as more selective filters are used, more time is required for analysis. Thus, this method may not be accurate for very brief sounds, such as some speech utterances. Manual filtering becomes a time-consuming project if a signal with a wide range of frequencies is to be analyzed. Recently, real time (spectrum) analyzers (RTAs) have become available that display the entire spectrum of a signal in a very brief amount of time. Currently, RTAs are available to perform analyses utilizing both of the procedures mentioned previously: by a mathematical means using the FFT and by a filtering method employing several narrow band filters simultaneously. The spectrum of the vowel /i/ is shown in Figure 3-3, as displayed on a commercially available real time analyzer. There is no means to determine the duration of this sample; also, errors can result in some instances if the sampling time of the device is not taken into account.

Spectrogram

The fruition of research at Bell Telephone Laboratories during the 1940s led to the development of the spectrograph, an instrument that shows the two characteristics of sound not paired heretofore: frequency and time (duration) (Koenig, Dunn, and Lacy, 1946). The (sound) spectrograph reveals frequency on the ordinate and time along the abscissa. Some intensity information is also available as a function of the darkness of the tracing, but it consists of a limited range. Thus, the display is, in a way, three dimensional as it were. The spectrographic representation (called a spectrogram) of the sentence "Joe took father's shoebench out," is seen in Figure 3-4. "Reading" any spectrogram without knowledge of its phonetic content is dubious (Fant, 1973); but if the speech sample is known, it is possible to identify the various phonemes. From the spectrogram it is practical to realize very accurate durational information, fairly precise frequency data, but only limited

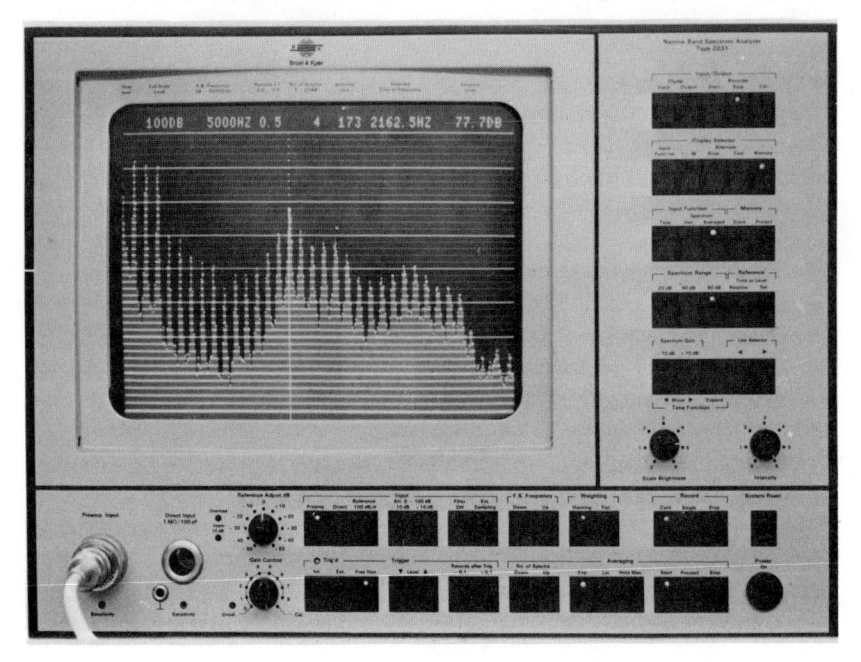

Figure 3-3. Spectrum of the vowel /i/ revealed on a real time (spectrum) analyzer.

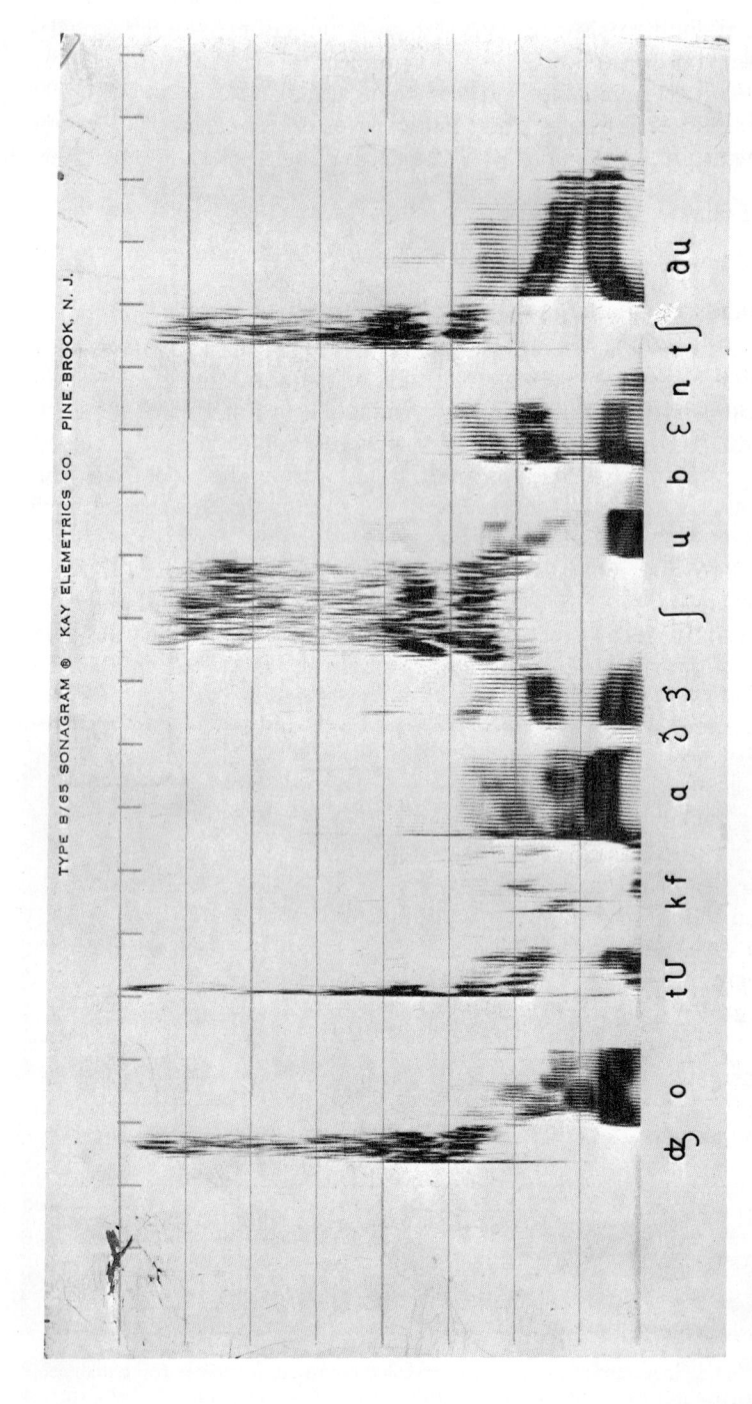

Figure 3-4. Spectrogram of the utterance "Joe took father's shoebench out." Note that the final /t/ in the word "out" was not uttered by the talker.

intensity resolution. The primary contributions afforded by the spectrograph have been to document the continuously changing acoustic structure of running speech, that is, the variations in frequency and intensity across time, and also to demonstrate the presence of coarticulation—"the overlapping of adjacent articulations" (Ladefoged, 1975, p. 48).

PRODUCTION OF SPEECH SOUNDS

The sounds of speech are produced by vibrations generated at the larynx and/or along the vocal tract, which consists of the mouth and associated structures such as the tongue, teeth, and lips. These phonemes are categorized according to where the sound is generated. The basic categories consist of vowels and consonants.

Vowels

The production of the vowel sounds is well understood, and models of how they are produced have been advanced. Fant (1970) indicates that there are three separate and independent components that affect vowel generation: 1) the complex waveform from the larynx (the source); 2) the resonating cavity of the vocal tract (the filter); and 3) the radiation of the sound leaving the cavity and being dispersed into the air. These units comprise the "source-filter" model.

The Source The sound source for vowel phonemes is the vibrating vocal folds in the larynx. They vibrate at average frequencies of about 120 and 220 Hz for adult males and females, respectively, and at higher frequencies (approximately 300 Hz) for young children (Fant, 1956). The waveform produced at the larynx is complex and quasiperiodic; for even though the patterns of vibration are highly repetitious, they are not exactly identical. Figure 3-5A illustrates the spectrum of the sound produced by the vocal folds. It can be seen that this sound is harmonically rich and, further, that the harmonics decrease first very rapidly and then more gradually in intensity as frequency increases. The harmonics decrease in intensity at a rate of approximately 12 dB per octave above about 250 Hz. This produces the decaying envelope observable in the top part of Figure 3-5. The sound generated at the larynx can be modified somewhat in intensity and fundamental frequency, but its overall characteristics remain rather constant. Stated otherwise, all the vowel sounds (as well as voiced consonants) are the result of essentially the same sound pattern being created at the larynx; the acoustic differences among vowels perceived during audition are caused by the effects of the filtering function of the vocal tract.

The Filter The vocal tract through which the sound vibrations travel after generation at the larynx and before expulsion into the air

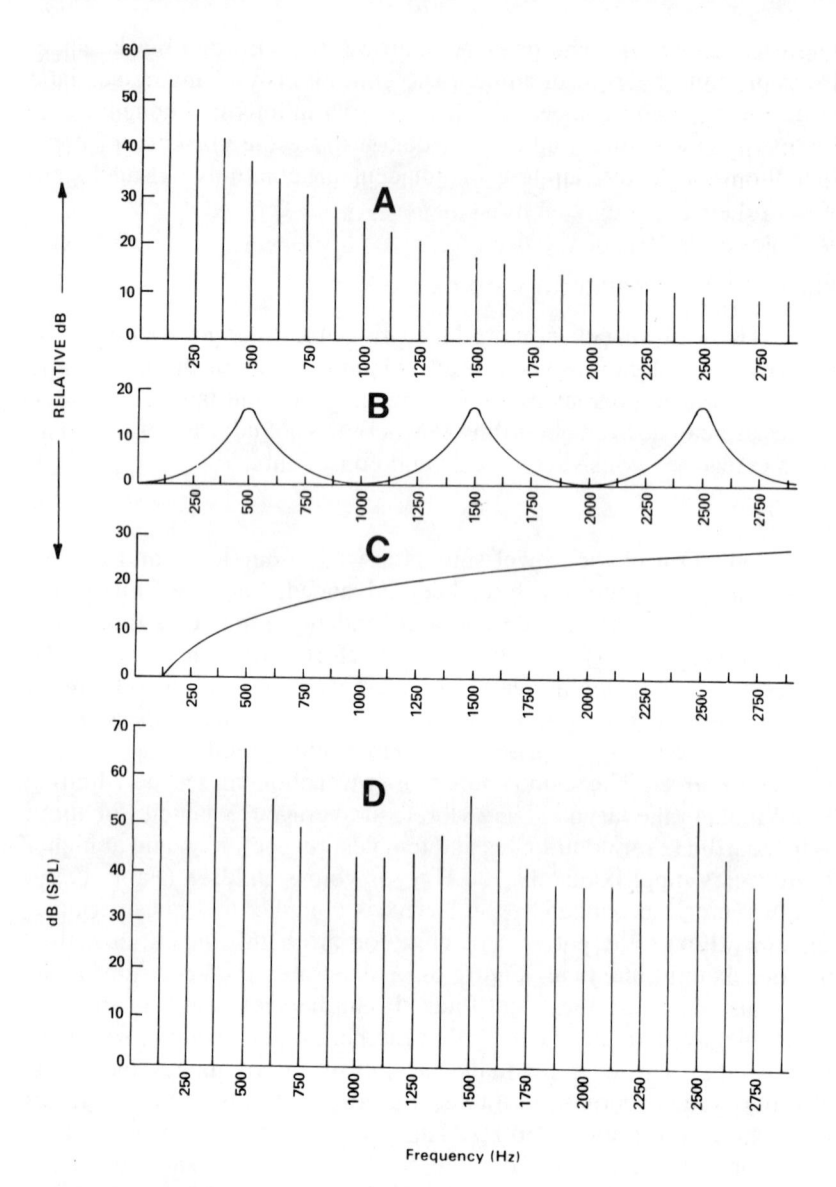

Figure 3-5. Components of the spectrum of the neutral vowel /ə/. A indicates the spectrum of the laryngeal source. B reveals the effect of the filter (vocal tract). C shows the radiation effect. D represents the spectrum of the vowel as it would exist in front of the talker's lips; that is, the sum of A, B, and C.

consists of a 17-cm tube in the average adult male. This tube, when unconstricted, a configuration present for the schwa /ə/, behaves like a quarter (¼) wavelength resonator, because the end in the larynx is essentially closed (at the glottis), while the other end is opened (at the lips). Consequently, sounds having wavelengths four times the length of the tube will be maximally resonated, or amplified, as will the *odd* multiples of this frequency. Inversely, this enclosure is a quarter wavelength of the resonated acoustic wave. For a tube 17 cm in length, the resonant frequencies, called formants, will be 500, 1500, 2500, Hz and so on. These formants are illustrated in Figure 3-5B.

Most vowels are formed with the vocal tract constricted: the tongue is moved toward the palate dividing the tube into two sections, one extending from the lips to the place of the constriction and the other extending from the constriction to the glottis. This latter tube, because it is largely closed at both ends, behaves like a half wavelength resonator. Thus, the overall resonant properties of the vocal tract depend on the interaction of both tubes as well as narrowing at the lips. In fact, the geometry of the entire vocal tract influences the formulation of the formants. Efforts to summarize the configurations for various vowels have resulted in the use of three parameters to specify these cavities: 1) the length of the tube measured from the glottis to the point of maximum constriction; 2) the radius of the tube at the point of greatest constriction; and 3) the ratio of the average cross-sectional area to the length of the tube of that portion near the lips (Stevens and House, 1955). Each vowel, therefore, has multiple, distinct formant frequency regions that are the result of the resonances in the tube (vocal tract). The formant of lowest frequency is labeled F_1, the next, F_2, etc. Whereas the frequency of F_3 remains fairly constant across most vowels, F_1 and F_2 vary considerably in frequency. Because adult females have on the average slightly shorter vocal tracts than males, their formant frequencies are lower by about 20 percent (Fant, 1973).

Specific formant frequencies associated with vowel sounds have been reported by Peterson and Barney (1952). One way to summarize these data is to describe them in order of place of articulation (anatomical point of maximum constriction) from the front to the back of the mouth. F_1 begins at a low value (low relative to the first formant of the unconstricted vocal tract, i.e., 500 Hz) for front vowels and rises to a high value for the mid vowels and then decreases again for the back vowels. F_2, on the other hand, almost continuously decreases from a high value (re: the unconstricted value of 1500 Hz) for the front vowels to a low value for the back vowels. This effect can be seen in Figure 3-6.

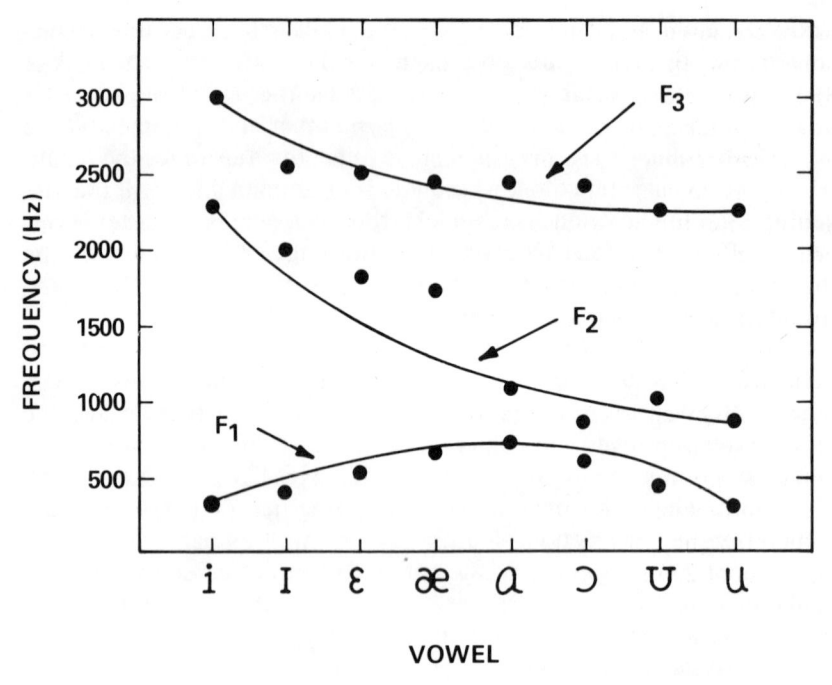

Figure 3-6. Variation in the first three formants across vowels.

Radiation The result of radiating the sound waves past the lips and into the air is to create a high frequency emphasis. Overall, the high-frequency components of speech sounds are accentuated at a rate of 6 dB per octave relative to the lowest frequency component, as depicted in Figure 3-5C.

Vowel Spectra A vowel, therefore, measured at a short distance in front of the lips, would have frequency-intensity characteristics contributed by the source, the filter, and the radiation. Each of these factors, as well as the final vowel spectrum, is illustrated in Figure 3-5 for the vowel /ə/. Note that the *only* sound source is at the larynx. Both the vocal tract and the radiation of the sound into the air serve to filter and thus modify the intensities of the frequency components generated at the larynx. The spectrum of the vowel, therefore, as measured in front of the lips, (Figure 3-5D) has an envelope affected by all three factors.

Consonants

Consonants may be voiced sounds, like vowels, or they may be unvoiced. Some of the voiced consonants are relatively similar to vowels from an articulatory viewpoint; consequently, their acoustic properties are also related. For purposes of describing acoustic composition, consonants may be divided into four categories: 1) approximants; 2) nasals; 3) fricatives; and 4) stops. Approximants and nasals are most like vowels in terms of their acoustic energy.

Approximants The approximants, /j, l, r, w/, can be analytically treated as vowels (Fant, 1973) in that they are formed according to the source-filter model discussed above. In short, they have resonant properties dependent upon the shape of the articulators and, in particular, the place of maximum constriction in the vocal tract. The first three formants decrease rapidly in amplitude and occur below approximately 3000 Hz.

Nasals The nasals, /m, n, ŋ/, are produced in a manner similar to that of vowels except, in addition to the vocal tract, the nasal cavity also serves as a resonator. Nasalized consonants, therefore, are characterized not only by more resonances than vowels but also by prominent antiresonances that cause reductions in the intensities of some formants. The net effect, referred to as the nasal murmur, is a strong F_1 at about 250 Hz, while F_2 is weak or absent, although higher weak formants exist.

Fricatives When the vocal tract is narrowed sufficiently, a turbulent airflow occurs, and a broad band noise results. These sounds, called fricatives, may be unvoiced or voiced. Two of them, /s/ and /ʃ/, are generated far enough posterior to the lips that the tube effect of the mouth creates distinct resonances. For /s/ the primary peak falls between 4000 and 7000 Hz, but for /ʃ/ it occurs at about 2000 Hz. In contrast, /θ/ and /f/ are formed so far forward in the vocal tract that the tube effect is inconsequential. As a result, the spectra of these sounds are very broad in frequency, with minor resonances between 7000 and 8000 Hz; they also are quite weak in intensity. The voiced cognates /z, ʒ, ð, v/ of the voiceless fricatives mentioned above have similar high-frequency spectra; however, there are high-intensity spectral components in the very low-frequency region below about 500 Hz (Minifie, Hixon, and Williams, 1973).

Stops Like the fricatives, the stops may be either unvoiced or voiced. The former consist of /p, t, k/, and the latter /b, d, g/. The stops are much shorter in duration than any of the other phonemes. The voiceless stops are created by a suspension of air flow through the vocal tract followed by a rapid opening which causes an explosive burst of sound. Because the stops cannot be produced in isolation, it is difficult to describe their spectra. In other words, if a consonant-vowel (CV) syllable consisting of a stop as the consonant is tape recorded, then by a cutting and splicing procedure it is possible to isolate the vowel but not the stop. An initial nondescript sound could be identified, but it does not convey the perceptual property of a stop. Available data indicate, however, that the labial pair /p/ and /b/ have the greatest energy between 500 and 1500 Hz; /t/ and /d/ have concentrated energy near 500 Hz and above 4000 Hz, whereas, energy predominates between 1500 and 4000 Hz for /k/ and /g/ (Halle, Hughes, and Radley, 1957).

Continuous Speech

Now that the acoustical properties of the various phonemes in American English have been described, it is appropriate to summarize and make some general statements about the acoustics of speech signals. The speech units commonly used for audiologic assessment are of at least syllabic size, as opposed to individual phonemes. One-syllable words are used most frequently due to the popularity of the monosyllabic word lists employed to test word recognition ability. Continuous speech of this nature often contains phonemic components that have markedly different characteristics from those discussed above for individual utterances of the various sounds. This fact by no means voids the aforementioned information; it only causes us to regard it within the proper perspective: namely, that the acoustic properties of phonemes change according to the context in which they are formed. This lack of acoustic invariance has significant implications and will be discussed subsequently in the section on perception. Furthermore, by examining spectrograms carefully (as in Figure 3-4), it can be observed that the frequency-intensity pattern also changes *within* individual phonemes because of the effect of coarticulation.

DIMENSIONS OF SPEECH

The overall intensity variation among phonemes in conversational speech is on the order of 25 dB. The most intense sounds are those vowels with their F_1 and F_2 close in frequency, such as /a/ and /ɔ/. The weakest vowel, /i/, is roughly 7 dB less intense and is equal to the most intense consonants, /l/ and /r/. The weakest phoneme, /θ/, has an intensity about 18 dB less than that of the strongest consonants. The relative intensities of several phonemes are listed in Table 3-1. A more complete inventory may be found in Levitt (1978).

The frequency content of speech sounds varies somewhat, depending on the sex and mannerisms (rhythm, rate, etc.) of the talker. The range often referenced is approximately 100 to 10,000 Hz. Few male fundamental frequencies are lower than 100 Hz, and the average intensity of frequency components higher than 10,000 Hz is more than

Table 3-1. Intensities of different speech sounds produced at conversational levels

Phoneme	Intensity (dB SPL)
ɔ	65
ɛ	61
i	58
l	58
ʃ	56
n	52
t̪	50
h	48
s	45
θ	40

Adapted from Levitt (1978).

50 dB less than those near 500 Hz, making them inconsequential if not inaudible.

When the average spectrum of a lengthy sample of speech is measured it appears like the one in Figure 3-7, which is called the long-time spectral average. From 100 to about 500 Hz, the average intensity rises a few decibels; then for frequencies above 500 Hz it falls rather steadily at a rate of about 10 dB per octave.

Frequently, one hears that vowels are low-frequency sounds, whereas consonants are high-frequency sounds. There is both truth

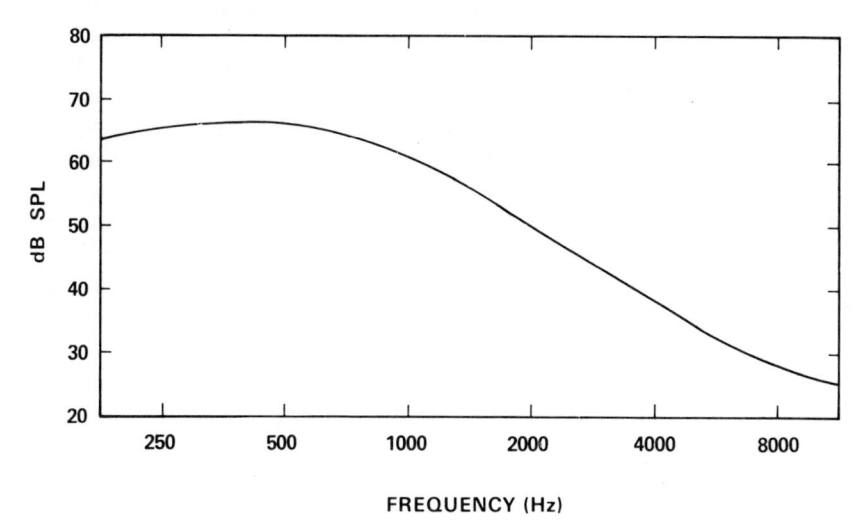

Figure 3-7. The long-time spectral average of speech.

and fallacy to this statement. Acoustically, both consonants and vowels are composed of a wide range of frequencies extending in most cases from a few hundred to several thousand Hertz. The low-frequency vowel versus high-frequency consonant dichotomy, however, has merit with regard to the range of frequencies important for perceptual purposes. Indeed, as will be seen below, the vowels require perception of only the lower frequency band (up to perhaps 2000 or 3000 Hz) for recognition, although reception of much higher frequencies (perhaps up to 8000 Hz) is necessary for complete understanding of all consonant sounds.

The duration of phonemes differs considerably among talkers and with changes in such factors as emotion and accent. In general vowels have durations in consonant-vowel-consonant (CVC) environments ranging from 160 to 350 msec (Fletcher, 1970), and these durations vary depending upon the specific context. Consonants vary much more in length with fricatives having durations comparable to vowels, whereas stops are generally much briefer. In summary, consonants endure from approximately 50 to 300 msec (Stevens and House, 1972).

The purpose of this section has been to summarize methods of analyzing speech signals and to review their acoustic properties. An extensive explication of the acoustics of speech may be found in a chapter by Levitt (1978). The reader is urged to consult this source for a more thorough treatment of this topic than could be provided herein.

COMMENTS ON PERCEPTION AND EARLY RESEARCH

The perceptual process involves the decoding and processing of the incoming stream of *acoustic* patterns by the auditory mechanism and their conversion into *linguistic* elements meaningful to the brain. The following discussion will concentrate on the recognition of short speech segments such as the monosyllabic words commonly used in hearing assessment. The role of memory, which is relevant especially to the consideration of longer speech elements such as sentences and paragraphs, will not be included; it has been discussed in detail by Norman (1969).

The early literature on perception has been summarized fully by Licklider and Miller (1951). Pertinent findings relate mainly to manipulations of the basic attributes of speech signals: frequency, intensity, and time.

Frequency

Documentation of the effects of frequency distortion has been provided by French and Steinberg (1947), who examined word recognition under conditions of high- and low-pass filtering. The latter condition is especially relevant because of its similarity to the effects of various high frequency sensorineural hearing disorders. Not surprisingly, discrimination performance decreases as the cutoff frequency (i.e., frequency above which filtering occurs) is lowered. Table 3-2 reveals the scores realized for several degrees of "hearing loss" simulated by filtering in this manner. A limitation to the analogy between these data and actual impairments is that here there is no attenuation at frequencies below the cutoff, so they relate only to cases in which hearing is normal in the low frequencies and deteriorates rapidly in the high-frequency range. Many sensorineural hearing losses, in contrast, slope across all frequencies. Another factor of import here is the nature of the word materials used, because performance varies differentially with the test employed, as is explained in Chapter 6. In summary, as increasingly more of the high frequencies are lost, poorer resolution of the consonants occurs with concomitant reductions in understanding.

Intensity

Intensity is a major factor in the perception of high-frequency speech sounds (see Figure 3-7). Gerber (1974) summarized this situation by indicating that whereas the frequency band from 1000 to 8000 Hz contributes 60 percent to speech intelligibility, it contains only 5 percent of the total intensity. Obviously, speech cannot be heard if the intensity is too low. The level required for near-perfect recognition varies with the nature of the speech material. For selected disyllabic words, such as those typically used for measuring the speech reception threshold, excellent understanding results at about 10 dB sensation level (SL), whereas monosyllabic words require 30–50 dB SL, depending on the test for individuals with normal hearing and greater SLs for the hearing impaired (Tillman, Carhart, and Wilber, 1963; Schwartz and Surr, 1979). At the other extreme, intensity levels that are too great may

Table 3-2. Effect of frequency distortion (low-pass filtering) on syllable recognition

Cut-off frequency	Performance (%)
8000	100
4000	90
2000	70
1000	30
500	10

Adapted from French and Steinberg (1947).

cause decreases in intelligibility. This concept is discussed in detail in Chapter 6.

Distortion related to excessive intensity of acoustic signals is called peak-clipping. Every physical and physiologic system has a limit to the maximal vibration which can be sustained, and if a signal exceeds this capacity, a distorted response results. The output of such a system will have a vibrational pattern in which the peaks are literally cut off, or clipped, resulting in the generation of harmonic distortion. Otherwise stated, when the mechanism is overdriven by a pure tone, a complex tone will be presented at the output. Licklider (1946) reported that 24 dB can be clipped from speech signals and only degrade understanding slightly (to 95 percent). This minimal reduction in score has led to considerable controversy regarding word recognition through hearing aids having harmonic distortion.

Time

Changes in the overall temporal dimension of speech materials have little effect on normal-hearing listeners, whereas selected subjects with sensorineural hearing impairment show a reduction in their ability to understand when the speech is time compressed 50 percent, that is, speeded up to twice its normal rate (Konkle, Beasley, and Bess, 1977). If the timing of speech is altered through interruption, the greatest deterioration in intelligibility occurs when the interruptions appear about once every second, that is, at a syllabic rate (Miller and Licklider, 1950). The significance of the syllable in perception will be explained later.

The consequence of the above discussion is that the speech signal is highly redundant to the normal-hearing person. It can be altered by frequency, amplitude, and time distortion and still remain largely intelligible (see Chapter 8 for further discussion of this topic). As a result, many hypacusic individuals with mild to moderate hearing impairments frequently function adequately given sufficient intensity (Bess and Townsend, 1977), because reception of a totally undistorted signal is simply unnecessary.

LEVELS OF PROCESSING

At first view one might consider speech perception as an operationally, though not neurologically, simple mechanism: acoustic waveforms enter the auditory system and are converted into linguistic messages. This concept is far too simplistic, as there are several steps to the perceptual process; and these are diagramed in Figure 3-8. They are: acoustic, phonetic, phonologic, syntactic, and semantic. Processing

```
┌─────────────┐
│  ACOUSTIC   │
└──────┬──────┘
       ▼
┌─────────────┐
│  PHONETIC   │
└──────┬──────┘
       ▼
┌─────────────┐
│ PHONOLOGIC  │
└──────┬──────┘
       ▼
┌─────────────┐
│  SYNTACTIC  │
└──────┬──────┘
       ▼
┌─────────────┐
│  SEMANTIC   │
└─────────────┘
```

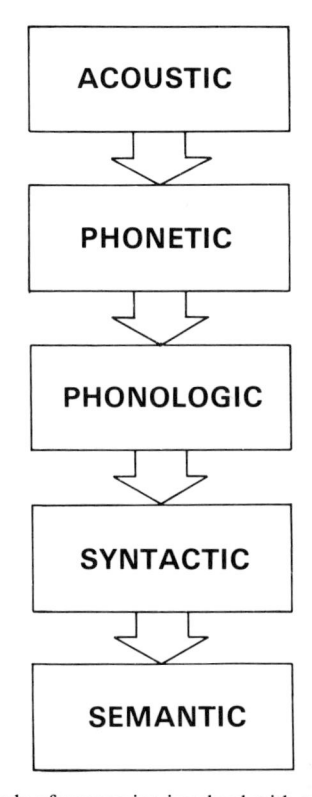

Figure 3-8. The levels of processing involved with speech perception.

through these levels proceeds in a partially serial and partially parallel manner (Studdert-Kennedy, 1976). At present, discussion is concerned primarily with the first two levels. How the auditory apparatus translates the frequency-intensity-time patterns into the phonetic percept has been the focus of a very extensive amount of research.

SPEECH MODE

A specialized kind of processing is believed to occur when the auditory system is exposed to speech as opposed to nonspeech stimuli, such as environmental sounds and melodies. Stevens and House (1972) have termed this method of analysis the *speech mode*.

Categorical Perception

Probably the most significant aspect of perception in the speech mode is a phenomenon called categorical perception. According to Studdert-

Kennedy (1976), it "... has provided basic evidence for the distinction between auditory and phonetic levels of processing" (p. 259). The human auditory system has a remarkable capability for distinguishing among tones differing in frequency and intensity; in fact its overall capacity has been estimated as exceeding 300,000 tones (Stevens and Davis, 1938). In contrast, a limited number (i.e., fewer than ten) of these same tonal stimuli can be repeatedly identified (Miller, 1956). When the stimuli resemble speech, however, the auditory system can discriminate no more categories than it can identify; in other words, discrimination performance decreases very significantly. Experiments with synthetically generated speech samples have shown that listeners are unable to discriminate changes in frequency, for instance, that are easily detected when the stimulus is not speech-like, such as mucical notes (Liberman et al., 1967). Thus, different processing techniques are utilized for speech and for nonspeech stimuli. Support for the concept of categorical perception of speech is not unanimous, as there are researchers who claim that this occurrence is related to the methodologies employed in the experiments that have led to this interpretation (Carney, Widin, and Viemeister, 1977).

Further impetus for the speech mode has been provided by studies revealing a lack of invariance in the speech signal and the presence of *phonetic* feature detectors medial to the peripheral portion of the auditory pathway.

The Syllable

A syllable consists of a vowel in isolation or, far more frequently, a vowel associated with one or more consonants. It should be emphasized that all languages are syllabic. In much of the literature, the syllable is regarded as the nucleus of speech. For example, Strange et al. (1976) reported that listening to vowels in a CVC context rather than in isolation improves the likelihood of perceiving them correctly, which suggests that the acoustic information of the entire syllable is considered by the listener. Studdert-Kennedy (1976) states that "... the basic *acoustic* unit of speech perception ... is roughly of syllabic length; ... perception entails the analysis of the acoustic syllable, by means of its acoustic features, into the abstract perceptual structure of features and phonemes. ..." (p. 253). Moreover, "... vowels are the rests between consonants" and they carry much of the suprasegmental information, like rhythm and stress (p. 270). In summary, Stevens and House (1972) have asserted that speech has "... certain dynamic or time-varying properties, among which are syllabic intensity fluctuations such as are associated with one of the most fundamental attributes of speech—the vowel-consonant dichotomy" (p.13).

Listening experiments have shown that consonants are subject to categorical perception, whereas vowels in isolation are perceived continuously. In other words, consonants are discriminated no better than they are identified, although vowels are discriminated much better than they are identified. The significance of these findings is that categorical perception is a type of behavior uniquely afforded to speech-like stimuli, especially syllables containing a stop consonant. The conclusion is twofold: 1) vowels in isolation are processed as nonspeech entities; and 2) speech-like vowel-consonant combinations are decoded in the speech mode.

DECODING ACOUSTIC PATTERNS

As speech signals enter at the lowest level of the system, the auditory stage, the physical manifestations are a three-dimensional matrix of frequency, intensity, and duration (time) patterns. The physical characteristics of these have been explored briefly; how the auditory mechanism utilizes these cues to implement the perception of speech remains to be discussed. There is abundant evidence to lead us to the conclusion that all of these parameters are used, either singly or in combination.

Implementation of Perception

Vowels Our knowledge of perception, in general, is best understood for the most intense and longest phonemes, the vowels. These have long been regarded as distinguishable on the basis of the frequencies of their lowest two or three formants (Delattre, et al., 1952). Recall from Figure 3-6 that each vowel has a fairly unique F_1-F_2 frequency duplex. Additionally, variability among talkers is slight enough that there is little overlap between the formant frequencies for most vowels (Peterson and Barney, 1952). Recent data, however, have suggested that the fine temporal structure of vowels may be of some import as well as their frequency contours (Scott, 1976).

Consonants Vowel-like consonants are decoded chiefly on the basis of the frequency shift in the onset of their formants (formant transitions), plus their steady-state formant frequencies (O'Conner et al., 1957). The same attributes pertain to the recognition of nasals (Mermelstein, 1977). Whereas relatively high intensity fricatives, like /s/ and /ʃ/ are perceived on the basis of their formant structures, fricatives such as /θ/ and /f/, which are of low intensity and broad spectrum, are difficult to hear under many circumstances; but cues are available from the F_2 transitions of adjoining vowels (Heinz and Stevens, 1961). Stops, in particular, are difficult to describe acoustically because their composition differs considerably with context; accordingly, much research has centered on the discovery of their perception. Because stops cannot be generated in isolation but must coexist with a vowel or vowel-like phoneme, a key to their perception has been found in the adjacent sound; that is, sufficient cues for perceiving a stop are the F_2 and F_3 transitions of the adjunct phoneme, which is often a vowel (Liberman et al., 1954). The extreme importance of the second formant transition has been stated by Liberman et al. (1967) as "probably the single most important carrier of linguistic information in the speech signal" (p. 434).

The experimental procedures used to derive these conclusions are worthy of brief consideration. Early work (circa the 1950s) centered on the analysis of frequency-intensity-time patterns of speech derived from the spectrograph. The pattern playback instrument permitted the reciprocal process: speech synthesis from spectrogram-like drawings of frequency-time representations. Thus, the complementary processes of analysis and synthesis have led to the understanding of many of the *minimal* acoustic cues necessary for the recognition of phonemes. Today, naturally, computer technology allows a more efficient means for both analysis and synthesis.

Invariance and Segmentation

There are two principle reasons why deciphering the link between the auditory and phonetic levels of perception has been so difficult. The first is that the sounds cannot be segmented: it is generally impossible to separate and identify phonemes at the acoustic level like "beads on a string" (Lieberman, 1977). One cannot cut a recorded tape into separate pieces and thereby isolate each sound that was heard when the intact tape was originally played. The second reason concerns the seeming lack of invariance in the acoustic signal. To explain, the *same* phoneme can be perceived from *different* acoustic patterns, depending on the speech sounds comprising the syllable(s). Furthermore, consider the differences in the formants of vowels spoken by a man, a woman, and a child. As indicated previously, these frequencies (and even the *ratio* of these frequencies) vary across vowels and among speakers. The listener must somehow normalize this information across talkers in order to permit proper identification. The quest for invariance is a topic of great interest among speech scientists, as this aspect of the speech signal has important implications for models of speech perception to be considered later. An extensive review of this subject may be found in Liberman et al. (1967).

Examples of Invariance Interestingly, as more sophisticated experimental techniques are being employed, examples of invariance are being discovered. One instance of an invariant, although complex, acoustic cue is voice onset time (VOT) (Studdert-Kennedy, 1976). This is the amount of time between the explosion of a stop consonant and the commencement of voicing in the ensuing vowel. It permits the distinction between voiced and unvoiced stops. Further evidence is supplied by Blumstein and Stevens (1979, 1980; Stevens and Blumstein, 1978) who found, using both natural and synthetic stimuli, invariant acoustic cues in the spectrum present at the instant of consonantal release for the perception of the place of articulation of stop consonants. Consequently, they relegate the long-honored formant transitions to a less important secondary role in perception. The discovery of invariant auditory segments in speech, together with experimental results demonstrating categorical perception for *nonspeech* stimuli, such as dual pure tones (Pisoni, 1977), has weakened the argument for a specialized processing mechanism sensitive exclusively to linguistic stimuli, that is, the speech mode. So, too, have studies regarding feature detectors as *auditory* rather than phonetic.

Feature Detectors

Physiologic studies on animals have contributed indications that neural feature detectors exist for the perception of certain kinds of stimuli. Lieberman (1977) reviews several findings, such as in the frog. More recent information has become available that extends the concept to the human auditory apparatus, specifically with regard to its potential for decoding phonetic features. An overview is presented by Abbs and Sussman (1971), who explain that the presence of such an arrangement may be in part responsible for man's success at evolutionary development. The methodology used to investigate this issue is this: if adaptation occurs after prolonged stimulation to a fixed stimulus, then specific neural detectors are believed to exist to facilitate that sensation. This paradigm has long been used in visual studies (Hochberg, 1964, 1972). Eimas and Corbit (1973) found such a result with speech-like stimuli in an experiment in which they selectively adapted subjects' *linguistic* feature detectors. Eimas, Cooper, and Corbit (1973) were more specific in stating that these detectors, which are responsive to VOTs, are present in the central speech processing mechanism. Evidence by Dorman, Raphael, and Liberman (1979) suggests that silence is a cue to the stop manner and that it is phonetic in nature. This interpretation was made based on the fact that variant acoustic cues yielded the same phonetic percept. In contrast, Tartter and Eimas (1975) found indications that voicing and place of articulation are mediated by specific detectors, but that they are sensitive to simple *auditory*, as opposed to strictly linguistic components of the stimuli. Thus, a controversy exists about the specific nature of feature detectors. Apparently, familiarity with language is not prerequisite, as similar inferences were reached after testing chinchillas; they seemed to be predisposed to respond in the same manner as human subjects to changes in VOTs (Kuhl and Miller, 1978).

Detectors in Infants Although evidence occurs to indicate that feature detectors exist in adults, speculation has arisen as to whether in infants this is a cognitive or innate function. Eimas et al. (1971) addressed this issue by testing infants 1 and 4 months of age to determine their ability to distinguish voiced versus unvoiced, synthesized initial stop-vowel syllables. Through an ingenious experimental method involving the measurement of sucking activity in response to the stimuli, they measured sensitivity to VOTs. They concluded that the infants, like adults, are clearly able to distinguish these voicing cues using inborn detectors. Eimas (1974) also looked at place of articulation distinctions (specifically, /b/ versus /d/ in the initial position) in young babies and found that they possessed the ability to note differences between these stimuli as well. He has concluded from this and other studies (Eimas, 1978) that infants' ". . . speech-analyzing mechanisms extract a phonetic message from the auditory representation" (p. 361). "Thus, the manner in which cues for place of articulation are perceived is linguistic . . ." (p. 364). Jusczyk (1977), moreover, demonstrated that infants can also distinguish the place of articulation of position-final stops. Although the adaptation procedure has enjoyed wide acceptance among researchers, its validity has been challenged. Elman (1979) posits that the results so widely obtained ". . . might be due. . . to changes at a higher, cognitive level of perception, rather than at the sensory level" (p. 190).

Type of Detector A fundamental issue of concern to investigators is whether the feature detectors responsive to cues revealing manner and place of articulation are acoustic or phonetic. If they are only auditory, then each phoneme must have basic isolable and identifiable properties. If phonetic, then the listener's speech production mechanism conceivably could mediate acoustic differences in terms of the constraints of his articulatory system. Data have been accumulating that suggest that feature detectors are responsive to acoustic characteristics of the speech signal and that recognition as a speech element is unnecessary (Blumstein, Stevens, and Nigro, 1977; Eilers, 1977; Ohde and Scharf, 1979; Wood, 1976). Sawusch (1977) hypothesizes two levels of processing: a peripheral analysis, which consists of feature detectors responsive to frequency patterns, and an unspecified type of central analysis. This interpretation is generally in harmony with that of Blumstein and Stevens (1979).

MODELS OF PERCEPTION

The decade of the 1970s yielded major advancements in the understanding of the speech perception process. To appreciate the significance, it is necessary to diverge momentarily to outline previous stages of work. The seemingly paramount obstacle of the past—the lack of acoustic invariance—led researchers to consider a neurologic link between an individual's speech perception and speech production mechanisms as the solution to this dilemma. Two major modes evolved. One was proposed by researchers associated with the Haskins Laboratories in New Haven, Connecticut and is termed the "Motor Theory" (see Liberman et al., 1967), whereas the other was espoused by Stevens and co-workers at Massachusetts Institute of Technology and is known as "Analysis by Synthesis" (see Cooper, 1972; Stevens, 1972).

The notable work by Eimas and Corbit (1973), employing the adaptation technique, heralded a new era in speech research and shifted the emphasis away from these earlier active models as well. (The term "active" was assigned because of the believed necessary participation of the speech production mechanism in perception.) Scores of studies have followed using the adaptation paradigm, as well as other methodologies, such as the measurement of evoked potentials (Wood, 1975).

It is now a widely accepted belief that there are neural property detectors that respond to acoustic stimuli. Just what acoustic properties of speech signals elicit these responses is currently a matter of controversy. Originally, Eimas and Corbit (1973), among others, interpreted their results as indicative of linguistic detectors which output phonemes in response to incoming acoustic patterns. More recently, there has been mounting evidence that they respond only to acoustic properties of the signal, like VOT, frequencies in the bursts of stop consonants, formant frequency transitions, and the like. This latter strategy, therefore, requires at least two stages of processing before the phonetic percept is realized.

It is interesting that after nearly 20 years, research efforts have begun to document a passive model of perception compatible with the work of Jakobson, Fant, and Halle (1963) on distinctive features. How seemingly simple speech perception would be if the auditory system analyzed the frequency-intensity-temporal patterns into a feature matrix which could uniquely select phonemes. Whether this approach will ultimately satisfy the rigors of scientific inquiry will hopefully be determined in the near future.

Speech perception is a significant and complex aspect of the field of speech science. This chapter has attempted to review past findings and current trends in the field. Those readers interested in a more complete discussion of this subject are referred to Borden and Harris (1980).

REFERENCES

Abbs, J. H., and H. M. Sussman. 1971. Neurophysiological feature and speech perception. J. Speech Hear. Res. 14:23–36.

Bess, F. H., and T. H. Townsend. 1977. Word discrimination for listeners with flat sensorineural hearing losses. J. Speech Hear. Disord. 42:232–237.

Blumstein, S. E., and K. N. Stevens. 1979. Acoustic invariance in speech production: Evidence from measurements of the spectral characteristics of stop consonants. J. Acoust. Soc. Am. 66:1001–1017.

Blumstein, S. E., and K. N. Stevens. 1980. Perceptual invariance and onset spectra for stop consonants in different vowel environments. J. Acoust. Soc. Am. 67:648–662.

Blumstein, S. E., K. N. Stevens, and G. N. Nigro. 1977. Property detectors for bursts and transitions in speech perception. J. Acoust. Soc. Am. 61:1301–1313.

Borden, G. L., and K. S. Harris. 1980. Speech Science Primer. Williams & Wilkins Company, Baltimore.

Carney, A. E., G. P. Widin, and N. F. Viemeister. 1977. Noncategorical perception of stop consonants differing in VOT. J. Acoust. Soc. Am. 62:961–970.

Cooley, J. W., and J. W. Tukey. 1965. An algorithm for the machine calculation of complex Fourier series. Math. Computers 19:297–301.

Cooper, F. S. 1972. How is language conveyed by speech? In J. F. Kavanagh and I. G. Mattingly (eds.), Language by Ear and by Eye, pp. 25–45. MIT Press, Cambridge.

Delattre, P. C., A. M. Liberman, F. S. Cooper, and L. J. Gerstman. 1952. An experimental study of the acoustic determinants of vowel color: Observations on one- and two-formant vowels synthesized from spectrographic patterns. Word 8:195–210.

Dorman, M. F., L. J. Raphael, and A. M. Liberman. 1979. Some experiments on the sound of silence in phonetic perception. J. Acoust. Soc. Am. 65:1518–1532.

Eilers, R. E. 1977. Context-sensitive perception of naturally produced stop and fricative consonants by infants. J. Acoust. Soc. Am. 61:1321–1336.

Eimas, P. D. 1974. Auditory and linguistic processing of cues for place of articulation by infants. Percept. Psychophysics 16:513–521.

Eimas, P. D. 1978. Developmental aspects of speech perception. In R. Held, H. W. Leibowitz, and H. -L. Teuber (eds.), Handbook of Sensory Physiology, pp. 357–374. Springer-Verlag, New York.

Eimas, P. D., W. E. Cooper, and J. D. Corbit. 1973. Some properties of linguistic feature detectors. Pecept. Psychophysics 13:247–252.

Eimas, P. D.,and J. D. Corbit. 1973. Selective adaptation of linguistic feature detectors. Cogn. Psychol. 4:99–109.

Eimas, P. D., E. R. Siqueland, P. Jusczyk, and J. Vigorito. 1971. Speech perception in infants. Science 171:303–306.

Elman, J. L. 1979. Perceptual origins of the phoneme boundary effect and selective adaptation to speech: A signal detection theory analysis. J. Acoust. Soc. Am. 65:190–207.

Fant, C. G. M. 1956. On the predictability of formant levels and spectrum envelopes from formant frequencies. In M. Halle, H. Lunt, and H. MacLean (eds.), For Roman Jacobson, pp. 109–120. Mouton, The Hague.

Fant, C. G. M. 1970. Acoustic theory of speech production. Mouton, The Hague.

Fant, C. G. M. 1973. Speech sounds and features. MIT Press, Cambridge.

Fletcher, S. G. 1970. Acoustic Phonetics. In F. S. Borg and S. G. Fletcher (eds.), The Hard of Hearing Child, pp. 57–84. Grune & Stratton, New York.

French, N. R., and J. L. Steinberg. 1947. Factors governing the intelligibility of speech sounds. J. Acoust. Soc. Am. 19:90–119.

Gerber, S. E. 1974. Introductory Hearing Science. W.B. Saunders Company, Philadelphia.

Halle, M., G. W. Hughes, and J.-P. A. Radley. 1957. Acoustic properties of stop consonants. J. Acoust. Soc. Am. 29:107–116.

Heinz, J. M., and K. N. Stevens. 1961. On the properties of voiceless fricative consonants. J. Acoust. Soc. Am. 33:589–596.

Hochberg, J. E. 1964. Perception. Prentice-Hall, Englewood Cliffs, N.J.

Hochberg, J. 1972. Perception II. Space and movement. In J. W. Kling and L. A. Riggs (eds.), Experimental Psychology, pp. 475–550. 3rd Ed. Holt, Rinehart, & Winston, Inc., New York.

Jakobson, R., C. G. M. Fant, and M. Halle. 1963. Preliminaries to speech analysis. MIT Press, Cambridge.

Jusczyk, P. W. 1977. Perception of syllable-final stop consonants by 2-month old infants. Percep. Psychophysics 21:450–454.

Koenig, W., H. K. Dunn, and L. Y. Lacy. 1946. The sound spectrograph. J. Acoust. Soc. Am. 18:19–49.

Konkle, D. F., D. S. Beasley, and F. H. Bess. 1977. Intelligibility of time-altered speech in relation to chronological aging. J. Speech Hear. Res. 20:108–115.

Kuhl, P. K., and J. D. Miller. 1978. Speech perception by the chinchilla: Identification functions for synthetic VOT stimuli. J. Acoust. Soc. Am. 63:905–917.

Ladefoged, P. 1975. A Course in Phonetics. Harcourt Brace Jovanovich, New York.

Levitt, H. 1978. The acoustics of speech production. In M. Ross and T. D. Giolas (eds.), Auditory Management of Hearing-Impaired Children, pp. 45–115. University Park Press, Baltimore.

Liberman, A. M., F. S. Cooper, D. P. Shankweiler, and M. Studdert-Kennedy. 1967. Perception of the speech code. Psychol. Rev. 74:431–461.

Liberman, A. M., P. C. Delattre, F. S. Cooper, and L. H. Gerstman. 1954. The role of consonant-vowel transitions in the perception of stop and nasal consonants. Psychol. Monograph 68:1–13.

Licklider, J. C. R. 1946. Effects of amplitude distortion upon the intelligibility of speech. J. Acoust. Soc. Am. 18:429–434.

Licklider, J. C. R., and G. A. Miller. 1951. The perception of speech. In S. S. Stevens (ed.), Handbook of Experimental Psychology, pp. 1040–1074. John Wiley & Sons, Inc., New York.

Lieberman, P., 1977. Speech Physiology and Acoustic Phonetics. MacMillan Publishing Company, New York.
Mermelstein, P. 1977. On detecting nasals in continuous speech. J. Acoust. Soc. Am. 61:581–587.
Miller, G. A. 1956. The magical number seven plus or minus two. Psychol. Rev. 63:81–97.
Miller, G. A., and J. C. R. Licklider. 1950. The intelligibility of interrupted speech. J. Acoust. Soc. Am. 22:167–173.
Minifie, F. D., T. J. Hixon, and F. Williams. 1973. Normal Aspects of Speech, Hearing and Language. Prentice-Hall, Inc., Englewood Cliffs, N.J.
Norman, D. A. 1969. Memory and attention. John Wiley & Sons, Inc., New York.
O'Conner, J. D., L. J. Gerstman, A. M. Liberman, P. C. Delattre, and F. S. Cooper. 1957. Acoustic cues for the perception of initial /w, j, r, l/ in English. Word 13:24–43.
Ohde, R. N., and D. J. Scharf. 1979. Relationship between adaptation and the percept and transformations of stop consonant voicing: Effects of the number of repetitions and intensity of adaptors. J. Acoust. Soc. Am. 66:30–45.
Peterson, G. E., and H. L. Barney, 1952. Control methods used in a study of the vowels. J. Acoust. Soc. Am. 24:175–184.
Pisoni, D. B. 1977. Identification and discrimination of the relative onset time of two component tones: Implications for voicing perception in stops. J. Acoust. Soc. Am. 61:1352–1361.
Sawusch, J. R. 1977. Peripheral and central processes in selective adaptation of place of articulation in stop consonants. J. Acoust. Soc. Am. 62:738–750.
Schwartz, D. M., and R. K. Surr. 1979. Three experiments on the California consonant test. J. Speech Hear. Disord. 44:61–72.
Scott, B. L. 1976. Temporal factors in vowel perception. J. Acoust. Soc. Am. 60:1354–1365.
Stevens, K. N. 1972. Segments, features, and analysis by synthesis. In J. F. Kavanah and I. G. Mattingly, (eds.), The Relationship between Speech and Reading, pp. 47–52. MIT Press, Cambridge.
Stevens, K. N., and Blumstein, S. E. 1978. Invariant cues for place of articulation in stop consonants. J. Acoust. Soc. Am. 64:1358–1368.
Stevens, K. N., and A. S. House. 1955. Development of a quantitative description of vowel articulation. J. Acoust. Soc. Am. 27:484–493.
Stevens, K. N., and A. S. House. 1972. Speech perception. In J. Tobias (ed.), Foundations of Modern Auditory Theory, Vol. 2, pp. 1–62. Academic Press, New York.
Stevens, S. S., and H. Davis. 1938. Hearing, Its Psychology and Physiology. John Wiley & Sons, Inc., New York.
Strange, W., R. R. Verbrugge, D. P. Shankweiler, and T. R. Edman. 1976. Consonant environment specifies vowel identity. J. Acoust. Soc. Am. 60:213–224.
Studdert-Kennedy, M. 1976. Speech perception. In N. Lass (ed.), Contemporary Issues in Experimental Phonetics, pp. 243–293. Academic Press, New York.
Tartter, V. C., and P. D. Eimas. 1975. The role of auditory feature detectors in the perception of speech. Percept. Psychophysics 18:293–298.
Tillman, T. W., R. Carhart, and L. Wilber. 1963. A test for speech discrimination composed of CNC monosyllabic words. Northwestern University

Auditory Test No. 4. Technical Documentary Report No. SAM-TDR-62-135, USAF School of Aerospace Medicine, Brooks Air Force Base.

Wood, C. C. 1975. Auditory and phonetic levels of processing in speech perception: Neurophysiological and information-processing analyses. Human Perception and Performance. J. Exp. Psychol. 104:3–20.

Wood, C. C. 1976. Discriminability, response bias, and phoneme categories in discrimination of voice onset time. J. Acoust. Soc. Am. 60:1381–1389.

CHAPTER 4

CALIBRATION MEASUREMENTS FOR SPEECH AUDIOMETERS

Dan F. Konkle and Thomas H. Townsend

CONTENTS

STANDARDS	56
Purposes	56
Development	57
THE SPEECH AUDIOMETER	59
CALIBRATION	61
General Measurement Considerations	62
Earphone Measures	64
Other Requirements	70
Loudspeaker Measures	71
Test Environment	76
CONCLUSION	76
REFERENCES	77

The process of interpreting speech audiometric findings typically is based upon comparing the responses for an individual listener either to standardized data for the same audiometric procedure, or to responses obtained previously for the same listener. Because this comparative approach to auditory assessment depends upon making repeated measurements for a specific test procedure, it is essential that such measures be obtained under similar listening conditions. Variables associated with the test procedure that can influence the listener's responses must be controlled so that test results reflect listener behavior rather than measurement artifact. The responsibility for controlling measurement variables rests with the audiologist and begins by insuring that the physical parameters of the stimuli (i.e., frequency, intensity, and time) can be delivered to the listener in the exact manner prescribed by the test procedure. This means that the instrument used to present stimuli, an audiometer, must be dependable and capable of presenting desired stimuli in the same manner in each trial.

The manufacturers of various audiometers design their equipment to operate precisely and dependably. Nevertheless, the findings of several published surveys suggest that audiometer performance often does not meet the electroacoustic specifications claimed by the manufacturer; therefore, frequently there are substantial differences in the electroacoustic outputs among different instruments (Eagles and Doerfler, 1961; Melnick, 1979; Thomas et al., 1969; Wilber, 1978). Such conditions must be avoided in speech audiometry because it is virtually impossible to obtain reliable and valid test results with malfunctioning equipment. Reasonable confidence in the comparison and interpretation of audiometric data and subsequent diagnostic and rehabilitative decisions depend upon the audiologist's assurance that the performance of an audiometer is within acceptable tolerance limits and has remained stable over time. It is critically important that the electroacoustic characteristics of an audiometer are compatible with those of other audiometers used to conduct the same test procedures.

Acceptable audiometer performance is verified by conducting routine electroacoustic measurements of the system's output. Should these measures indicate that the audiometer is functioning improperly, the instrument must be adjusted so that it conforms to established specifications. This process of measurement and adjustment is termed calibration. Calibration thus implies two related but different functions: 1) the measurement of instrument performance to determine whether it meets certain designated specifications (i.e., criteria); and 2) the process of making adjustments or modifications of the instrument so that it complies with designated criteria.

The information presented in this chapter is focused on the former definition: the measurement of electroacoustic performance of speech audiometers to determine compliance with existing national standards. Because the purpose of measuring the electroacoustic output of an audiometer is to document the instrument's performance consistent with published criteria, the first section of this chapter considers the purposes and development of national standards. Next, the components and functions of a speech audiometer are described, followed by a detailed discussion of the measurements that must be made to confirm accurate audiometer performance. Finally, consideration is given to additional standards that are important to speech audiometry and the topic of sound field speech audiometry is discussed.

STANDARDS

The following discussion of the purposes and development of standards emphasizes the importance of standardization as a dynamic process. Standards must not restrict technological advancement, nor should they inhibit the development of new assessment procedures. In order to realize fully the implications associated with these concepts, it is necessary to understand both the general purposes and the procedure followed in the development of a national standard.

Purposes

Standards serve many purposes vital to the development and advancement of a modern technological society. The process of standardization provides a commonality among manufacturers and service providers that permits an orderly transfer of goods and services from provider to consumer. One need only contemplate briefly the chaos that could result without an accurate method of defining distance, speed, or mass, among other important factors. Although economic concerns probably account for the primary motivation for the development of most standards, other factors also serve to stimulate standardization. Motivational factors in the area of audiology, for example, include standardized nomenclature and units of measurement that simplify the exchange of data among facilities and related professions. Specific to instrumentation, consumer protection and safety are promoted through the process of standardization because audiometers used to assess hearing are manufactured in a uniform and quality-controlled manner (Sanders, 1972). Standardization thus permits a means to compare data obtained using different audiometers from various hearing centers, so long as each instrument performs consistently in a manner specified by an accepted standard.

Development

It was noted previously that standards are developed in response to a need. Motivation for a standard can arise from any number of sources either within the private sector or through governmental sanction. In the United States, the organization responsible for the development of standards is the American National Standards Institute (ANSI). ANSI is a private organization rather than a governmental agency, and, although responsible for developing and maintaining standards, ANSI does not actually write or revise specifications. Rather, ANSI delegates this responsibility to various organizations, usually technical or professional societies. In the area of acoustics, the Acoustical Society of America (ASA) holds the Secretariat for American National Standards Committee S3 on Bioacoustics. The scope of this committee is defined as: "Standards, specifications, methods of measurement and test, and terminology in the fields of psychological and physiological acoustics, including those aspects of general acoustics, noise, and shock and vibration which pertain to biological safety, tolerance, and comfort" (ASA, 1980; p. iv). Included within this scope is the development of specifications for both pure tone and speech audiometers.

The ASA is a professional and scientific society whose membership is open to any individual with an interest in acoustics. Committee S3 on Bioacoustics, however, actually is comprised of individuals not only with technical backgrounds, but also representatives from the manufacturing and consumer communities, governmental agencies and persons with a general interest in the area of standardization. This diverse membership allows several viewpoints to be expressed during the formation of a standard and thus minimizes the influence of special interest groups in structuring a standard that may restrict development of new technology or assessment procedures. Although the entire membership of Committee S3 usually is not involved directly in writing a specific standard, each member reviews a proposed standard prior to its adoption by the ASA and ANSI. The actual standard is drafted by a subcommittee, or working group, assigned by Committee S3. The working group (WG) responsible for audiometric standards, for example, is WG S3-35. This group not only must devise new standards when necessary, but also is required to review existing standards at least every five years. When an existing standard is reviewed, the working group makes one of the following recommendations: 1) to reaffirm the standard as written; 2) to revise the entire, or part, of the standard; or 3) to withdraw and abandon the standard. Regardless of whether the working group has drafted a new standard or reviewed an existing standard, either the draft or recommendation is forwarded to Committee S3 where a "substantial consensus" of the membership, usually by written ballot, must be reached prior to approval. Because this process requires that all conflicts be resolved, the development or revision of a standard often is a time-consuming task. This does not mean that all members of S3 must vote affirmatively before acceptance, but that conflicts concerning the wording or specifications of a proposed standard must be resolved if it is to become a published document. Finally, both the ASA and ANSI must approve the proposed standard before it is published as an American National Standard. Once published, however, compliance with a national standard is not mandatory, nor does the existence of a standard preclude manufacturing or using instruments that do not conform to the standard's specifications. Nevertheless, ANSI standards often become authoritative and they commonly are cited by industry, technical and professional societies, and national, state, and local governmental agencies. It is important, therefore, that a standard reflect the consensus of a majority of providers and consumers directly concerned with its applications.

The development of national specifications for audiometers has been an ongoing process since the early 1950s. Before that time, national standards for audiometers did not exist; although the Council on Physical Medicine and Rehabilitation of the American Medical Association periodically published minimal requirements for acceptable audiometers. These documents served as unofficial standards from 1937 until the early 1950s and provided specifications for pure tone diagnostic and screening instruments as well as speech audiometers. The first national standard concerned with audiometers dealt with pure tone devices and was published in 1951 by the American Standards

Association[1] (ASA-Z24.5, 1951). This document was followed 2 years later by a national standard for speech audiometers (ASA-Z24.13, 1953). It is interesting that despite substantial advancements in technology and developments in audiologic assessment procedures, these two documents remained the only national standard for audiometers for almost 20 years. It was not until 1969 that a revision of these two standards was published (ANSI-S3.6, 1969; R-1973). The primary reason for this delay was a failure of the S3 committee membership to reach consensus concerning acceptable criteria for standard reference threshold levels. The specifics of this controversy represent the exception rather than the rule and are beyond the scope of this chapter (interested readers are directed to Davis, 1970 for an historical account of this controversy). It should be noted that the ANSI S3.6, 1969 (R-1973) standard is in effect at the time of this writing (1982). This standard, however, has been under revision by the S3-35 working group for the past several years and a new version should be published in the near future. Readers are advised of this situation so they may order the new standard when it is published by writing to:

> Standards Secretariat
> Acoustical Society of America
> 335 East 45th Street
> New York, New York 10017

THE SPEECH AUDIOMETER

ANSI-S3.6 (1969; R-1973) defines four types of pure tone and two types of speech audiometers. These distinctions imply that the pure tone and speech audiometers are different instruments. Indeed, early audiometers were not designed to present both pure tone and speech stimuli. Rather, if one wanted to conduct both pure tone and speech audiologic assessments, it was necessary to have two different audiometers—one for speech and another for pure tone testing. This is the reason initial standards were developed independently for pure tone (ASA-Z24.5, 1951) and speech (ASA-Z24.13, 1953) audiometric systems. The current generation of audiometers, however, contains circuitry that permits presentation of both pure tone and speech signals. Moreover, many of the components in current audiometers are used jointly for presenting both types of stimuli. Because the circuitry as-

---

[1] The American Standards Association was responsible for the standards program in the United States before ANSI. In 1966, the name of the American Standards Association was changed to the United States of America Standards Institute (USASI), and three years later (1969) was renamed ANSI.

sociated with the presentation of either pure tone or speech signals shares many of the same electronic components, it is convenient to describe first the fundamental elements of a pure tone system and then to compare the additional components necessary to present speech stimuli. This is illustrated by the block diagrams shown in Figure 4-1.

The basic components of a pure tone audiometer (Figure 4-1A) usually consist of: 1) two input sources (an oscillator and noise generator), with associated controls to select specific pure tone frequencies (frequency switch) or noise spectra derived from various filter networks (spectrum switch); 2) an input selector to determine the source of choice (i.e., pure tone, noise, or both); 3) a tone switch to present and interrupt the signal; 4) an attenuator to control the intensity of the signal; and 5) an output selector to direct stimuli to a transducer (i.e., earphones, a bone vibrator, or loudspeaker). Comparison of these components to those shown in Figure 4-1B, a combination pure tone and speech audiometer, reveals the principle differences between the two systems. These include: 1) provision to accept one or more additional input sources (e.g., a microphone, tape player, and/or a phonograph turntable); 2) a level control (potentiometer) and 3) a volume unit (VU) meter. Not shown in either Figure 4-1A or B are the various amplifiers that are common to all audiometers. The purpose of the additional input sources is to allow the conversion of acoustic energy contained

A. PURE TONE AUDIOMETER

B. PURE TONE & SPEECH AUDIOMETER

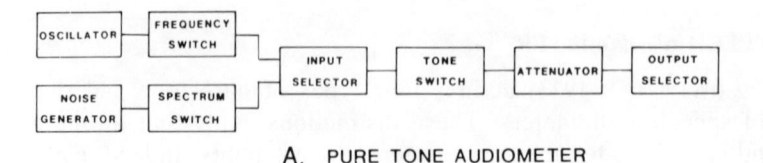

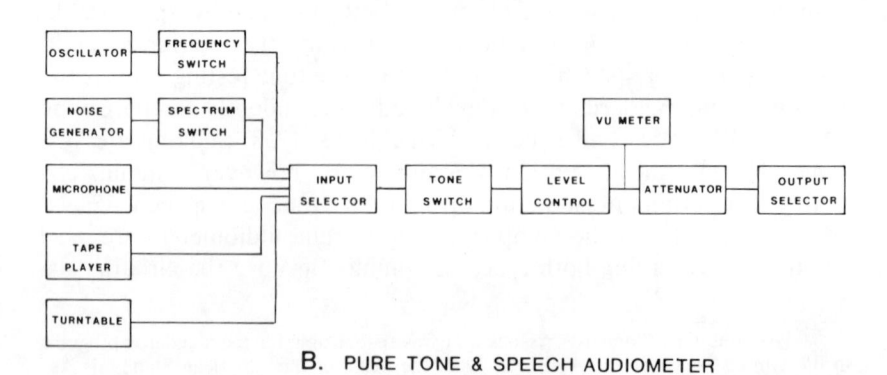

Figure 4-1. Block diagrams showing the basic components of a pure tone audiometer (A) and a combination pure tone and speech audiometer (B). Both diagrams are conceptual and do not represent a specific design for any particular audiometer.

in the spoken speech signal into electromagnetic energy that can be controlled and processed by the audiometer. This is accomplished for live voice presentations by a microphone, or for recorded presentations by storing the spoken message either on audio tape or a phonograph disc. The function of the level control and VU meter, however, is not as obvious. Recall from Chapter 3 that speech stimuli are complex acoustic signals whose physical parameters (i.e., intensity, frequency, and temporal patterns) change rapidly with time. The relative relationships among these parameters can be preserved for repeated presentations by recording stimuli on tape or disc. Whereas recorded stimuli are recommended for speech audiometry because they promote standardization, it should be recognized that the overall intensity levels of different recordings can vary considerably. This means that input intensities to the audiometer also vary regardless of whether the clinician uses live voice or recorded presentations. Thus, in order to accommodate clinicians with different voice intensities, as well as tapes or discs recorded at various overall intensity levels, it must be possible to adjust the audiometer so that input signals represent the same intensity level. The level control is used either to increase or decrease the relative intensity of varied input signals to a common reference read from the VU meter. This process maintains the intensity calibration of the audiometer (to be discussed subsequently) because all input signals, regardless of their overall intensities, are adjusted to the same reference level. Furthermore, this practice avoids overloading the amplifiers in the remainder of the system, thus preventing distortion. Note that the level control and VU meter are placed in the circuitry before the attenuator in order to maintain constant intensity inputs that are not influenced by the attenuator setting. Changing the attenuator will not affect the adjusted intensity level of the input signal because the level control and VU meter are inserted into the circuitry before the attenuator; that is, the VU meter will remain at reference (i.e., 0 dB VU) regardless of the position of the attenuator. The remaining components of the audiometer are essentially the same for both pure tone and speech presentations. In summary, most pure tone and speech audiometers currently are housed in the same instrument and often share many of the same components. The primary additional components for a speech audiometer consist of extra input sources, a volume control and VU meter.

CALIBRATION

Recall that calibration previously was defined as a process of measurement and adjustment (i.e., making corrections in signal output parameters), and that the focus of this chapter is on the measurement of speech audiometer performance. This does not imply that the adjustment process is less important than performance measurements, nor does it suggest that the audiologist can ignore responsibility in the area of adjustment. Even though other persons with expertise in audiometer calibration may actually make the measurements and adjustments, the audiologist ultimately is responsible for determining that such procedures have been performed correctly. In the final analysis the audiologist is accountable for the reliability and validity of audiologic test results, and this goal can only be realized when an adequately calibrated audiometer is used for audiologic assessment.

Calibration of a speech audiometer requires the measurement of several electroacoustic and electronic output parameters. The procedures used to make these measurements are described in detail in section 5.0 of ANSI S3.6, 1969 (R-1973): *American National Standard Specifications for Audiometers*. The following discussion does not cite these specifications verbatim, nor is a step-by-step procedure presented to make each measurement. Rather, the subsequent sections of this chapter contain explanations of the principle features of ANSI S3.6 that pertain specifically to speech audiometers. Readers interested in a complete description of ANSI S3.6, including measurements for both pure tone and speech audiometers, are directed to Melnick (1979) and Wilber (1978) as well as directly to the ANSI S3.6 standard.

General Measurement Considerations

In addition to electroacoustic measurements of audiometer performance, there are several general considerations that are important to the calibration process. First, the individual performing the calibration should be completely familiar with the operation of the instruments used to make calibration measurements. Equally important, however, is complete familiarization with the audiometer to be calibrated. As noted previously, the current generation of clinical audiometers is designed to present both pure tone and speech signals. These units often contain a variety of switches that can be activated to present sophisticated stimuli used for various audiologic tests. Some of these switches may serve a dual purpose, depending upon the type of stimuli presented to the output transducer. If these switches are not positioned correctly, the audiometer may not function in the desired mode and thus, calibration measurements will not reflect the instrument's true performance. The manufacturers of audiometers and instrumentation used for calibration provide manuals that describe the operation and set-up procedures that apply to their particular equipment. Clearly, one should read these manuals thoroughly before conducting calibration measurements.

Another consideration is the general requirements specified for all audiometers in section 3.0 of ANSI S3.6. Contained in this section is information related to audiometer identification (i.e., name and serial number), power supply voltage and frequency, appropriate earphones and earphone cushions, headbands, safety requirements, and instrument warm-up time. Although most of these specifications do not require measurement, many provide important information for the purpose of calibration. Most of the audiometers manufactured for use in the United States, for example, are designed to operate on a power supply of 120 volts with a frequency of 60 Hz. It would not be proper, therefore, to attempt calibration of such an instrument with a substantially different power supply. Indeed, such a practice could result in severe damage to the audiometer.

Before electroacoustic calibration, the audiometer should be inspected visually and a listening check performed. Visual inspection can reveal abnormalities such as worn earphone cushions, loose or misaligned dials, broken switches, and frayed, cracked, or broken earphone cords. These deficiencies should be corrected before calibration. Listening to the output of the audiometer while manipulating the attenuator, switching the output selector from the right to left earphone, or pulling lightly on the earphone cord often can indicate malfunction. If one hears an excessive level of background noise mixed with the speech signal, fails to perceive a notable change in loudness as the attenuator is altered, receives an intermittent signal as the earphone cords are manipulated, or if the signal does not alternate between earphones with appropriate switching of the output selector, the audiometer is not functioning in a proper manner. Although a listening check cannot determine if a speech audiometer complies with ANSI S3.6, it can indicate potential problem areas that need correction (i.e., faulty earphone cords, a broken attenuator or output selector, etc.). Hence, a visual and listening check of the audiometer should be conducted as part of each calibration.

A final general consideration important to the calibration process is the type of equipment used to make electroacoustic measurements. Whereas calibration of pure tone audiometers requires an array of instruments to measure output signals, calibration of speech audiometers must include additional equipment to provide controlled input signals. Input stimuli must be directed through the entire audiometer and thus either need to be recorded (i.e., on tape or disc) or presented as sound field stimuli to the audiometer's microphone. The specific instruments necessary to present input signals and to make output measurements have been described previously (see Dirks, Morgan, and Wilson, 1976; or Melnick, 1973; 1979) and will not be given further consideration in this chapter. It is important, however, to consider briefly the methods used to obtain calibration measurements.

Speech stimuli can be presented to a listener either by earphones, a bone vibrator, or a loudspeaker. The majority of speech audiometric procedures are conducted via earphone or loudspeaker presentations. ANSI S3.6, 1969 (R-1973) only stipulates specifications for speech audiometers when signals are transduced by an earphone. The standard does not provide specifications for sound field testing when stimuli are presented via a loudspeaker. The following discussion, therefore, pertains to earphone measurements. Consideration of sound field calibration is contained in a later section.

Earphone Measures

When the output of an audiometer is directed to an earphone, both electrical and acoustical measurements are necessary for calibration. Figure 4-2 schematically illustrates a convenient arrangement that allows both electrical and acoustical measurements to be made at the same time. The majority of measurements are made acoustically by placing the earphone on an acoustic coupler with dimensions consistent with those specified for a National Bureau of Standards (NBS) 9-A coupler. The NBS 9-A coupler consists of a hard-walled cavity terminated at one end by a calibrated microphone, and has a volume of 6 cm^3 when the earphone in conjunction with the earphone cushion is placed over the other end. It is important that the earphone is placed carefully on the 6 cm^3 cavity so the diaphragm of the earphone is

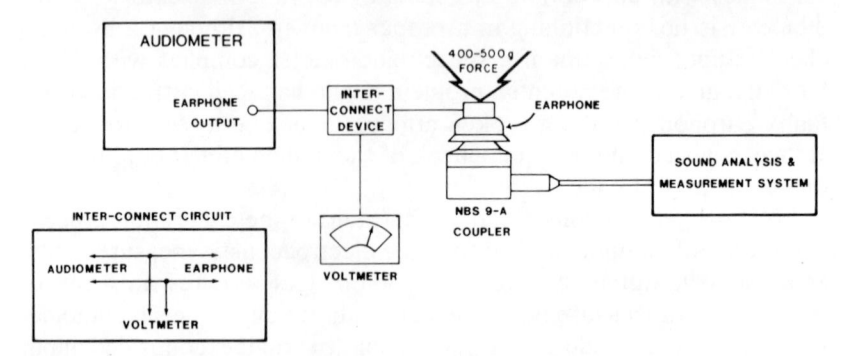

Figure 4-2. Schematic illustration of an arrangement that allows convenient measurement of both the electrical and acoustic outputs of an audiometer. Note that the inter connect device has two outputs (i.e., one to the earphone and the other to a voltmeter) that are connected in parallel. This means that electrically the two outputs are connected at the same point; that is, the input to the earphone. Thus, use of a high-impedance vacuum tube or digital voltmeter to make electrical measurements will not result in an additional load on the earphone output. See text for further discussion of this arrangement.

centered over and parallel with the diaphragm of the microphone, and that the earphone is loaded (e.g., weighted) by a 400- to 500-gram force. Given this arrangement, the acoustic output from the earphone is measured as the intensity generated in the 6 cm^3 cavity at the surface of the microphone. The microphone, of course, is connected to instrumentation appropriate for sound measurement and analysis. Electrical measurements are made across the input to the earphone with the input line (i.e., earphone wire) loaded either by the earphone or an electrical simulation of the earphone. When electrical calibration measurements are made, it is incorrect to disconnect the earphone from the audiometer and simply plug the voltmeter, or some other electrical measurement device, into the earphone jack. Rather, either the earphone must remain connected to the audiometer, or the audiometer must be loaded (i.e., connected) with an electrical network that simulates the effect of the earphone when it is attached to the audiometer and placed on a NBS 9-A coupler. This requirement can be accomplished easily by using an interconnect device with the simple circuitry shown in Figure 4-2. Such a device is inexpensive and can be built with only a basic knowledge of electronics. The device is plugged into the earphone output jack of the audiometer, thus allowing both the earphone and voltmeter to be plugged into the interconnect device (see Figure 4-2). In this manner, correct electrical measurements may be made because the audiometer is loaded by the earphone, and acoustical measurements can be obtained at the same time without disrupting the position of the earphone on the NBS 9-A coupler.

The methods for making electrical and acoustical earphone measurements just described are specified by ANSI S3.6, 1969 (R-1973). The revision of this standard currently under review is not expected to change these methods. It is probable, however, that the new ANSI document will specify several measurements that are not included in the current standard. Consequently, these probable changes are discussed, in general, after first describing the measurements currently required to specify audiometer performance.

Frequency Response The frequency response of a system refers to the relative differences in gain as a function of frequency. Gain is defined as the dB difference between input and output intensities. A flat frequency response generally is considered a highly desirable characteristic; that is, the amount of gain is equal for the various frequencies measured. ANSI S3.6 specifies the frequency response for speech audiometers over a range from 200 to 4000 Hz—a bandwidth that approximates that of speech. The gain at frequencies within this range must not exceed the gain at 1000 Hz by more than ±5 dB. Otherwise stated, the frequency response must not vary by more than 10 dB over the range from 200 to 4000 Hz. A further restraint placed on audiometers that use recorded inputs is that gain shall not rise by more than 10 dB relative to the 1000-Hz gain for frequencies below 200 or above 4000 Hz. Frequency response is measured for recorded inputs with a constant-intensity sine wave recording of various frequencies (either tape or disc, depending on the input mode) with the VU meter adjusted to a standard reference position. For the microphone input mode, however, various pure tones are presented via sound field at an intensity of approximately 74 dB sound pressure level (SPL) at the microphone. Generating these signals requires an external array of equipment consisting of an oscillator, attenuator, and loudspeaker in addition to a calibrated microphone and sound analyzer. A more convenient approach that has been used successfully in the authors' laboratories is to place the audiometer's microphone in a commercially available hearing aid test box. Hearing aid test systems usually are capable of delivering constant intensity pure tone signals within the range necessary for speech audiometer calibration. The VU meter, as with recorded inputs, is adjusted to a standard reference position. Regardless of the input mode, frequency response is determined with the hearing loss dial (i.e., attenuator) adjusted to 60-dB hearing level (HL).

Reference Sound Pressure Level The reference sound pressure level of a speech audiometer is specified relative to the output intensity of a 1000-Hz pure tone rather than a speech signal. This manner of specification is used because it is impractical to integrate the fluctuating intensities associated with speech into a single value. Thus, the sound pressure level of speech is defined as the level of a 1000-Hz tone having an amplitude equal to the average intensity of speech as displayed on a VU meter. Consequently, when the volume control of a speech audiometer is adjusted so that an input speech signal peaks the VU meter at the standard reference position, the audiometer's output level will be at the same intensity as measured for the 1000-Hz calibration tone. Recorded speech materials, therefore, should be preceded by a 1000-Hz tone that is recorded on the tape or disc at an intensity equal to the average amplitude of the speech signal.

The reference sound pressure level for a speech audiometer will vary as a function of the specific earphone used to transduce the stimuli. ANSI S3.6 currently specifies reference sound pressure levels for only two earphones: the Western Electric Type 705-A and the Telephonics Type TDH-39. The reference level for the TDH-39 earphone mounted in a MX-41/AR cushion (ANSI only recommends the MX-41/AR earphone cushion) is 20 dB SPL, whereas the reference level for the 705-A is 19 dB SPL. Both these earphones, however, have been replaced by newer models. Consequently, the new ANSI standard probably will define the reference sound pressure level of a speech audiometer as 12.5 dB above the pure tone reference test threshold at 1000 Hz for the specific earphone and associated earphone cushion used by the audiometer. Because this is a reasonable criterion that applies equally to a variety of different earphones, it is recommended that calibration measurements for reference sound pressure level employ the forenoted 12.5-dB definition.

In order to determine the proper reference sound pressure level for a given earphone, therefore, it first is necessary to establish the reference test threshold value for 1000 Hz. These values are provided for several different earphones in the current ANSI specifications, and these data probably will be expanded to other earphones with publication of the new standard. For a TDH-39 earphone mounted in a MX-41/AR cushion, for example, the 1000-Hz reference test threshold is specified in ANSI S3.6 as 7 dB SPL. Thus, the reference sound pressure level for speech using this earphone/cushion combination is 19.5 dB SPL (i.e., 12.5 dB plus 7 dB equals 19.5 dB SPL). The speech reference sound pressure levels for other earphone/cushion arrangements, however, may vary because pure tone reference threshold levels for 1000 Hz may be different. Measurement of the reference sound pressure level for speech is conducted in the same manner as frequency response measures. The 1000-Hz input tone, whether recorded or presented to the microphone at approximately 74 dB SPL, is adjusted to the reference VU position and the attenuator is set to 60 dB HL. Given these conditions and the aforementioned TDH-39 earphone in a MX-41/AR cushion, the intensity measured from the 6 cm^3 coupler should be 79.5 dB SPL (i.e., 60 dB HL attenuator plus 7 dB 1000 Hz reference test threshold level plus 12.5 dB speech reference sound pressure level equals 79.5 dB SPL). The permissible tolerance for this measurement is ±3 dB.

Attenuator Linearity The current ANSI standard stipulates that the attenuator of a speech audiometer should range from 0 to 100 dB and be capable of delivering signals in increments of 2.5 dB or less. The measured output of the audiometer for a 1000-Hz tone with the attenuator set at 0 dB HL must equal the reference sound pressure level. Moreover, the difference between any two sequential attenuator settings must not differ by more than 1 dB from the numerical difference between the settings. This means that if the attenuator is changed from a setting of 50 to 55 dB HL, the measured difference in output must be 5 dB, ±1 dB, or between 4 and 6 dB. These measurements must be made electrically at the input to the earphone, and the earphone must be placed on the 6 cm^3 coupler, or the earphone may be replaced by a load that electrically simulates the earphone. A simple and effective means to make electrical measurements was described at the outset of this section (see Figure 4-2).

Distortion Although there are several types of distortion, the current ANSI standard for speech audiometers only requires the measurement of harmonic distortion using specific pure tone frequencies (e.g., 250, 500, 1000, 2000, and 4000 Hz). The harmonics of the input stimuli must be at least 40 dB or more below the intensity of the fundamental frequency. The input tones are presented to the audiometer in the same manner as that described for previous measurements; however, the volume control is adjusted to provide a VU reading of 6 dB greater than the standard reference level, and the attenuator is set to provide maximum output. The intensity of each fundamental frequency measured at the output must be at least 25 dB above the level of any associated higher harmonic.

Noise The purpose of this measurement is to determine the intensity ratio of the output signal relative to the intensity of electrical background noise produced by all components (including input sources) in the speech audiometer circuitry. This ratio must be at least +50 dB. In other words, signals processed by the audiometer must be at least 50 dB above the level of the electrical background noise. In order to determine this value, it is necessary to make two measurements. First, the acoustic output of the audiometer is measured for a 1000-Hz input tone presented as noted for previous measurements, except the tone is presented at 85 dB SPL for the microphone input. The volume control is set to give a standard VU reference reading and the attenuator is adjusted to 100 dB HL. Second, the acoustic output of the audiometer is measured without presenting the input tone, but with all other settings maintained. For recorded input modes, either the tape recorder is activated without tape crossing the pick-up heads or the phonograph turntable is allowed to rotate with the pick-up arm placed in the rest position. For the microphone input mode, the microphone remains on but it is shielded (as much as possible) from environmental noise. The intensity difference (in dB) between the first (input signal present) and the second (input signal off) measures must be at least 50 dB.

Masking In order to meet current ANSI S3.6 requirements a speech audiometer must provide a masking noise that is able to mask a 60-dB HL speech signal. The standard does not specify an acoustic spectrum for the masking noise. Instead, the ANSI document recommends that the masker be a broadband noise covering a frequency range from 250 to 4000 Hz. The maximum acoustic output of the masker must not exceed 120 dB SPL as measured in a 6 cm^3 coupler. Moreover, the intensity of the masking noise has to be adjustable in steps of 5 dB or less over a range at least 40 dB below the 60-dB HL criterion noted above.

VU Meter A speech audiometer must be equipped with a meter for monitoring the relative level of input stimuli. Recall that the function of this meter, in conjunction with the level control, is to adjust the level of the input signal to a standard reference, and that the meter must be connected in the speech circuit before the attenuator. It follows, therefore, that the intensity output of the audiometer will remain in calibration only when the input signal is made to peak at the standard VU reference level. A representative VU meter is illustrated in Figure 4-3. Observe that the dB scale of the VU meter extends from −20 dB at the left to +3 dB on the right and that the meter is indicating a value of 0 dB VU. The 0-dB VU point commonly is used as a standard reference level, although other levels may be used as long as that same level is maintained as the standard reference for subsequent presentations of stimuli. The S3.6 standard, however, states that the characteristics of this meter shall be dictated by another standard— ANSI C16.5, 1954: *Volume Measurements of Electrical Speech and Program Waves*. The most significant portions of this document relate to the frequency response and dynamic characteristics of the VU meter. Specifically, the frequency response must not vary by more than 0.2 dB between 35 and 10,000 Hz, nor by more than 0.5 dB between 25 and 16,000 Hz. The dynamic characteristics must be such that the indicating pointer must reach 99 percent of its reference deflection (i.e., the standard reference level) in 270 to 330 msec after an impulse signal is applied. Furthermore, the pointer shall then overswing the standard reference level by 1.0 to 1.5 percent. Realistically, it is extremely inconvenient to make measurements of the VU meter to determine whether it meets these very stringent criteria. The meter

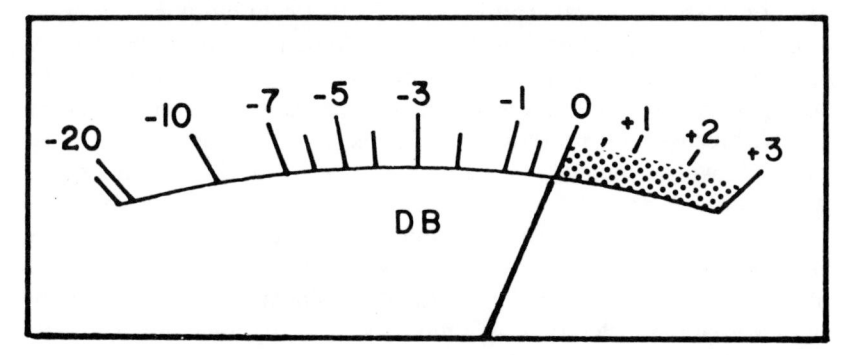

Figure 4-3. Schematic illustration of a volume unit (VU) meter. See text for a discussion of the function and calibration measurements related to this audiometer component.

circuit, for example, must be electrically isolated within the audiometer so that other components of the audiometer do not influence the performance of the VU meter. Also, most facilities do not have the instrumentation necessary to resolve the required reading from the VU meter to a fraction of a decibel. In addition, a gated strobe light, or some similar device, must be employed to measure the dynamic characteristics. Given these problems, the performance of the VU meter seldom is tested during the calibration of a speech audiometer. This is a most unfortunate circumstance because the intensity calibration of the audiometer depends directly on this component.

Other Requirements

The reliability and validity of speech audiometric measurements depend upon the application of standardized procedures. This is best accomplished when standardized, recorded speech materials are used in conjunction with a calibration signal (i.e., a 1000-Hz calibration tone). The current ANSI S3.6 document, however, only provides specifications for disc recordings. Because recorded stimuli are important to standardized speech audiometric procedures, it is expected that the revised draft of ANSI S3.6 will not only contain criteria for disc recordings, but also for magnetic reel-to-reel and audio cassette tape recordings. In all probability, these specifications will be provided through reference to other existing ANSI standards, or to standards developed by other organizations.

There are several other aspects associated with the proposed revision of ANSI S3.6 that deserve brief consideration. Recall that the current ANSI standard specifies that earphone measurements be made using the MX-41/AR cushion. The new standard most likely will permit using other supra-aural-type cushions similar in design to either the MX-41/AR or the newer Telephonics 51 cushions. Regardless of the specific cushion, however, it is expected that calibration of earphones using supra-aural cushions will continue to be made using the NBS 9-A coupler. Calibration procedures for alternative air conduction transducers (i.e., earphones mounted in circumaural headsets designed for use with or without supra-aural cushions, insert earphones, etc.) also probably will be included in the new standard with the stipulation that manufacturers provide reference equivalent threshold sound pressure levels obtained from specified loudness balance procedures. Calibration measurements for these alternative air conduction sources probably will be required using an artificial ear similar to that specified by the International Electronics Commission (IEC) publication 318-1970: *An IEC Artificial Ear, of the Wide Band Type, for the Calibration of Earphones Used in Audiometry.*

Perhaps the most substantial changes expected in the new ANSI document will relate to masking stimuli. It is expected that masker amplitude spectra will be specified (i.e., broadband or speech spectrum, or both), that reference intensity levels will be expressed in decibels HL relative to effective masking levels (see Chapter 9 for a discussion of effective masking level), and that tolerances and masking level ranges will be redefined. The new standard probably will not be expanded to include speech audiometry conducted via sound field presentations, although WG S3-35 is considering an appendix to the new standard that will address this area. Although an appendix is not considered part of a national standard, it typically provides suggested measurements and criteria to assist standardization. Some of the suggestions advanced by WG S3-35 for sound field speech testing are reviewed in the next section.

Loudspeaker Measurements

Sound field speech audiometric measures have become a vital aspect of speech audiometry. As stressed previously, however, the current ANSI standard does not address the issue of sound field calibration, nor does it appear that the revised standard will specify performance characteristics for speech audiometers that transduce stimuli through a loudspeaker. This is unfortunate because sound field speech testing often is a routine clinical procedure, especially for testing young children and for the selection and evaluation of hearing aids. This situation is confounded further by a paucity of experimental data to draw upon for clarification of a rather complex issue. Nonetheless, the new ANSI standard is expected to contain an appendix that provides calibration guidelines for sound field speech audiometry. Before examination of suggested sound field calibration procedures, however, a brief review is provided of several pertinent acoustical terms and concepts.

Terminology There are two types of spaces into which speech stimuli may be introduced during sound field testing: 1) a free field; and 2) a reverberant field. A free field is an environment in which there are insignificant reflections of sound waves from the surfaces, or boundaries of the room. A common term for such a room is an anechoic chamber. An anechoic chamber, however, does not necessarily constitute a free field for all frequencies; that is, such a room will be anechoic for a given frequency range, but significant reflections will be present for frequencies outside this range. A picture of an anechoic chamber is shown in Figure 4-4. All structures that are not anechoic are reverberant rooms. This means that sound waves are reflected off the walls, ceiling, and floor to various degrees depending upon the "hardness" or "softness" of the respective surfaces. A room with

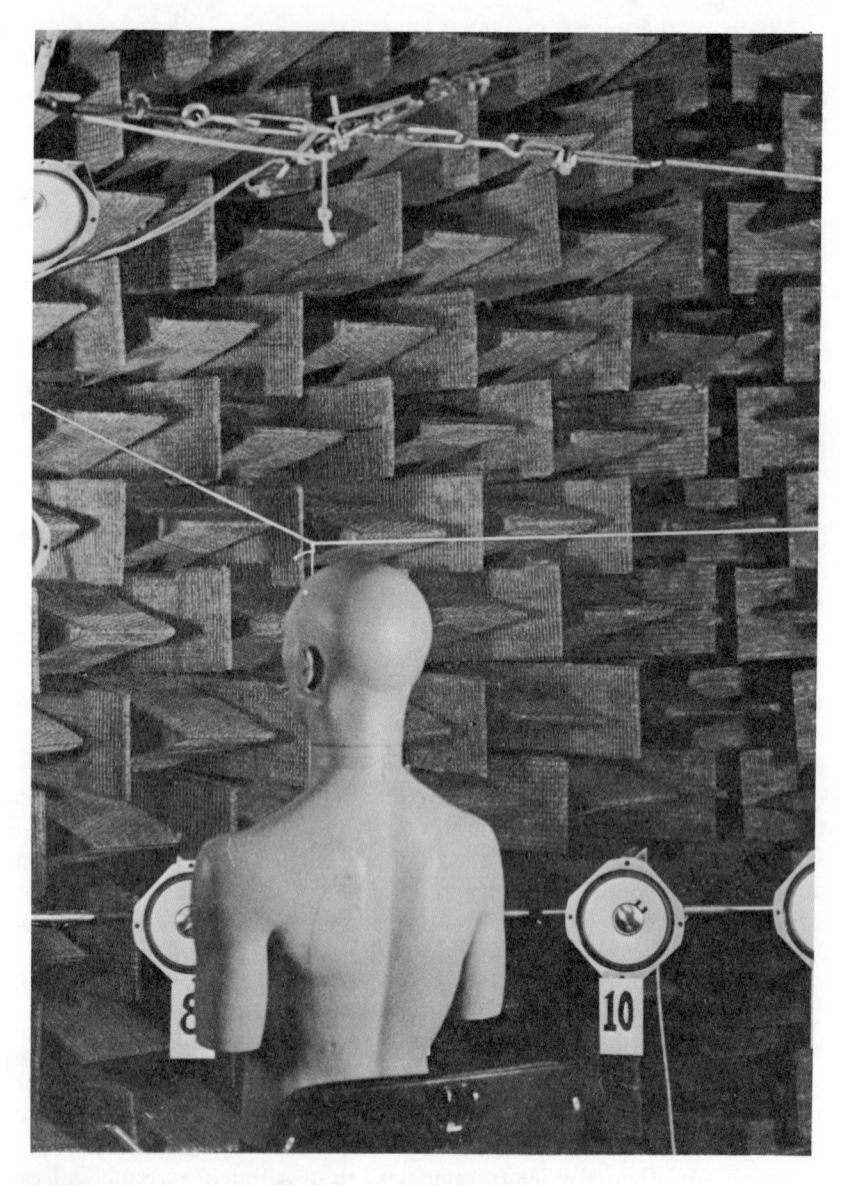

Figure 4-4. Picture of an anechoic chamber. Note that the walls, ceiling, and floor are comprised of wedge-shaped structures. The wedges are constructed of highly sound-absorbent material and are oriented at alternate right angles. Such construction results in insignificant reflection of sound waves.

smooth marble walls, for example, will be more reverberant than one in which walls are treated with acoustic tiles or draperies. The degree of reverberation also depends upon the size and configuration of the room, the relative location of the sound source (i.e., loudspeaker), any furniture or objects placed in the room, and the point at which sound measurements are made. Commercially available prefabricated or custom-built audiometric test rooms represent reverberant rather than free fields. In audiology the term *sound field* has been adopted to refer to the presentation of stimuli in these environments via a loudspeaker. It is important that the term sound field is not confused with free field. Indeed, these two environments usually represent two completely different conditions.

The importance of the foregoing explanation is that the reverberant characteristics of the sound treated audiometric test room affect the signals delivered by the loudspeaker. The effect will vary, depending upon the acoustic parameters of the stimuli. The influence is so profound for pure tones that the intensity of such stimuli cannot be specified accurately because of standing waves. Standing waves are caused by phase differences between the sound wave propagated directly from the loudspeaker and the wave that is reflected from a boundary (i.e., the walls, ceiling, furniture, etc.). Such differences, of course, result in substantial variations in the intensity of the signal when it is measured at different locations within the room. Consequently, pure tones cannot be used to determine audiometer performance (i.e., frequency response, reference sound pressure level, harmonic distortion, etc.) for loudspeaker outputs. Conversely, quasiperiodic signals like speech or aperiodic stimuli such as noise can be used successfully in the sound field because these signals do not form significant standing waves. The intensity of speech, however, fluctuates rapidly and thus noise stimuli provide the best signals for calibration measurements of the sound field.

Minimal Audible Pressure and Minimal Audible Field One of the most critical issues in sound field testing concerns the appropriate intensity to use as the reference sound pressure level. Recall that for earphone presentations this level was specified as 12.5 dB above the pure tone reference test threshold level at 1000 Hz. In 1933, Sivian and White obtained pure tone thresholds from a small group of listeners for signals presented via earphones and a loudspeaker located in an environment that had the characteristics of a free field. Their results, averaged across frequencies, indicated that about 6 dB greater intensity was required to reach threshold for the earphone compared to the loudspeaker condition. Sivian and White termed the earphone listening condition minimal audible pressure (MAP), and the free field condition minimal audible field (MAF). The difference between MAP and MAF thresholds became known as the "missing 6 dB" and was the topic of several subsequent investigations using speech rather than tonal stimuli (Breakey and Davis, 1949; Dirks, Stream, and Wilson, 1972; Stream and Dirks, 1974; Tillman, Johnson, and Olsen, 1966; Tillman et al., 1973). A summary of the findings from these investigations is presented in Table 4-1. The data shown in this table reveal similar results for the various studies, despite differences in specific test materials, subjects, earphones, and field listening conditions. Examination of the data indicate two important trends. First, the differences between MAP and MAF thresholds decreased as the angle of incidence (i.e., azimuth) defining the loudspeaker location relative to the midsagital plane of the listener's head decreased. For a 0° azimuth (e.g., loudspeaker located directly in front of the listener and at an equal distance from both ears), for example, the MAP - MAF difference ranged from 2.7 to 3.5 dB among four different investigations; whereas, for a 60° azimuth the MAP - MAF difference was reported as 7.0 dB by both Dirks et al. (1972) and Stream and Dirks (1974). Second, there appears to be a reduction in the MAP - MAF threshold difference when data are obtained in a sound field compared to a free field. Tillman et al. (1966) and Dirks et al. (1972) each reported a 7.5 dB difference in MAP - MAF thresholds for a 45° loudspeaker azimuth when field data were obtained in an anechoic environment. Tillman et al. (1973), however, found only a 4.4 dB MAP - MAF difference when field thresholds were measured in a standard audiometric test room.

The reasons for the MAP - MAF difference (i.e., the missing 6 dB) have been explained by Killion (1978) This apparent discrepancy results because of measurement artifacts associated with stipulating the intensity of earphone- and loudspeaker-transduced signals, and does not relate to the biomechanics of the human ear. The influence of loudspeaker location (i.e., azimuth) is best explained by changes in real ear canal SPL that result from various external and ear canal resonances that fluctuate as a function of altered sound source location (Shaw, 1975). Despite available data and the resolution of the MAP - MAF controversy, however, appropriate reference sound pressure levels for use in sound field testing remain unspecified. Although it seems apparent that a reference level of 7 dB less than the earphone reference sound pressure level may be reasonable for speech assessments conducted in a free field, this difference may be too great for sound field testing. Based on the limited data of Tillman et al. (1973) (see Table 4-1), a difference of only 3.5 to 4.5 dB may more closely approximate the appropriate reference sound pressure level for speech testing in a sound field. Clearly, additional experimental data are necessary before this level can be defined and specified in a national standard.

Table 4-1. Summary of several investigations that examined monaural thresholds for minimal audible pressure (MAP) and minimal audible field (MAF) listening conditions

Investigation	Test conditions	Loudspeaker azimuth[a]	Threshold difference (MAP-MAF)	Subjects
Breakey and Davis (1949)	Earphone; unspecified (non-anechoic) field	0	3.4[b]	Normal hearing
Tillman, Johnson, and Olsen (1966)	Earphone; anechoic chamber	45	7.5	Normal hearing and sensorineural hearing loss
Dirks, Stream, and Wilson (1972)	Earphone; anechoic chamber	0 30 60 90	2.8 5.6 7.0 6.6	Young sophisticated listeners; hearing status unspecified
	Earphone; anechoic chamber	0 45	3.5 7.5	Normal hearing
Tillman, et al. (1973)	Earphone; sound-treated test booth	45	4.4	Normal hearing
Stream and Dirks (1974)[c]	Earphone, anechoic chamber	0 30 60 90	2.7 5.6 7.1 6.7	Normal hearing

[a] Reported in degrees relative to the midsagital plane of the listener's head.
[b] Reported in decibels.
[c] Also reported binaural MAP and MAF data.

In the meantime, it is recommended that the reference sound pressure level for sound field speech measures be 13 dB SPL for loudspeakers located between 30° and 60° azimuth, and 16 dB SPL when loudspeakers are situated between 0° and 30° azimuth. These levels should be calibrated using a speech spectrum noise similar to that shown in Figure 9-6. This stimulus should be directed to the input of the audiometer in the same manner described for earphone calibration, the VU meter should be adjusted to the same reference position, and the attenuator set to 60 dB HL. The stimulus, of course, is transduced by a loudspeaker the intensity of which is measured by placing a calibrated microphone at the approximate position to be occupied by the listener's head. The listener, however, should not be in the sound field at the time calibration measurements are made. These criteria and measurement procedures are expected to be similar to those suggested in the forthcoming revision of ANSI S3.6. Until this document is published and consensus is reached concerning sound field calibration procedures and criteria, audiologists are encouraged to use a consistent reference sound pressure level for sound field speech testing, and as an absolute minimum report this value on the audiogram.

Test Environment

The level of noise present in an audiometric test room must not interfere with speech audiometric assessments. Permissible levels of noise during audiometric testing are specified as a national standard—ANSI S3.1, 1977: *Criteria for Permissible Ambient Noise During Audiometric Testing*. This standard indicates the maximum noise level that can be tolerated across a rather broad frequency range for testing conducted both with and without earphones. Measurements are to be made using either a one-octave or one-third-octave filter, the output of which leads to a sound level meter or measuring amplifier. In addition, noise levels within a very narrow frequency range centered around each audiometric test frequency are to be measured. For details of the measurement procedure as well as permissible noise levels, the reader is referred directly to the standard (ANSI S3.1, 1977). Measurements of noise levels are to be included as part of audiometric calibration.

CONCLUSION

This chapter has focused on the calibration of audiometers used for speech audiologic assessment. The content of the chapter is intended to supplement current national standards. Space restrictions have precluded a detailed discussion of each standard related to audiometric calibration. Pertinent standards, however, have been cited in the text.

The reader should obtain copies of these documents and develop an understanding of both the measurement procedures and tolerance criteria necessary for proper calibration. Although it is recognized that some audiologists may prefer to contract (i.e., purchase) calibration services, complete understanding of the calibration process often can minimize expensive audiometer down-time and unnecessary repairs. Moreover, the reliability and validity of audiometric measures depend upon using calibrated audiometers. As is emphasized in this chapter, there simply is no excuse for ignorance of calibration requirements and procedures on the part of audiologists.

REFERENCES

Acoustical Society of America. 1980. Catalog of Acoustical Standards, ASA Catalog 2. Acoustical Society of America, New York.
American National Standards Institute. 1954. Volume Measurements of Electrical Speech and Program Waves, ANSI-C16.5-1954. American National Standards Institute, Inc., New York.
American National Standards Institute. 1970. American National Standard Specifications for Audiometers, ANSI-S3.6-1969 (R-1973). American National Standards Institute, Inc., New York.
American National Standards Institute. 1977. Standard Criteria for Permissible Ambient Noise During Audiometric Testing. ANSI-S3.1-1977. American National Standards Institute, Inc., New York.
American Standards Association. 1951. American Standard Specifications for Audiometers for General Diagnostic Purposes, Z24.5-1951. American National Standards Institute, Inc., New York.
American Standards Association. 1953. American Standard Specifications for Speech Audiometers, Z24.13-1953. American National Standards Institute, Inc., New York.
Breakey, M. R., and H. Davis. 1949. Comparisons of thresholds for speech: Words and sentence tests; receiver vs. field and monaural vs. binaural listening. Laryngoscope 59:236–250.
Davis, H. 1970. Audiometry: Pure tone and simple speech tests. In H. Davis and R. S. Silverman (eds.), Hearing and Deafness, 3rd Ed., pp. 179–220. Holt, Rinehart & Winston, New York.
Dirks, D. D., D. E. Morgan, and R. H. Wilson. 1976. Experimental audiology. In C. A. Smith and J. A. Vernon (eds.), Handbook of Auditory and Vestibular Research Methods, pp. 498–547. Charles C Thomas Publisher, Springfield, Ill.
Dirks, D. D., R.W. Stream, and R. H. Wilson. 1972. Speech audiometry: Earphone and sound field. J. Speech Hear. Disord. 37:162–176.
Eagles, E. L., and L. G. Doerfler. 1961. Hearing in children: Acoustic environment and audiometric performance. J. Speech Hear. Res. 4:149–163.
International Electrotechnical Commission. 1970. An IEC Artificial Ear of the Wideband Type, for the Calibration of Earphones Used in Audiometry, IEC-318. American National Standards Institute, New York.
Killion, M. C. 1978. Revised estimate of minimum audible pressure: Where is the "missing 6 dB." J. Acoust. Soc. Am. 63:1501–1508.

Melnick, W. 1973. Psychoacoustic instrumentation. In J. Jerger (ed.), Modern Developments in Audiology, pp. 253-300. 2nd Ed. Academic Press, Inc., New York.

Melnick, W. 1979. Instrument calibration. In W. F. Rintelmann (ed.), Hearing Assessment, pp. 551-586. University Park Press, Baltimore.

Sanders, T. R. B. 1972. The Aims and Principles of Standardization. International Organization for Standardization, Geneva.

Shaw, E. A. G. 1975. The external ear: New knowledge. Scand. Audiol. 5(Suppl.):24-50.

Sivian, L. J., and S. D. White. 1933. On minimum audible sound fields. J. Acoust. Soc. Am. 4:288-321.

Stream, R. W., and D. D. Dirks. 1974. Effect of loudspeaker position on differences between earphone and free-field thresholds (MAP and MAF). J. Speech Hear. Res. 17:549-568.

Thomas, W. G., M. J. Preslar, R. Summers, and J. L. Steward. 1969. Calibration and working condition of 100 audiometers. Public Health Rep. 84:311-327.

Tillman, T. W., W. O. Olsen, M. C. Killion, M. G. Block. 1973. MAP versus MAF for spondees: Nothing's really missing. Paper presented at the convention of the American Speech and Hearing Association, October 12-15, Detroit.

Tillman, T., R. Johnson, and W. Olsen. 1966. Earphone versus sound field threshold sound pressure levels for spondee words. J. Acoust. Soc. Am. 39:125-133.

Wilber, L. A. 1978. Calibration, pure tone, speech and noise signals. In J. Katz (ed.), Handbook of Clinical Audiology, pp. 81-97. Williams & Wilkins Company, Baltimore.

CHAPTER 5

MEASUREMENTS OF AUDITORY THRESHOLDS FOR SPEECH STIMULI

Richard H. Wilson and Robert H. Margolis

CONTENTS

THRESHOLD AS A MEASURE OF PERFORMANCE	79
Threshold and the Psychometric Function	79
Detection Versus Recognition	82
Vocabulary	87
HISTORICAL RETROSPECTIVE	89
MEASUREMENT PROCEDURES	93
Physical Characteristics of Speech Stimuli	93
Stimulus Materials	99
Procedures for Estimating Thresholds for Speech	105
Special Considerations with Difficult-to-Test Subjects	109
DETERMINANTS OF SPEECH RECOGNITION THRESHOLDS	111
Relations between Thresholds for Pure Tones and Speech	111
Masking and the Speech Recognition Threshold	113
Masking Level Difference for Spondaic Words	113
Speech Recognition Thresholds in Sound Field	116
COMMENT	119
REFERENCES	122

Measurements of auditory thresholds for speech stimuli are used routinely in the clinical evaluation of patients with hearing impairment. In this chapter, speech threshold measurements are considered as a special case of the more general psychophysical problem of establishing relationships between human performance and stimulus dimensions. The relationships between threshold measurements and various psychometric functions are discussed. The history of clinical speech threshold measurement is reviewed and measurement procedures are developed. From considerations of the nature of such measurements in normal and hearing-impaired subjects, the clinical utility of speech threshold measurements is evaluated.

THRESHOLD AS A MEASURE OF PERFORMANCE

Threshold and the Psychometric Function

The term *threshold* can be defined in several ways. In the strictest sense, a threshold is the value of a stimulus dimension, usually intensity, above which the stimulus always elicits a response and below which there is never a response. Because *always* and *never* are difficult to establish, it is necessary to redefine threshold in terms of measurable probabilities. A substantial body of literature exists that deals with an examination of response probabilities in an attempt to settle the controversy of the existence of a true sensory threshold. (For discussions of the various threshold theories, see Green and Swets, 1966; and Swets, 1961.)

Whether the concept of a true sensory threshold finds support in physiologic and psychophysical experiments, it is possible to agree on an operational definition for the measurement of threshold. In psychoacoustic experiments, for example, threshold often is defined as the stimulus level resulting in some proportion of correct responses. Viewed in this way, a threshold is simply a point on a *psychometric function*. A psychometric function is a graph relating a measure of performance to a stimulus dimension. Consider the psychometric function illustrated in Figure 5-1. The ordinate represents the percentage of correct responses in a two-alternative forced choice (2AFC) paradigm. The signal was a 1000-Hz pure tone, presented in one of two observation intervals, and the subject had to decide which interval contained the signal. Both observation intervals contained a background noise so that the subject's task was to discriminate between signal plus noise and noise alone. Because the signal always occurred in one of the two intervals, a score of 50 percent represents chance performance. The data in Figure 5-1, therefore, range from 50 to 100 percent. It is difficult to determine a point on this function that represents a "true" threshold, that is, a level that separates chance performance from errorless performance. Consequently, it is conventional to define threshold as the signal intensity level resulting in a performance level (like 75 percent), which is midway between chance performance and errorless performance. Defined in this manner, the threshold for the 1000-Hz tone presented in a background noise with a pressure spectrum level[1] of 40 dB is approximately 50 dB sound pressure level (SPL), a signal-to-noise ratio of 10 dB. It is important to remember that the selection of a performance level for the purpose of operationally defining threshold is purely arbitrary. In choosing a different definition of threshold (a different performance level) it is

---

[1] The spectrum level of a specified signal at a particular frequency is the level of that part of the signal contained within a band of unit width, centered at the particular frequency. Ordinarily this has significance only for a signal having a continuous distribution of components within the frequency range under consideration. The term *spectrum level* cannot be used alone but must appear in combination with a prefatory modifier, for example, pressure, velocity, voltage, power (ANSI-S3.20-1973, p. 51).

Auditory Thresholds for Speech Stimuli 81

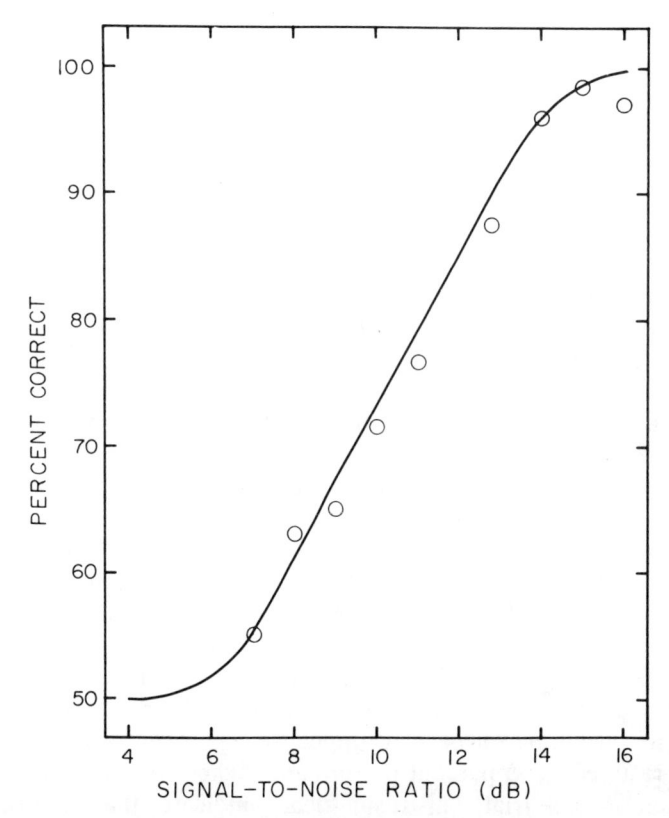

Figure 5-1. Psychometric function for a detection task. The signal was a 1000-Hz tone presented in noise. The ordinate represents the percentage of correct responses in a two-alternative forced-choice experiment. The subject's task was to determine which of two observation intervals contained the signal. Because on each trial the signal occurred in one of the two observation intervals, a score of 50 percent represents chance performance. As the signal-to-noise ratio was increased from 4 to 16 dB, performance increased from chance to nearly errorless performance. (From Green and Swets, 1966)

important to consider the slope of the psychometric function, that is, the change in performance for a given change in signal intensity. The slope of the function in Figure 5-1 is about 5 percent per decibel. If we redefine threshold as the 90 percent performance level, then the signal-to-noise ratio at threshold from Figure 5-1 would be 13 dB.

In clinical practice it often is important to compare two thresholds. If, for example, we are interested in observing the effect of a remedial procedure, we could measure threshold before and after the treatment. A threshold difference, then, is simply an indication of the difference in the positions of two psychometric functions. The effect that the treatment may have on the slopes of the psychometric functions is ignored if only a threshold difference is obtained. The treatment might influence the function in such a way that the slope and/or the maximum score may change as well as, or independently of, the performance level operationally defined as threshold. Thus, threshold estimates must be considered as incomplete indices of the relationship between signal intensity and performance.

Detection Versus Recognition

The experiment that produced the results in Figure 1 was a *detection* experiment. The subject only had to identify the *presence* of the stimulus without being required to identify any of its characteristics. In the classical detection experiment, the signal to be detected is identical from trial to trial. A different kind of detection experiment is one in which the signal may vary from trial to trial. In this type of experiment the subject is asked to detect the signal regardless of which signal is selected from a set of possibilities. An experiment of this type was described by Green and Swets (1966, p. 283). First, the sound pressure level of a 500-Hz tone that resulted in 95 percent performance was determined. The SPL resulting in 95 percent performance for a 1000-Hz tone was similarly determined. Then the experiment was repeated, but this time the subject did not know which of the two signals would be presented on each trial. When the signals were randomly selected from trial to trial, performance dropped to 73 percent, even though the signals resulted in 95 percent performance when the same signal was presented on each trial. This result clearly indicates that performance is critically dependent upon the subject's a priori knowledge of the signal.

Thus far, two kinds of detection experiments have been discussed, one in which the signal is the same on each trial, and another in which the signal is selected from a set of possible signals. Consideration now will be given to the *recognition* experiment. The task of the subject in the recognition experiment is not only to detect the presence of a signal, but also to identify which of the set of possible signals occurred.

It is logical that recognition would be more difficult than detection. Although this is usually a fair generalization, the relationship between detection and recognition is a complicated one. For example, Lindner (1968) demonstrated that the difference between detection and recognition was critically dependent on the subject's response criterion. He was able to demonstrate that, with proper manipulation of instructions, subjects could actually recognize a stimulus even though they reported that the stimulus was not detected. The point here is that differences in performance for detection and recognition tasks are dependent on many nonsensory variables that make one experimental result difficult to predict from the other. The subsequent discussion illustrates how these observations relate to threshold measurements with speech stimuli.

Figure 5-2 presents three psychometric functions from a single subject, representing results of the three kinds of experiments just discussed. In these experiments, however, the stimuli were selected from those speech stimuli commonly used for clinical threshold measurements, namely, the 36 spondaic words that constitute the Central Institute for the Deaf (CID) W-1 test (Hirsh et al., 1952) recorded by Technisonic Studios. Two types of detection experiments were conducted, one in which the stimulus word was identical from trial to trial and one in which the stimulus word was different on each trial. Note in Figure 5-2 that the slope of the function was much steeper when a

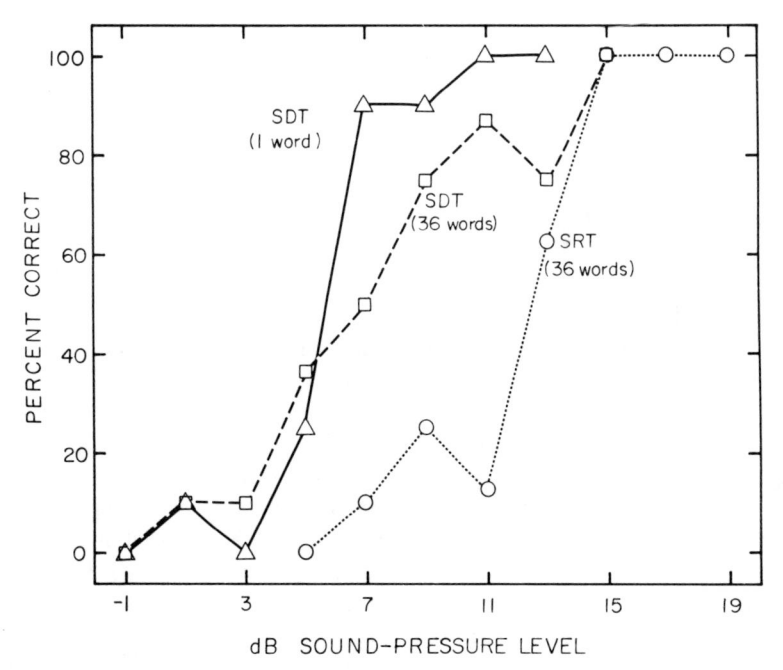

Figure 5-2. Psychometric functions from one subject in three types of experiments. Speech detection threshold (SDT) (1 word): the stimulus, identical from trial to trial, was the CID W-1 recording of the word *birthday*, presented at 8 intensity levels employing a method of constant stimuli. The subject's task was to indicate whether the word was detectable after the carrier phrase "say the word . . ." that was presented 10 dB higher than the stimulus word. SDT (36 words): the stimuli were the 36 spondaic words that constitute the CID W-1 recording. The subject's task was to indicate whether the word following the carrier phrase was detectable, but this time the word was different on each trial. Speech recognition threshold (SRT; 36 words): again the stimuli were the 36 spondaic words of the CID W-1 recording, but the subject's task was to repeat the word correctly.

single stimulus was used on each trial as compared to the function where 36 words were used as stimuli. The slope of a psychometric function is an indication of the degree of homogeneity of the difficulty of the stimuli. In the 36-word detection experiment, some words become detectable at lower levels than others, that is, the words are not homogeneous. In the one-word detection experiment, the stimulus word was identical on each trial, representing the greatest possible homogeneity. The difference in slope for the one-word and 36-word psychometric functions, then, is expected because of differences in homogeneity of detectability. The homogeneity of test items used for clinical threshold assessment with speech stimuli is discussed further in a subsequent section of this chapter.

In the speech recognition threshold (SRT) data shown in Figure 5-2, the subject was required to identify which of the 36 spondaic words was presented on each trial. The listener in this experiment was very familiar with the list of words that constituted the stimulus set. If a "naive" subject had been used, one who was not familiar with spondaic words, a different psychometric function may have resulted because of the subject's unfamiliarity with the materials (Pollack, Rubenstein, and Decker, 1959; Tillman and Jerger, 1959). Consequently, differences in subjects' knowledge of the stimulus material influence recognition performance just as the two detection psychometric functions in Figure 5-2 represent a difference in performance due to familiarity with the stimuli.

It is possible to extract a threshold from each of the psychometric functions in Figure 5-2. Note that, unlike Figure 5-1, the data in Figure 5-2 span a range from 0 to 100 percent. This is due to the fact that the data shown in Figure 5-1 were obtained in a *forced choice* experiment in which 50 percent represented chance performance. The data in Figure 5-2 were obtained with a method of constant stimuli in which a response was not required unless the subject knew that a stimulus occurred (detection) or could identify the word (recognition). If threshold is arbitrarily defined as the sound pressure level resulting in 50 percent performance, then speech detection thresholds would be measured at 6 dB SPL for one-word and 7 dB SPL for 36-word procedures. Note, however, that the two psychometric functions differ substantially in slope. If a different arbitrary definition of threshold were selected, the difference between the two threshold estimates would vary. In fact, performance at low intensity levels was actually better for the 36-word experiment than for the one word experiment. This is probably due to the fact that *some* of the 36 words could be detected at a lower sound pressure level than the word selected for the one-word experiment.

The psychometric function obtained in the speech recognition experiment lies to the right of those resulting from the detection procedures, indicating that more sound pressure is required to recognize the words than to detect them. If threshold were defined as the 50 percent performance level, a speech recognition threshold of 12.5 dB SPL is obtained. The difference between detection and recognition thresholds for this subject was about 6 dB.

Several investigators have measured thresholds for detection and recognition of speech stimuli (Beattie, Edgerton, and Svihovec, 1975; Beattie, Svihovec, and Edgerton, 1975; Chaiklin, 1959; Hawkins and Stevens, 1950; Hirsh, 1952; Thurlow et al., 1948). In each of these experiments, however, the stimuli used for the detection measurements were different from those used to measure recognition. Due to differences in stimuli and procedures, the relationship reported between detection and recognition thresholds for speech stimuli cannot be expected to be the same from one experiment to the next. Furthermore, Thurlow et al. (1948) suggested that this difference may not be the same for hearing-impaired subjects and normal listeners. Most investigators agree that, on the average, the threshold for the detection of speech for subjects with normal hearing is about 6 to 10 dB lower than the threshold for the recognition of speech.

The difference between detection and recognition thresholds demonstrates that more energy is required to recognize a stimulus than to detect it. Two factors probably account for this 6- to 10-dB difference. First, even for stimuli with constant intensity levels (e.g., pure tones), more energy is required to provide the information necessary to select a response from a set of alternatives than is needed for the detection of the stimulus. The exact amount of increased energy required for recognition relative to detection is dependent upon the specific characteristics of the stimuli (MacMillan, 1971; 1973). However, the special nature of speech stimuli results in a second determinant of the difference between detection and recognition. The levels of the individual speech sounds that comprise a speech sample can vary over a substantial range. Fletcher (1929) reported that the most intense vowel may be 25 dB more intense than the softest consonant. The average difference between vowel energy and consonant energy is about 13 dB. Thus, the detection threshold for speech most likely relates to the intensity level at which the vowels become detectable (Licklider and Miller, 1951). In order to recognize the speech sample, the level must be increased so that the vowels become recognizable, and enough consonant information is obtained to allow the recognition of the word. The important point is that these measures are dependent upon stimulus material, procedures, and subject selection, so that it is not possible to state the difference between speech detection and speech recognition thresholds with a single number that is applicable to all situations. Rather, a threshold measurement is an estimate of only one point on a psychometric function. Differences in stimulus materials, procedures, and the state of the auditory system may affect psychometric functions resulting from detection and recognition tasks in complex ways. The threshold estimate, therefore, should be regarded as a crude estimate of the position of the psychometric function, which does not completely describe the subject's performance.

At times it is desirable to combine individual psychometric functions into a single function that represents the performance of a group. Care must be taken when developing such a function since it is possible, and probably not uncommon, to combine individual data into a group function that does not accurately describe the performance of any of the members of the group. Two examples of incorrectly averaged psychometric functions are illustrated in Figure 5-3. In each example, five individual psychometric functions are represented. The "average" psychometric functions, were obtained by calculating mean performance for each value of signal magnitude. In the example given in the top panel of Figure 5-3, the individual functions are linear with equal slopes but the "average" function has a slope that is uncharacteristic of the slopes for the individual functions. In the example given in the bottom panel, the "average" function is nonlinear, whereas each individual function is linear. In each case, the "average" function does not represent accurately the performance of the group.

A representative average function can be obtained as follows. If the individual functions are linear, as in the examples shown in Figure 5-3, an average function can be constructed from the mean slope and the mean Y-intercept of the individual functions. The results would be identical to the individual functions marked c in Figure 5-3 and would represent accurately the performance of the group. Another way to calculate the group function is as follows. For each value of performance level (percent correct), the mean signal magnitude is determined at which that performance level is achieved. For example, the average signal magnitude required for 5 percent performance is determined; then 10 percent, and so on. These average values can be fit with an appropriate function, linear or nonlinear, to represent accurately the average psychometric function. Figure 5-4 presents individual psychometric functions for a detection task and two estimates of the "average" performance. The "function of mean" is the best predictor of subject performance at a given signal level. In contrast, "mean of function" is the best predictor of the slope of an individual subject function.

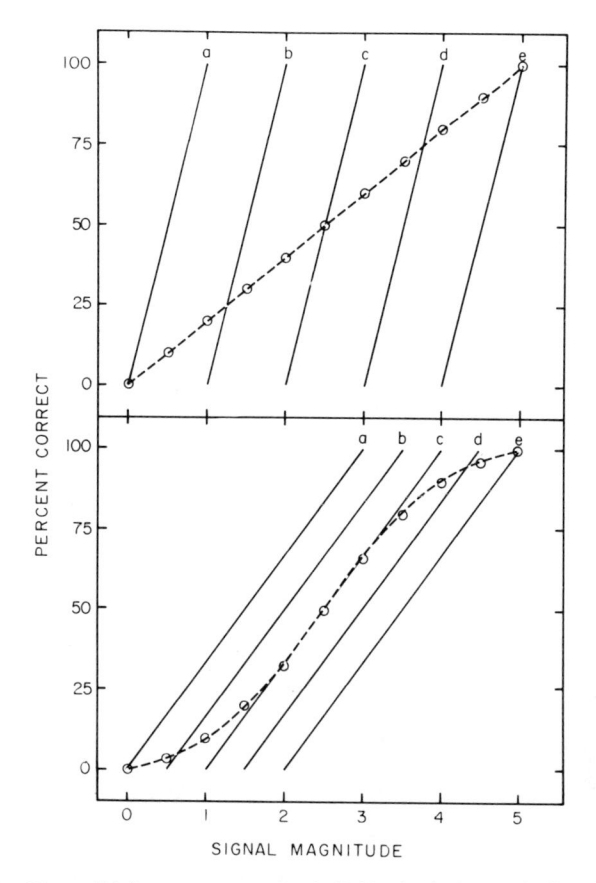

Figure 5-3. The *solid lines* represent the individual psychometric functions for five subjects. The *dashed lines* represent the average of the performance scores (percent correct) for each value of signal magnitude and do *not* accurately represent the data. A representative average psychometric function can be obtained by averaging the signal magnitudes required for each performance level. In each case, the resulting average function would be identical to the individual function (c) and would accurately characterize the data.

Vocabulary

In the foregoing discussion we have tried to relate performance measures for speech stimuli to classical psychophysical experiments. Many terms have been used to describe these measurements which are, at times, in conflict with well-accepted usage. The result is confusion between audiologic usage and the terminology used in related (and older) disciplines.

The term *speech detection threshold* is appropriately descriptive and consistent with the psychophysical use of the term detection. Other

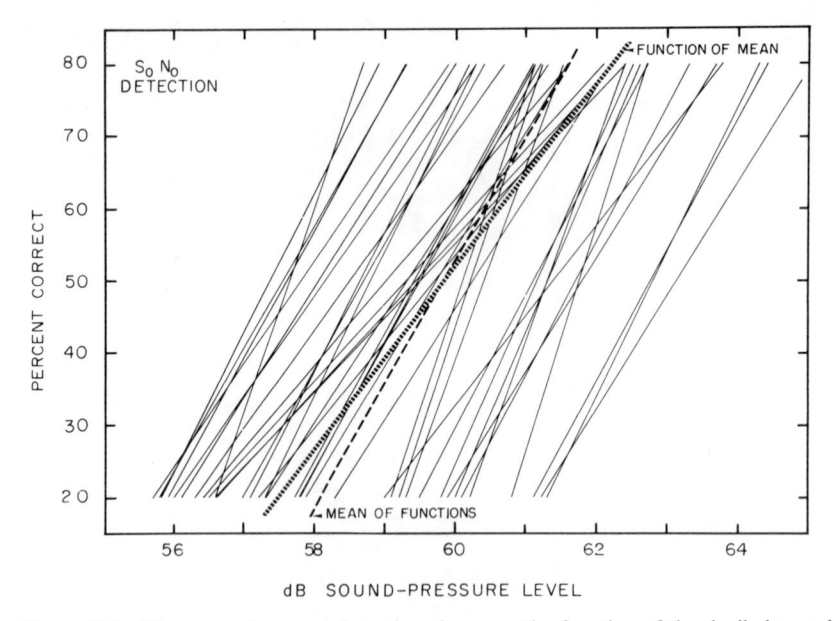

Figure 5-4. The percent correct detection shown as the function of the decibel sound pressure level of the CID W-1 spondaic words. The data were obtained with the S_0N_0 masking level difference paradigm in 70 dB SPL speech spectrum noise. The thin lines are the linear regressions generated by the data from each of 36 listeners. The mean of functions is the mean function derived by averaging the sound pressure levels required for each performance level. The function of the mean is the mean function derived by averaging the percent correct for each sound pressure level.

terms that have been used to describe the same type of measurement are *speech awareness threshold* and *threshold of audibility*. The term awareness refers more to the psychologic set of the observer than to the nature of the task, and the term audibility is less specific than detection.

The two most commonly used auditory tests employing speech stimuli are usually referred to as the *speech reception threshold* and the *speech discrimination test*. The only difference between the two tests is the selection of the dependent and independent variable. In a threshold measurement, the performance level (independent variable) is selected by the experimenter and the sound pressure level of the signal (dependent variable) that results in the selected performance level is sought. The measurement commonly referred to as speech discrimination represents the reverse situation, in which the signal level is the independent variable and the performance level is the dependent variable. The task of the subject is identical in both the reception and discrimination task—to recognize speech stimuli. Accordingly, the term *recognition* could appropriately describe both types of tests.

The term *speech reception threshold*, introduced by Hughson and Thompson (1942), is nonspecific in that reception could refer to detection, recognition, or discrimination. The term *spondee threshold*, recently recommended by the subcommittee on Speech Audiometry of the American Speech-Language-Hearing Association (ASHA) Committee on Audiometric Evaluation (1979) is specific with regard to the type of stimulus commonly employed, but is nonspecific with respect to the aspect of performance being measured, namely, recognition.

The term *discrimination* is commonly used to describe experiments in which the subject makes comparative judgments of two or more stimuli. *Intelligibility* properly refers to a characteristic of a system or of a particular speech sample (Owens and Schubert, 1968). *Articulation* refers to one aspect of the speech production process. These three terms have been used to describe the percentage of words correctly recognized at a specified intensity level. The use of the term *recognition* to describe these measurements was used as early as 1929 by Fletcher, and recently by several investigators (Bilger and Wang, 1976; Cramer and Erber, 1974; Erber, 1969, 1971, 1974; Schultz, 1972). Olsen and Matkin (1979) recommended the use of the term *recognition* in preference to the several other words that have been used. We suggest the term *speech recognition threshold* (first used by Feldmann, 1960) to describe the measurement commonly referred to as the speech reception threshold. Similarly, *speech recognition score* could be used to describe the test usually referred to as speech discrimination. The term could be made more specific by substituting for the word *speech*, the exact type of test materials used, for example, *syllable recognition score, word recognition score*, or *sentence recognition score*. The use of these terms will facilitate communication with other disciplines by reducing ambiguity in our own vocabulary.

HISTORICAL RETROSPECTIVE

The use of speech stimuli in the assessment of the status of the auditory mechanism was advocated and debated among otologists in the late 1800s. The following excerpt from Gruber (1891) demonstrates how speech was used in the "estimation of the hearing capacity for speech" (pp. 131-132):

> Oscar Wolf considers this the most perfect method of testing the hearing power, inasmuch as it embodies the most delicate shades in the pitch, intensity, and character of sound. Hartmann thinks, on the con-

trary, that the test is too complicated to insure accuracy. In any case it is indispensable, from the fact that nearly every patient seeks relief from disability in respect of it, and therefore for social intercourse. It is desirable, in estimating the degree of perception for speech, to test first of all both ears simultaneously, even though only one be affected; proceeding afterwards to the examination of each in turn. A separate examination of the hearing power should be made for each ear, even if previous testing by the watch and the tuning-fork has indicated an equally diminished hearing capacity on both sides; since experience shows that the perception for speech is not always deficient in the same measure as that for simple noises and tones. Cases indeed occur in which conversation is best heard on that side on which the watch and tuning-fork are not perceived so well as on the other, and vice versa. The repetition of the test-words gives the best control for the perception of them (Dennert).

Interest in utilizing speech to test "hearing power" was facilitated by several scientific inventions that enabled the evolution of speech audiometry as we know it today. First, in 1876 Alexander Graham Bell developed a transducer that converted sound energy into electrical energy, and vice versa. Second, Thomas Edison patented the phonograph in 1877. Shortly after this invention Lichtwitz (1889) wrote *On the Application of the New Edison Phonograph to General Hearing Measurement* (Hawley, 1977), which suggested applications of the phonograph in measuring the hearing of speech. Several years later Bryant (1904), apparently independently, reported a similar application of the phonograph. Another important development occurred in 1883 when Edison devised the vacuum-tube principle (termed "the Edison effect") that made possible the development of electronic amplifiers.

During the early 1900s, these and other inventions led to the development of electroacoustic communication systems. Because these systems were used for speech communication, speech materials were devised to evaluate their communicative efficiency. Fletcher and Steinberg (1929) reported the use of 49 lists each with 50 simple interrogative or imperative sentences. For example, from list 1, "Why are flagpoles surmounted by lightning rods?" and "Explain why the name stringbean is appropriate." Various responses to these sentences were required from the listener. Often when evaluating communication systems, the listener repeated the sentences, whereas at other times the listener was asked to answer the question or comment on the sentence material.

Jones and Knudsen (1924), in an alliance of otology and physics, developed an audiometer ("Audio-Amplifier") that generated tones by the "audion bulb" (vacuum tube) to test both air and bone conduction thresholds. They also utilized two audion bulbs as an amplifier of whispered and conversational voice. The speech circuit was able to provide low pass or high pass speech spectrum characteristics. The authors stated that they were unaware of other instruments at that time that incorporated bone conduction and speech testing capabilities. Jones and Knudsen (1924) then proceeded to describe their experience with the speech circuit.

> At first, tests were made for the conversational voice and the whisper, with a simple vacuum-tube amplifier. Two old ladies, about equally deaf, were the first ones tested. It was found that one of them heard perfectly the ordinary conversational speech and even the whisper, with the use of the amplifier. The other one not only did not hear better with the instrument, but heard better without the amplification. Careful functional tests, auditory and vestibular, showed that the first one had good internal ear function; the second one, impaired internal ear function. A series of patients was then tested. In these patients the nature of the hearing impairment was carefully studied by the usual functional tests. It seemed that the following tentative conclusions could be drawn: Those with conductive lesions can hear very well with the use of the amplifier; those with perceptive lesions can not hear so well, and in many instances are much annoyed by the use of the amplifier. (From Jones and Knudsen, *The Laryngoscope*, 34:675, 1924.)

Perhaps this was the first speech recognition experiment performed on individuals with hearing impairment in which electronic devices were employed to control the intensity of the speech stimulus.

The Western Electric 4A audiometer, incorporating the phonograph, also was introduced in 1924 (Feldmann, 1960). Disc recordings of two-digit sequences, reproduced in descending intensity level, could be presented simultaneously to groups of up to 40 listeners. The 4A was used mainly as a screening audiometer.

Hughson and Thompson (1942) reported the results of a 3-year study in which "speech reception thresholds" were established on patients with a variety of hearing impairments. The materials from the 49 lists of sentences developed by Fletcher and Steinberg (1929) were delivered to the patient via monitored live voice. Hughson and Thompson required the patient to repeat the sentence verbatim. A bracketing technique was used to establish threshold, defined as the degree (in decibels) of attenuation for speech "below which the subject can no longer repeat at least two thirds of the sentences correctly" (p. 531). Hughson and Thompson concluded from their findings that the speech test was useful and that "frequencies above and below 512 and 2048 have little significance in the subject's ability to understand speech" (p. 540).

During World War II, Hudgins et al. (1947) working at the Harvard Psycho-Acoustic Laboratory (PAL) introduced the spondaic word as the stimulus material for measuring "the loss of hearing for speech."

The spondaic words were selected to satisfy the following four criteria: "(1) familiarity, (2) phonetic dissimilarity, (3) normal sampling of English speech sounds, and (4) homogeneity with respect to basic audibility" (p. 58). In selecting the spondaic-stress pattern of disyllabic words in preference to other patterns (e.g., trochaic and iambic), Hudgins et al. (1947) were the first to develop speech stimuli that continue to be used to measure the auditory threshold for speech. They produced disc recordings of 84 spondaic words, two lists of 42 words, and six randomizations of each list. The carrier phrase "Number one . . ." preceded each word and a 1000-Hz tone was recorded for instrument calibration. Two methods were devised to present the words to subjects. The first of these was called PAL Auditory Test No. 9. In this test, the words were recorded in sets of six with each successive set recorded 4 dB below the preceding set. PAL Auditory Test No. 9, therefore, provided a range of 24 dB of attenuation across the 42 words. The spondaic words also were recorded without the built-in attenuation (PAL Auditory Test No. 14). At the same time, PAL Auditory Test No. 12, which utilized simple questions with one-word answers (e.g., "What month comes after January?"), was developed. PAL Auditory Tests No. 9 and No. 12 were used in the Aural Rehabilitation Service at Deshon General Hospital as the materials for testing recognition thresholds for speech stimuli (Hirsh, 1947).

Hudgins et al. (1947) arbitrarily defined the threshold for speech as the intensity level resulting in 50 percent correct responses. For convenience, the threshold could be determined from either a tabular or a graphic procedure in which decibel values were designated for the corresponding number of correct responses. Psychometric functions obtained with normal-hearing subjects with the spondaic word materials had a slope of approximately 10 percent per decibel between the 20 and 80 percent correct points. The Hudgins et al. study provided the basic guidelines and principles that still are utilized in establishing auditory thresholds for speech.

After the recordings of PAL Auditory Test No. 9 had been in use for several years, Hirsh et al. (1952) at the Central Institute for the Deaf (CID) reported a revised version of the test (CID Auditory Tests W-1 and W-2). Three factors led the CID group to develop and record shortened versions of PAL Auditory Test No. 9. First, it was "reported informally" that the Auditory Test No. 9 lists did not produce equivalent thresholds for normal subjects. Second, the 84 spondaic words that comprised PAL Auditory Test No. 9 were not homogeneous with respect to the threshold of recognition, that is, some words became recognizable at lower intensity levels than others. Third, the advent of magnetic recording tape made it possible to record a test word once and then copy and splice the original for needed replications.

Initially, the 84 spondaic words from PAL Auditory Test No. 9 were rated by judges for their familiarity. The words judged most familiar then were recorded. Listening experiments were performed and the pool of words was reduced further to 36 spondaic words (given in Table 5-1) by eliminating the words that were the easiest and most difficult. Six randomizations of the 36 words were recorded utilizing the carrier phrase "Say the word . . .". Psychometric functions obtained with the 36 words revealed some differences that were attributed to the minimally different levels, as judged on a VU meter, at which the words were recorded. Finally, the 36 words were re-recorded from the master with the levels of some words adjusted ±2 dB in order to make the words more homogeneous with respect to intelligibility. Mean recognition thresholds obtained with the final CID W-1 recordings were 20 or 21 dB SPL for groups of experienced or inexperienced listeners, respectively. A second version (CID Auditory Test W-2) of these 36 spondaic words was recorded with 3 dB of attenuation for every three words. The Hirsh et al. (1952) study provided the list of 36 spondaic words that is used throughout the country for establishing auditory thresholds for speech stimuli.

MEASUREMENT PROCEDURES

Physical Characteristics of Speech Stimuli

The acoustics of speech are discussed in detail in Chapter 3. In this section we will describe some of the acoustic properties of the speech stimuli most commonly used for measuring auditory thresholds, namely, spondaic words.

In Figures 5-5 and 5-6 the spondaic words *birthday* and *sunset* are represented three ways. The upper panels present the *pressure waveforms* recorded from an earphone (TDH-49) mounted in a standard 6-cc coupler (NBS-9A). This representation provides an approximation of the pressure wave that would be present at the tympanic membrane. Certain characteristics of these speech stimuli are evident from observations of the pressure waveforms. The most obvious characteristic is the variation in sound pressure that occurs with time. If the root mean square (rms) sound pressures associated with various speech sounds within a spondaic word were measured individually, differences as great as 25 dB between the most intense vowel and the softest consonant would be seen (Fletcher, 1929).

Table 5-1. The 36 spondaic words employed in the disc recording of the CID W-1 lists and their threshold of recognition. The first two columns give the sensation levels at which the threshold of recognition was observed in two studies. The third column is the mean sensation level derived from the first two columns. The fourth and fifth columns give the decibel corrections obtained with a VU meter and computer, respectively. The final two columns represent the sensation level and sound pressure level at which the threshold for the words would have been attained if the words were recorded at the same level. The 21 spondaic words included in the bracket are the homogeneous words (defined by ± 1 standard deviation, column 6) if the words were recorded at the same level.

	Sensation level[a] (1)	Sensation level[b] (2)	Mean of 1 and 2[c] (3)	VU meter dB correction (4)	Computer dB corrections (5)	Sum of 3 and 5 (6)	dB SPL (7)
hotdog	5.0[c]	3.8[c]	4.40	−1	−1.42	2.98	16.44
iceberg	4.8[c]	4.0[c]	4.40	0	−1.39	3.01	16.47
airplane	4.7[c]	4.2[c]	4.45	−1	−1.39	3.06	16.52
workshop	2.7	2.8	2.75	+1	+1.07	3.82	17.28
northwest	5.2[c]	6.2[c]	5.70	−1	−1.84	3.86	17.32
birthday	6.3[c]	5.6[c]	5.95	−2	−2.08	3.87	17.33
playground	4.5[c]	4.6[c]	4.55	0	−0.64	3.91	17.37
baseball	3.0	3.0	3.00	+1	+1.18	4.18	17.64
hardware[d]	3.5	4.9[c]	4.20	0	+0.34	4.54	18.00
duckpond	8.3	10.1	9.20	−2	−4.42	4.78	18.24
cowboy	4.3[c]	5.0[c]	4.65	+2	+0.48	5.13	18.59
whitewash	7.2[c]	7.8[c]	7.50	−1	−2.31	5.19	18.65
sidewalk	6.0[c]	6.5[c]	6.25	+1	−0.94	5.31	18.77
sunset	6.2[c]	6.2[c]	6.20	0	−0.88	5.32	18.78
oatmeal	7.0[c]	7.6[c]	7.30	−1	−1.48	5.82	19.28
railroad	4.8[c]	6.5[c]	5.65	0	+0.37	6.02	19.48
drawbridge	8.2	4.8[c]	6.50	+1	−0.07	6.43	19.89
eardrum	6.9[c]	6.1[c]	6.50	0	+0.20	6.70	20.16
schoolboy	8.5	6.9[c]	7.70	−1	−0.75	6.95	20.41

farewell	6.3[c]	8.0[c]	7.15	−1	−0.12	7.03	20.49
horseshoe	7.8[c]	8.6	8.20	−1	−1.13	7.07	20.53
greyhound	7.0[c]	6.0[c]	6.50	+1	+0.62	7.12	20.58
pancake	7.7[c]	8.0	7.85	−1	−0.53	7.32	20.78
toothbrush	7.5[c]	8.0[c]	7.75	0	−0.40	7.35	20.81
inkwell	8.8	7.0[c]	7.90	+2	−0.38	7.52	20.98
woodwork	4.3[c]	4.8[c]	4.55	+2	+3.11	7.66	21.12
mousetrap	7.7[c]	7.7[c]	7.70	+1	+0.25	7.95	21.41
armchair	7.5[c]	4.4[c]	5.95	+2	+2.30	8.25	21.71
stairway	6.3[c]	8.0[c]	7.15	0	+1.56	8.71	22.17
padlock	8.3	8.0[c]	8.15	0	+0.78	8.93	22.39
daybreak	8.3	6.6[c]	7.45	+1	+1.75	9.20	22.66
headlight	8.3	8.6	8.45	+1	+1.07	9.52	22.98
mushroom	10.3	7.7[c]	9.00	0	+0.81	9.81	23.27
hothouse	12.7	10.9	11.80	−2	−1.93	9.87	23.33
doormat	8.3	6.8[c]	7.55	+1	+3.06	10.61	24.07
grandson	12.2	8.4	10.30	0	+0.32	10.62	24.08
Mean	6.8	6.5	6.59			6.54	20.00
SD	2.3	1.9	1.92			2.25	2.25

[a] Sensation level at which the threshold of recognition was observed in the study by Bowling and Elpern (1961).
[b] Sensation level at which the threshold of recognition was observed in the study by Curry and Cox (1966).
[c] Spondaic words identified as being homogeneous by respective authors.

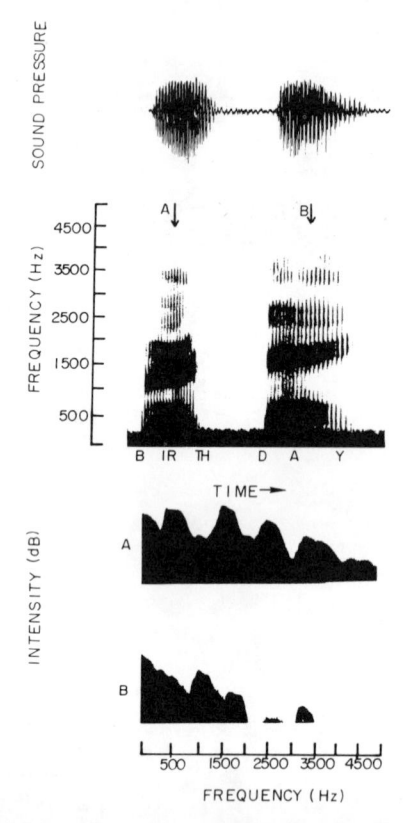

Figure 5-5. Three representations of the acoustic characteristics of a spondaic word. Top: the acoustic waveform of the word *birthday*. The CID W-1 recording of the word was presented by a TDH-49 earphone to a NBS-9A coupler and microphone. The output of the microphone was recorded in digital form by a computer and reproduced on an oscillograph. Middle: a spectrogram of the electrical output of the tape recording used to reproduce the word *birthday*. Bottom: amplitude cross sections of the steady state portions of the vowels in *birthday*. These are power spectra taken at the times indicated by the arrows in the middle panel.

One way to characterize the fluctuations in the intensity level of a waveform is the *crest factor*. The crest factor is the ratio of the peak pressure to the rms pressure. The crest factor of a sinusoidal waveform, for example, is 1.4 or 3 dB. A speech waveform has a much higher crest factor because the peaks are much higher than the rms pressure. The crest factors of the speech waveforms in Figures 5-5 and 5-6 are 3.0 (9.5 dB) and 2.6 (8.3 dB), respectively. The effects of transducing a wide band signal like speech through a typical earphone used in audiometry include restricting the bandwidth and reducing the crest factor. If these crest factors had been determined in a sound field rather

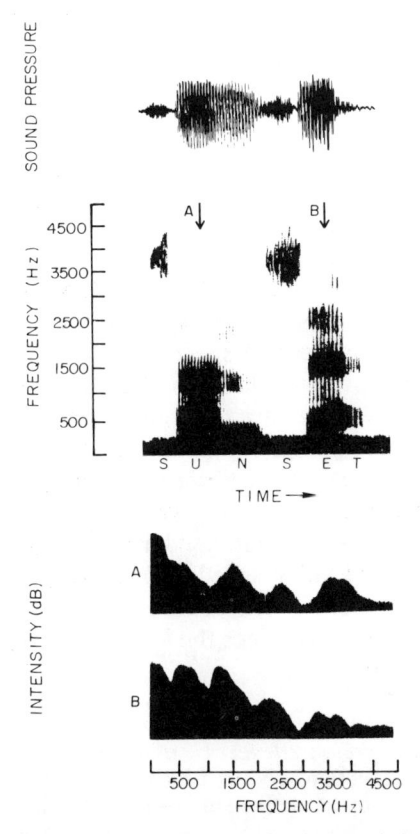

Figure 5-6. Three representations of the acoustic characteristics of a spondaic word. Top: the acoustic waveform of the word *sunset*. Middle: a spectrogram of the electrical output of the tape recording used to reproduce the word *sunset*. Bottom: Amplitude cross sections of the steady state portions of the vowels in *sunset*. Details as in legend to Figure 5-5.

than from the output of an earphone, crest factors as high as 14 dB could be obtained (Wathen-Dunn and Lipke, 1958).

The middle panels of Figures 5-5 and 5-6 are *speech spectrograms* for the words *birthday* and *sunset*. Note the substantial differences that are evident in the patterns for the two words. The physical differences among spondaic words, evident in the spectrograms, result in differences in detectability and intelligibility. This heterogeneity is responsible for many of the characteristics of speech detection and speech recognition measurements. For example, the slopes of the psychometric functions in Figure 5-2 are determined, in part, by the heterogeneity of the stimuli. The problem of homogeneity is discussed in the next section.

The lower panels of Figures 5-5 and 5-6 are *amplitude cross sections* taken during the steady-state portion of the vowels. These displays are power spectra corresponding to the points in time indicated by the arrows in the middle panels of the figures. The peaks in the power spectra correspond to the formant energy that is represented by the dark bars in the spectrogram. If these power spectra were taken at regular time intervals during the speech sample, it would be evident that the power spectrum of speech changes rapidly with time. Thus, speech is a highly variable signal both in the time domain, as illustrated by the pressure waveforms, and in the frequency domain, as indicated by the spectrograms and power spectra.

Because sound pressure level is the dependent variable in any threshold measurement, precise determination of this quantity is crucial if thresholds for speech stimuli are to be measured accurately. Because the sound pressure of speech is changing constantly, as indicated in the upper panels of Figures 5-5 and 5-6, it is a difficult quantity to specify. The current standard governing the specification of the sound pressure level of speech stimuli for audiometric purposes is the American National Standard Specifications for Audiometers (S3.6-1969). That standard defines the sound pressure level of a speech stimulus as follows (p. 15):

> ... the sound pressure level of a speech signal at the earphone is defined as the rms sound pressure level ... of a 1000 Hz signal adjusted so that the VU meter deflection produced by the 1000 Hz signal is equal to the average peak VU meter deflection produced by the speech signal.

One problem with this definition is that "average peak VU meter deflection" is difficult to determine. In order to understand the meaning of a VU meter deflection it is necessary to consider the characteristics of a VU meter. In 1954 the American Standards Association defined the ballistic characteristics of a VU meter (C16.5-1954) as follows: if the meter were fed a sinusoidal signal with an instantaneous rise-fall time, the needle must move to "0 VU" in 300 msec (± 10 percent) with an overshoot between 1 and 1.5 dB. Any meter that does not conform to these time constant and overshoot characteristics is not a standard VU meter. Because speech is a rapidly changing signal, the ballistics of the meter introduce a certain amount of "distortion" to the meter's representation of the signal. Any "peak deflection" is determined both by the level of the input signal and by the ballistics of the meter. The effect of the ballistic characteristics of the meter is dependent on the temporal structure of the waveform. For a steady state signal (e.g., a pure tone) a VU meter measures the rms voltage applied to its input terminals. The rms transformation is a type of average, so that the VU meter reading at any instant in time is an average determined over some time interval. A "peak deflection" for a speech signal, therefore, is an average that is "distorted" by ballistic characteristics that cannot follow accurately rapid changes in level. "Average peak VU meter deflection," then, is an average of a number of averages, each of which is not precisely accurate.

The advent of laboratory digital computers offers a more precise method of measuring the level of a speech sample. The entire sample (or any part of it) can be analyzed by a computer that can determine the rms level associated with the entire word or the desired part of the word. The authors utilized this computer technique to determine the rms sound pressure of each of the CID W-1 spondaic words from the disc recordings (Technisonic Studios) played through a TDH-49 earphone mounted on a standard earphone coupler (NBS-9A). The relative sound pressure level of each word then was computed with reference to the mean rms sound pressure. The results of these measurements, presented in Table 5-1 (column 5), demonstrate that when presented at the same attenuator setting, the actual rms sound pressure for the 36 spondaic words vary over a 7.53 dB range (-4.42 dB to 3.11 dB). The data from the rms procedure can be compared to the peak levels estimated by visual observation of the VU meter (Table 5-1, column 4). The two methods are in reasonable agreement ($r = 0.75$), although differences in measured rms sound pressure and "peak VU meter deflection" can exceed 2 dB. The remainder of the data in Table 5-1 is discussed in the next section.

Stimulus Materials

An important concept regarding stimulus word materials was given by Kruel, Bell, and Nixon (1969). They stated that "tests ought not be thought of as the written lists of words but as recordings of these words" (p. 287). The characteristics of any spoken test materials vary substantially across speakers and across utterances from a single speaker, so that stimulus characteristics can only be defined precisely for a given utterance or recording. Although the high redundancy[2] and information content of spondaic words tend to decrease the variability in difficulty across repeated utterances of the same word, the Kruel et al. (1969) warning should be considered in the determination of the detectability and intelligibility of these words.

The variability associated with a threshold estimate is inversely related to the slope of the psychometric function. Consequently, it is

---

[2] Redundancy may be defined as ". . . a property of languages, codes, and sign systems which arises from a superfluity of rules, and which facilitates communication in spite of all the factors of uncertainty acting against it" (Cherry, 1966, p. 19).

desirable for threshold estimation to choose stimuli for which the psychometric function is steep. Two characteristics contribute to the steepness of the function for spondaic words. First, the 36 words constitute a limited or "closed set" of materials that are familiar to the listener. Because a relatively closed set is involved, the number of response alternatives is reduced substantially.

Second, because the spondaic words are familiar two-syllable words, the correct recognition of one of the syllables can produce correct recognition of the entire word. Here, prior knowledge of the words should enable the listener to fill in the syllable that is not recognized, thereby providing correct recognition of the word. In other words, the spondaic words are so redundant that only minimal auditory cues are necessary for correct recognition.

The remainder of this section includes a discussion of the homogeneity and presentation modes of the spondaic words incorporating both the philosophy advocated by Kruel et al. (1969) and the concept of redundancy and information as they relate to the speech recognition threshold. Finally, considerations of the response mode of the listener are described.

Homogeneity If the spondaic words were homogeneous with respect to recognition, then each word would become recognizable at the same stimulus presentation level. Unfortunately, this is not the case, as many studies have demonstrated (Beattie et al., 1975; Bowling and Elpern, 1961; Conn, Dancer and Ventry, 1975; Curry and Cox, 1966; and others). The reasons for the lack of homogeneity among the spondaic words are sometimes subtle, even among the CID W-1 recordings that have had the intensity "adjusted" in an attempt to attain homogeneity.

Familiarity with the spondaic words is an important factor in determining the degree of intelligibility. Better performance is achieved when the observer knows the stimulus material for which he is listening (Pollack et al., 1959; Tillman and Jerger, 1959). There are two aspects to familiarity. The first is how familiar the observer is in general with the target words, that is, the more the listener uses the target word, the more familiar he is with it. The second is whether or not the listener knows that the target word is a member of the set of test items. These relationships are obvious in the data of Conn et al. (1975) that are shown in Table 5-2. As can be seen, the familiarization process produced a differential effect on the intelligibility of the CID W-1 spondaic words. *Baseball* and *sunset*, for example, were recognized correctly the same number of times, regardless of whether or not the listeners were familiarized with the test items. With other words (e.g., *duckpond* and *drawbridge*), a substantial difference can be noted between the

Table 5-2. A comparison of the number of correct responses to unfamiliarized and familiarized spondaic words from the CID W-1 recordings

	Correct responses		
Spondaic word	Unfamiliarized	Familiarized	Difference
baseball[a]	22	23	1
airplane[a]	19	21	2
iceberg[a]	18	21	3
sunset[a]	18	18	0
hardware	17	24	7
armchair[a]	16	17	1
playground[a]	16	18	2
stairway[a]	16	16	0
woodwork	16	22	6
workshop	16	21	5
birthday[a]	14	14	0
eardrum[a]	14	18	4
doormat[a]	13	13	0
northwest[a]	13	17	4
railroad[a]	13	17	4
grandson[a]	12	16	4
sidewalk[a]	12	16	4
farewell[a]	11	12	1
mousetrap[a]	11	15	4
mushroom[a]	11	15	4
whitewash	11	19	8
horseshoe	10	9	1
hotdog	10	19	9
oatmeal	10	18	8
pancake	10	15	5
cowboy	9	20	11
daybreak	8	14	6
toothbrush	8	14	6
drawbridge	7	18	11
greyhound	7	14	7
inkwell	7	18	11
schoolboy	7	12	5
padlock	6	14	8
duckpond	3	16	13
headlight	3	11	8
hothouse	1	6	5

From Conn et al. (1975). Reprinted with permission.

[a] Spondaic words with 11 or more unfamiliarized correct responses and with different values less than 4.5. These words qualify for the list for obtaining spondaic word thresholds without familiarization.

familiarized and unfamiliarized conditions. The results of the Conn et al. (1975) study indicate that better homogeneity of the spondaic words is achieved when the listener has been familiarized with the list of words.

Another factor contributing to the heterogeneity of test stimuli is that the differences in the total energy contained in each spondaic word and in each syllable are different, even when the syllables of the words produce equal peak values on the VU meter. This energy difference is the result of the variety of sounds composing the words and the silent intervals within the words. Differences in durations among the words, which vary from speaker to speaker, also contribute to heterogeneity.

The homogeneity with respect to recognition of the CID W-1 recordings of the spondaic words has been the subject of two investigations (Bowling and Elpern, 1961; Curry and Cox, 1966). The procedures in both studies were essentially the same in that the 36 words were presented in an ascending intensity order from -10 dB hearing level to an intensity level at which 100 percent correct recognition was achieved. The recognition threshold for each word was expressed in decibels relative to the lowest attenuator setting at which any word was recognized. At this point, it should be recalled that the words on the CID W-1 recordings are *not* recorded at the same intensity level, relative to the 1000-Hz calibration tone. As was mentioned earlier, in an attempt to attain better homogeneity on the final master recording of the CID W-1 lists, some words were recorded unchanged, amplified 2 dB and recorded, or attenuated 2 dB and recorded. The two studies that investigated homogeneity (Bowling and Elpern, 1961; Curry and Cox, 1966) did not take into account the different word levels that characterize the CID W-1 recordings. Table 5-1 lists the 36 spondaic words along with homogeneity data from the two studies, and indicates (^{c}) the words found to be homogeneic in the respective studies. Nineteen of the 36 spondaic words were included in the subset of homogeneous words by both investigations.

A more useful index of homogeneity would relate the intelligibility of each word that would be achieved if the words had been recorded at equal intensity levels. To accomplish this, the data from the two aforementioned studies were averaged, the results of which are presented in column 3 of Table 5-1. The previously described computer technique was used to compute the rms voltage of the recorded CID W-1 words. The individual rms voltages were transformed into decibel variation with regard to the mean rms for the 36 words. These values are given in column 5 of the table. The correction values (column 5) were then added to the mean decibel sensation level of recognition for each word (column 3), thereby defining the decibel sensation level for each spondaic word (column 6) that would have resulted if the words had been recorded at equal intensity levels. The mean was a 6.54-dB sensation level with a 2.25-dB standard deviation (SD) and a 7.64-dB range. Defining homogeneity of recognition as ±1 standard deviation, 21 words were identified (within the bracket) that were homogeneous when recorded at equal levels. Of the 21 homogeneous words, 14 words also were considered homogeneous by both Bowling and Elpern (1961) and Curry and Cox (1966). Finally, in Table 5-1, the threshold of recognition of each word in decibels sound pressure level (column 7) is estimated by assuming that the mean (6.54 dB) sensation level is equal to the 20-dB SPL (ANSI S3.2-1969) reference threshold level and scaling the values for the individual words. When viewed in this manner, the thresholds for the 36 recorded CID W-1 spondaic words range from 16.44 dB SPL (*hotdog*) to 24.08 dB SPL (*grandson*). In contrast, the thresholds of the homogeneous words range only from 18.00 dB SPL (*hardware*) to 22.17 dB SPL (*stairway*).

Recently, Young et al. (1982), using the Northwestern recording of the 36 CID spondaic words, generated psychometric functions for each word. The words were presented in 2-dB increments from 10 to 26 dB SPL. Thresholds for the words ranged from 15.2 dB SPL (*hotdog*) to 21.6 dB SPL (*greyhound*). The mean for all the words was 18.7 dB SPL (SD, 1.5 dB). Twenty-six of the words were ±1 standard deviation of the mean and were defined as equally recognizable. The authors also considered the slopes of the individual psychometric functions, which ranged from 6.1 percent/dB (*farewell*) to 20.6 percent/dB (*schoolboy*). Utilizing slope as criteria for homogeneity, 22 words were within ±1 standard deviation. Only 15 words were homogeneous with respect to both threshold and slope criteria.

In summary, the homogeneity of the commonly used 36 CID spondaic words varies with different speakers recording the materials. Because the ranges of threshold for understanding spondaic words are typically 6 to 8 dB (see Table 5-1, columns 1, 2, 3, and 7), audiologists using recorded words should confirm the homogeneity of their materials. Once the homogeneity of the spondaic words has been determined, then the audiologist can decide whether or not changes in the lists are warranted to attain better homogeneity of the spondaic words.

Presentation Mode The spondaic words can be presented to the listener by either monitored live voice (MLV) or a recording (disc or magnetic tape). For standardization purposes, recorded materials are preferred. In contrast, monitored live voice procedures allow greater flexibility and may save time when testing certain types of patients (e.g., pediatric or geriatric populations). As discussed earlier, both the sound pressure level and the ballistic characteristics of the VU meter must be calibrated. Finally, it is important to note the mode of presentation of the spondaic words or other speech materials on the audiogram form.

A second variable that pertains to the presentation mode is the intensity direction from which threshold is approached. The three basic choices are descending, ascending, or a combination descending-ascending procedure (bracketing). The descending approach has been advocated by Hirsh et al. (1952), Hudgins et al. (1947), and Tillman and Olsen (1973). Chaiklin, Font, and Dixon (1967) suggested that the ascending approach was useful with patients having suspected pseudohypacusis. Both Jerger et al. (1959), and Newby (1958) have described bracketing techniques that can be used to estimate the speech recognition threshold. As pointed out by Chaiklin and Ventry (1964), however, these bracketing procedures are "too general and unsystematic" and they omit "too many important procedural details" (p. 53).

The use of a carrier phrase (e.g., "Say the word," as with the CID W-1 recordings) before the presentation of the spondaic words serves to define the listening interval for the observer. In general, observers demonstrate better performance when the listening interval is defined than when the interval is not defined. The recordings of the spondaic words that do not incorporate a carrier phrase (e.g., Auditec of St. Louis) present the words at a fixed interval, e.g., one word every 5 seconds. With most listeners this periodicity of the word presentation provides adequate definition of the listening interval. Considering the redundancies present in the spondaic words, it is doubtful that recognition thresholds obtained with and without a carrier phrase are substantially different.

The size of the attenuation steps employed in the speech recognition threshold procedure is another variable that has been studied. Usually, 2-dB or 5-dB attenuation steps are used because most audiometers provide one of these step sizes. Chaiklin and Ventry (1964) and Wilson, Morgan, and Dirks (1973) reported that these two attenuation steps produce differences that are small enough that either the 2-dB or 5-dB step sizes can be used.

Routinely, all 36 spondaic words are not utilized to establish the speech recognition threshold. With some patients, for example, young children, the audiologist can present only a few spondaic words that are appropriate for the patient. Here again, familiarity of the stimulus material with regard to language abilities should be of primary concern.

When this situation occurs, the audiologist should note on the audiogram which "selected spondaic words" were used.

Response Mode Conventionally, the listener responds to the presentation of a spondaic word by repeating (orally) the test word. This can be considered a verbal-recall response mode because the listener must recall the word from the familiarized set of 36 words. With some patients, for example, those with expressive aphasia and young children, it may be necessary to modify the response mode by having the patient point to a picture or object from a set of alternatives that depict the stimulus word.

The pointing response is an identification response based on a restricted number of choices (typically 4 to 6) in contrast to the verbal-recall response in which the choice is drawn from a substantially larger number of words (usually 20 to 36). Although the task is still one of recognition, the two response modes can result in different performances. For example, in a recent study with monosyllabic words (Wilson and Antablin, 1980), the 50 percent correct point on the psychometric function was 5 dB lower with the identification-recognition task as compared with the verbal-recall recognition task. The difference between the two response modes with spondaic words, however, is probably not as large. For clinical purposes, the speech recognition thresholds for spondaic words that are established with the identification response probably can be considered equivalent to thresholds established with the verbal-recall response. A definitive answer to this question, however, awaits research.

Procedures for Estimating Thresholds for Speech

Currently, there is no American National Standards Institute standard in which a speech recognition threshold protocol is defined. The need for a standard procedure was emphasized by Tillman and Olsen (1973) who pointed out that a systematic procedure ". . . confines all clinicians to the same operational definition of threshold, and thus reduces variability in estimates of the speech reception threshold produced by variations in this definition" (pp. 45-46). Tillman and Olsen (1973) revived the speech recognition threshold technique (for spondaic words) originally used by Hudgins et al. (1947) with the PAL Auditory Test No. 9 and subsequently incorporated into the CID Auditory Test W-2 by Hirsh et al. (1952), and urged that the procedure be considered for standard implementation in the clinical setting.

The speech recognition threshold protocol just mentioned has the following four features: 1) spondaic words that are familiar to the listener; 2) a descending intensity approach to threshold; 3) a threshold defined as 50 percent correct; and 4) a scoring process in which each spondaic word is assigned a decibel value. Regarding these last two features, Wilson et al. (1973) observed that the computational procedure involved in the speech recognition threshold technique was based on a long-standing statistical precedent, the Spearman-Kärber method (Finney, 1952). Thus, for audiologists requiring speech recognition threshold information, a systematic technique is available that has a statistical basis. The procedures are described below. (See Wilson et al., 1973, for further details.)

Test Procedure The estimation of the speech recognition threshold involves, basically, four steps. In step 1 the patient is familiarized with the spondaic words. This is achieved by presenting the materials at a comfortable listening level and having the patient repeat the words. The words that are not recognized by the patient should not be used in the test procedure.

In step 2 an initial presentation level is established so that the majority of test words can be presented at intensity levels that are close to the level of the final speech recognition threshold. The initial presentation level is estimated by presenting one spondaic word at each 10-dB decrement starting 30 to 40 dB above the estimated threshold, which can be determined from the pure tone thresholds. When one word is missed, a second word is presented at the same intensity level. The test run is initiated 10 dB above the intensity level at which two words are missed.

In step 3 the search for the speech recognition threshold involves the presentation of two spondaic words at each 2-dB decrement. The following two conditions must be met in the course of the procedure: 1) five of the first six words presented must be repeated correctly, and 2) the test run terminates when five of six words are missed. (Other combinations of words per presentation level and decibel decrements can be employed and are discussed in the next section.)

In step 4 the hearing threshold level (HTL; 50 percent correct) then is calculated by subtracting the number of correct responses during the test run from the initial presentation level. A correction factor of one is added to the difference to compensate for the extra word (decibel) included in the initial presentation level. The intensity level derived represents the speech recognition threshold. The derivation of the formula for calculating the speech recognition threshold is presented below.

Figure 5-7 (left panel) illustrates a portion of the worksheet the authors have found useful in the clinical application of this speech recognition threshold procedure. (For convenience, each worksheet includes 24 copies of the form.) The initial presentation level (step 2)

Auditory Thresholds for Speech Stimuli

INTENSITY		INTENSITY				INTENSITY					
0		40	✓	✓		0					
8		8	✓	✓		5					
6		6	✓	✗		0					
4		4	✓	✓		5					
2		2	✗	✓		0					
0		30	✓	✗		5					
8		8	✗	✗							
6		6	✗	✗		0					
4		4				85	✓	✓	✓	✓	✓
2		2				0	✓	✗	✓	✗	✓
0		0				75	✗	✗	✗	✗	✗
8		8				0					
6		6				5					

Figure 5-7. An example of the spondaic word threshold worksheet found to be useful in the clinic. The left panel is designed for 2-dB decrements whereas the right panel is used with a 5-dB decrement protocol. See text for a discussion of the examples included on the worksheet. (From Wilson et al., 1973; reproduced with permission.)

is specified in the *Intensity* column with the correct responses (✓) or incorrect responses (✗) being recorded at the corresponding presentation levels. Immediately, from the worksheet, it is apparent when the criterion for test initiation and termination (step 3) have been satisfied, and threshold derivation (step 4) can be completed. The protocol of the threshold computation is the focus of the following section.

Derivation The data generated by the speech recognition threshold procedure just described are amenable to a statistical treatment initially described by Spearman (1908) in England and independently by Kärber (1931) in Germany. This statistical protocol, termed the Spearman-Kärber method (Finney, 1952) is expressed in the following formula (the mathematical derivation is found in the previous three references):

$$T_{50\%} = i + \tfrac{1}{2}(d) - \frac{d(r)}{n} \tag{1}$$

where $T_{50\%}$ is the speech recognition threshold defined as the 50 percent point on the psychometric function, i is the initial presentation level, d is the size of the decrement in stimulus level (dB), r is the total number of correct responses, and n is the number of words presented per decibel decrement. For cases in which $d = n$, formula 1 can be reduced to:

$$T_{50\%} = i + \tfrac{1}{2}(d) - r \tag{2}$$

This formula (2) is applicable to the data generated by the speech recognition threshold procedure described in the previous section. The derivation of threshold (step 4) was accomplished using this reduced formula. Applying formula 2 to the data given in Figure 5-7 (left panel) where the decibel decrement (d) is equal to the number of words per decibel decrement (n), we are given $i = 40$ dB HTL, $d = 2$ dB decrements, and $r = 9$ correct responses. By substituting in formula 2 we have

$$T_{50\%} = 40 + 1 - 9 \tag{3}$$

$$T_{50\%} = 32 \text{ dB HTL} \tag{4}$$

Variations in this speech recognition threshold method are appropriate, especially considering the clinical audiometers in use today. The two words per 2-dB decrement protocol is well suited for instruments with 2-dB step attenuators. Audiologists with audiometers having 5-dB step attenuators, however, will find their efforts to attain 2-dB decrements demanding and tedious. For these clinicians, the following substitutions are recommended and may be incorporated into the speech recognition threshold procedure: 1) 5-dB decrements; 2) five words per decibel decrement; 3) termination of the test when all words at an intensity presentation level are incorrect; and 4) threshold determination based on a correction factor ($\tfrac{1}{2}(d)$) of 2 instead of 2.5 (see Wilson et al., 1973 for the rationale for this choice). An example of this modification of the procedure is provided in Figure 5-7 (lower right panel) where $i = 85$ dB HTL, $d = 5$ dB decrements, $r = 8$, and $n = 5$. By substituting in formula 2 we have

$$T_{50\%} = 85 + \tfrac{1}{2}(5) - 8 \tag{5}$$

$$T_{50\%} = 79.5 \text{ dB HTL} \tag{6}$$

Finally, for audiologists utilizing combinations in which the decibel decrement and the number of words per decibel decrement are not equal, the following serves as an example.

Given: $i = 72$ dB HTL, $d = 3$-dB decrements, $r = 12$ correct, and $n = 5$ words per decrement, then substituting in formula 1 we have

$$T_{50\%} = 72 + \tfrac{1}{2}(3) - \frac{3(12)}{5} \tag{7}$$

$$T_{50\%} = 72 + 1.5 - 7.2 \tag{8}$$

$$T_{50\%} = 66.3 \text{ dB HTL} \tag{9}$$

These three examples demonstrate the procedure for applying the Spearman-Kärber method to data generated by the speech recognition threshold protocol described in the previous section, that is, two words per 2-dB decrement, the adaptation of the statistical procedure for other values of d and n, and the revisions necessary to utilize the statistical method when unequal parameters of d and n are needed.

Special Considerations with Difficult-to-Test Subjects

The usual procedure utilized to establish a speech recognition threshold is to have the patient repeat (orally) the spondaic word that was presented through the earphone. There are patients on whom this simple procedure will not work, namely, young children with limited expressive language skills and some adults with acute communicative problems, such as expressive aphasia, glossectomee, and laryngectomee. Information concerning the threshold for speech can be obtained from most of these individuals by changing the presentation and/or response modes to coincide with the performance abilities of the patient. Here, there are no strict rules and the ingenuity of the audiologist is paramount. There are, however, several practical considerations that assist in the evaluation of these patients with limited expressive skills. (For a detailed discussion, see Olsen and Matkin, 1979.)

First, the receptive language skills of the patient must be assessed informally. Is the patient able to repeat all or some of the spondaic words? Only those words that are repeatable by the patient, referred to as selected spondees, should be used in the test procedure. If none of the spondaic words are repeatable by the patient, then other speech materials must be considered, for example, common nouns.

When the stimulus materials have been selected, the next step is to determine the appropriate components that comprise the presentation mode. For flexibility and expediency, monitored live voice and 5-dB attenuation steps may be helpful. Also, the use of a carrier phrase, "show me" or "point to," is suggested as a means of defining the listening interval. Presentation of the stimulus materials through earphones is preferred, but for those patients who will "not tolerate" the earphones, sound field[3] testing must be employed.

The response mode also must be decided. Because we are concerned with patients who are unable to respond orally, the response task must be modified to a pointing response in which pictures or

---

[3] Sound field is defined as a listening environment in which the boundaries (e.g., floor, ceiling, and walls) and other structures (e.g., table and chairs) influence the frequency region of interest.

objects are used to represent the stimulus materials. To avoid confusion, only four to six items should be in the visual field of the patient. Further modification of the response mode may be necessary with patients having motor problems.

Even though the materials, presentation mode, and response mode tentatively can be determined, modifications in one or all of these test parameters may have to be made throughout the test procedure. Once an estimate of the threshold for speech has been obtained, the pertinent information about the test parameters should be recorded on the audiogram. Interpretation of the test results must be made with caution and restricted to the task at hand.

Finally, some individuals may respond to speech stimuli but not to tonal stimuli. In addition, some individuals may respond at lower presentation levels to speech stimuli than to tonal stimuli. For those patients unable to perform the picture-pointing response, and to respond to pure tone stimuli, behavioral unconditioned or conditioned techniques[4] with speech stimuli can be used (for a further discussion see Eisenberg, 1976; and Northern and Downs, 1978). The conditioned technique involves an ascending presentation of speech stimuli (nonsense syllables or words) via earphones or sound field. A response is recorded when there is an alteration in the ongoing behavioral (e.g., play) or physiologic (e.g., heart rate or sucking) activities of the child that coincides with the stimulus presentation. The following three behavioral conditioning techniques are available: 1) visual reinforcement audiometry (VRA); 2) conditioned orienting response (COR); and 3) tangible reinforcement operant conditioning assessment (TROCA). With these techniques, speech detection levels are established in sound field (VRA, COR, or TROCA) or under earphones (TROCA). As discussed previously, limited information can be inferred from the speech detection task. First, no information is obtained regarding the speech recognition performance of the patient. Second, because speech is a complex signal in which low frequency energy (vowels) predominates (Fletcher, 1929), no frequency-specific information is obtained from speech detection thresholds. Third, data from sound field testing may reflect only the better ear. Considering these limitations, interpretation of results obtained with behavioral unconditioned and conditioned techniques in a speech detection paradigm must be made with caution.

---

[4] With both of these behavioral techniques, pure tone stimuli (frequency and/or amplitude modulated tonal complexes) are preferred because they provide frequency selective information, whereas speech stimuli do not.

DETERMINANTS OF SPEECH RECOGNITION THRESHOLDS

Relations between Thresholds for Pure Tones and Speech

A considerable effort has been directed toward determining the relationship between auditory thresholds obtained with pure tone and speech stimuli. Clinicians who were involved in the development of materials for speech audiometry naturally were interested in the relationship between thresholds for speech and results from the more accepted procedure of measuring thresholds for pure tones. Because these investigators were interested in obtaining information about the patient's ability to understand speech, their threshold measurements using speech stimuli were *recognition* thresholds rather than detection thresholds. Consequently, it is important to keep in mind that the comparison that was made in these studies was that of a *recognition threshold* for speech and *detection thresholds* for tones. Although the two measures are mutually dependent upon many auditory processes, the fundamental difference in the nature of the task inevitably complicated the relationship.

Several early investigators compared pure tone thresholds and speech recognition thresholds and concluded that the two measurements of auditory sensitivity were highly correlated (Carhart, 1946; Fowler, 1941; Hughson and Thompson, 1942). Carhart (1946) advocated the use of the three-frequency (512, 1024, and 2048 Hz) pure tone average for predicting the recognition threshold for sentence material or for spondaic words. After considerable scrutiny by later investigators, the three-frequency pure tone average (now 500, 1000, and 2000 Hz) has survived as the most popular method of evaluating the relationship between pure tone and speech recognition thresholds.

Fletcher (1950) and several later investigators (Carhart and Porter, 1971; Graham, 1960; Harris, Haines, and Myers, 1956; Quiggle et al., 1957) evaluated various multiple regression equations and compared them with simpler averaging procedures. All of the methods could be used to predict speech recognition thresholds from pure tone thresholds with some degree of precision. In general, the statistically more complicated regression procedures were not remarkably better at predicting speech recognition thresholds than the simpler averaging procedures. The three-frequency pure tone average appears to be an adequate prediction method, although it systematically overestimates the speech recognition threshold for many patients with high-frequency sloping audiometric configurations. Carhart and Porter (1971) recommended averaging pure tone thresholds at 500 and 1000 Hz and subtracting 2 dB from the average as a method that appeared to be adequate regardless of audiometric configuration. For making more precise predictions they derived separate regression equations for each of five audiometric configurations.

Two important limitations of the relationship between pure tone sensitivity and speech recognition thresholds must be emphasized. First, due to the success of the three-frequency pure tone average in predicting speech recognition thresholds for spondaic words, some investigators and clinicians have dubbed 500, 1000, and 2000 Hz as the "speech frequencies" (e.g., Newby, 1979, among others). This terminology is dangerously misleading because it leads to the erroneous conclusion that "the frequencies above 2000 Hz are 'expendable' in the sense that they are not important in communication by speech" (Newby, 1979, p. 344). This conclusion is surprising in view of early evidence that frequencies above 2000 Hz contribute substantially to understanding speech both in quiet (French and Steinberg, 1947) and in noise (Kryter, Williams, and Green, 1962). As early as 1929, Fletcher pointed out that frequencies above 3000 Hz are as important for recognizing syllables as are the frequencies below 1000 Hz. Davis (1970) specified the important range for understanding everyday conversational speech as 400 through 3000 Hz. Recent physiologic evidence (Kiang and Moxon, 1974) suggests that high-frequency auditory channels may be responsible for encoding speech in noisy situations, whereas lower-frequency (and lower-threshold) channels may be masked by the noise. The relationship between the speech recognition threshold for spondaic words and the three-frequency or two-frequency pure tone average must be interpreted with consideration for the differences between the task of recognizing items from a small set of materials and the more complicated problem of speech communication. Although the pure tone average may predict (± 6 dB) the speech recognition threshold, it does not assess adequately communicative ability or disability (see Chapter 11 for a discussion of this concept).

A second limitation in the use of pure tone thresholds for predicting speech recognition thresholds lies in the effect of auditory pathology on speech recognition thresholds. Because the recognition of speech is a much more complicated process than the detection of a tone, certain auditory pathologies will inevitably influence the two measures differentially. Patients who suffer severe disturbances in speech communication ability may demonstrate substantial disparities between pure tone thresholds and speech recognition thresholds. Intracranial tumors that exert pressure on the auditory nerve commonly result in marked deficits in word recognition ability (Dirks et al., 1977; Flower and Viehweg, 1961; Jerger and Jerger, 1971; Johnson, 1968; Parker,

Decker, and Gardner, 1962). One effect of this type of lesion is to elevate the speech recognition threshold more than the pure tone average. Flower and Viehweg (1961) presented an extreme example in which a patient had a two-frequency (500 and 1000 Hz) pure tone average of 18 dB hearing level (HL), a speech detection threshold of 14 dB HL, but was unable to repeat spondaic words at the maximum output of the speech audiometer. Patients having less severe difficulties with word recognition may manifest similar, though less marked, disparities between pure tone thresholds and speech recognition thresholds.

Pseudohypacusis is another source of disparity between pure tone and speech thresholds (Ventry and Chaiklin, 1965). Usually the disparity is in the opposite direction from the difference produced by retrocochlear disease, that is, the pseudohypacusic patient usually has lower speech recognition thresholds than the pure tone results would predict. Presumably, this disparity is related to the patient's inability to match accurately the loudness of the speech stimuli to pure tones (see Rintelmann, 1979 for further discussion of this topic).

Masking and the Speech Recognition Threshold

When establishing a speech recognition threshold on an ear for which the threshold is poorer than the threshold for the opposite (nontest) ear, masking the nontest ear may be necessary. Precisely, the critical interaural difference is between the stimulus presentation level via air conduction to the poorer ear and the bone conduction threshold of the better ear. When this difference is >50 dB (Liden, 1954; Snyder, 1973), the nontest ear may perceive the test signal and thereby influence the test results. To minimize such influences, masking must be applied to the nontest ear.

Due to the complex nature of the spectral characteristics of speech, the responses to speech stimuli presented in noise are more difficult to predict than are the responses to pure tones in noise (Fletcher, 1940; Fletcher and Munson, 1937; Hawkins and Stevens, 1950; Sanders and Rintelmann, 1964). Empirical masking data for speech (Hawkins and Stevens, 1950; Hirsh and Bowman, 1953; Wilson, Stream, and Dirks, 1973), based on a paradigm in which the speech and noise were presented to the same ear (ipsilateral masking), are available to assist the audiologist in formulating masking guidelines for use with spondaic words. The details of masking employed with speech stimuli are provided in Chapter 9.

Masking Level Difference for Spondaic Words

An interesting application of the speech recognition threshold in noise is with the *masking level difference* (MLD) phenomenon, which is designed to assess the status of the central auditory nervous system at the level of the brainstem. (Chapter 8 details the use of the MLD test with patients having suspected central auditory dysfunction.) Before describing the MLD as related to spondaic words, it is instructive to consider an example of the masking level difference as it relates to low frequency pure tones (see Levitt and Voroba, 1974, for a discussion of MLD).

In the MLD paradigm, both the signal (S) and the masking noise (N) are presented binaurally to the listener through earphones. The task is to establish detection thresholds for the signal in noise for the two signal conditions. The two signal conditions are illustrated in Figure 5-8 where the pure tone signals delivered to the left ear and to the right ear are depicted. Consider first the upper panel of Figure 5-8 in which the phase difference between the two signal waveforms is 0°. This is the *homophasic* (S_o) condition. The subscript *o* indicates that there is no phase difference between the signals. In the lower panel of Figure 5-8, the signal waveforms have an opposite phase relation-

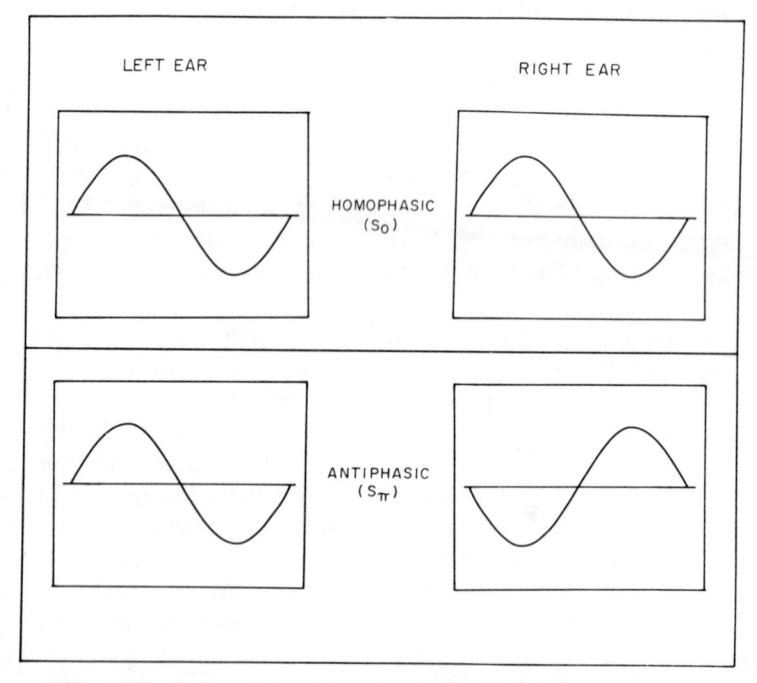

Figure 5-8. An illustration of the phase relationship between the signals employed in the masking level difference (MLD) paradigm. The signal waveforms in the upper panel have the same phase relationship, that is, in phase, between the left and right ear (S_0). The signal waveforms in the lower panel have opposite phase relationships, that is, they are 180° out of phase (S_π).

ship. This second signal condition, in which the signals are 180° *out of phase*, is called *antiphasic* (S_π), the subscript π indicating the 180° phase difference between the signal waveforms. In the MLD paradigm, binaural thresholds in noise are established for the signal in these two phase configurations (S_o and S_π). The decibel difference between the two thresholds is the masking level difference (also referred to as the binaural release from masking). The example below with a 500-Hz signal illustrates the MLD effect.

First, continuous broadband or narrowband noise is presented binaurally to the listener. Because the noise is presented in phase to the two ears it is designated N_o. Then the threshold for the in-phase 500-Hz signal (S_o in Figure 5-8) is established in the noise. This condition is termed S_oN_o because both the signal and the noise are in phase at the two ears. If broadband noise were presented at 70 dB SPL, then a realistic threshold for the 500-Hz signal would be 38 dB SPL. Finally, the phase of the signal is reversed in one ear relative to the other and the threshold measurement is repeated. This antiphasic condition is designated $S_\pi N_o$ because the 500-Hz signal is out of phase at the ears, whereas the noise is in phase at the ears. Again, with the 70 dB SPL broadband noise, a reasonable threshold for $S_\pi N_o$ would be 27 dB SPL.

The masking level difference for the example just presented with a 500-Hz tone in 70 dB SPL broadband noise is expressed as follows:

MLD = homophasic (S_oN_o) threshold − antiphasic ($S_\pi N_o$) threshold

MLD = 38 dB SPL − 27 dB SPL   (10)

MLD = 11 dB

In this example, the threshold for the homophasic condition (S_oN_o) is attained at a higher sound pressure level than is the threshold for the antiphasic condition ($S_\pi N_o$). This relationship between the thresholds attained for the two 500-Hz signal conditions is characteristic of the MLD phenomenon in the low frequencies. Specifically, for normal-hearing young adults the homophasic threshold should be at a higher sound pressure level than the antiphasic threshold. Finally, it should be noted that various phase combinations of the signal and noise can be used, for example, S_oN_o, $S_\pi N_o$, S_oN_π, and $S_\pi N_\pi$; however, the two conditions described in the example are most commonly used in the clinic situation.

The speech MLD involves the binaural presentation of spondaic words embedded in binaural noise in each of two speech phase conditions. In the homophasic condition, both signals (speech and noise) at the ears are in phase (S_oN_o). In the antiphasic condition, the speech signal is 180° out of phase, whereas the masking noise is in phase ($S_\pi N_o$). The data in Table 5-3 were obtained from 16 young adults. Speech recognition thresholds were established for two phase conditions ($S_o N_o$ and $S_\pi N_o$), in 70 dB SPL speech spectrum noise (~40 dB pressure spectrum level). The thresholds obtained for the two conditions are given in Table 5-3 along with the 7.5-dB MLD that resulted from the lower threshold being obtained when the spondaic words were out of phase ($S_\pi N_o$) as compared to in phase ($S_o N_o$). The MLD reported in Table 5-3 is representative of the MLD for spondaic words using a 50 percent correct criterion. As has been shown by Levitt and Rabiner (1967a, b), the magnitude of the MLD is dependent, among other things, upon the response task, increasing from 6 to 8 dB (recognition threshold) to 11 to 13 dB (detection threshold).

The clinical application of the MLD phenomenon generally is restricted to the assessment of central auditory nervous system lesions. In the future, however, the MLD technique in conjunction with physiologic data, for example, brainstem auditory evoked potentials (BAEP), may provide useful information about subtle brainstem lesions. For example, Novak (1977) suggested that the MLD may be sensitive in differentiating among the subgroups of presbycusis. Here again, further study is needed.

Speech Recognition Thresholds in Sound Field

The majority of audiologic testing is performed by presenting the signal to the patient through earphones. There are certain situations, however, in which the signal must be presented to the patient through a loudspeaker. This arrangement, referred to as *sound field testing*, is utilized in hearing aid evaluations and with children on whom earphone testing is precluded for various reasons. These two listening conditions (i.e., earphone versus sound field) are very different and, therefore, separate considerations and calibration rules must be applied to each.

Table 5-3. The mean and standard deviation (SD) for the spondaic word thresholds established in two masking conditions for normal hearing young adults

Condition	Mean (dB SPL)	SD (dB SPL)
$S_0 N_0$	64.6	1.1
$S_\pi N_0$	57.1	1.4
MLD	7.5	1.1

The binaural masker was 70 dB SPL speech spectrum noise. The mean MLD in dB also is shown. (From Carr, 1979; unpublished data.)

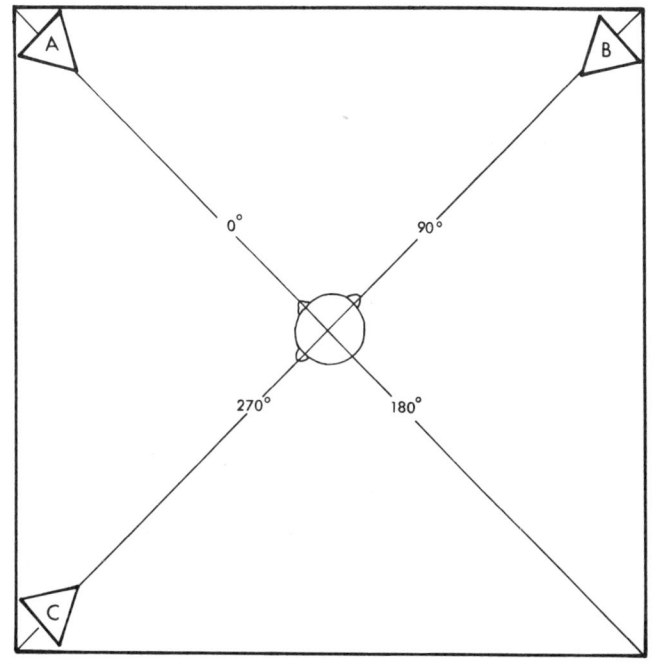

Figure 5-9. The azimuth notation utilized to document the relationship between the listener and loudspeakers (A, B, and C) in sound field. 0° is to the front, 90° is to the right, 180° is to the back, and 270° is to the left of the listener. (From Dirks and Wilson, 1980; reproduced with permission.)

Before proceeding, however, it is necessary to understand the terminology that is used with reference to sound field.

The threshold for speech in a sound field is dependent on the type of test materials and the room acoustics, including the physical arrangement of the test environment, that is, the location of the loudspeaker in regard to the test ear. Conventionally, the location of the loudspeaker is specified as an azimuth position in degrees with 0° indicating that the loudspeaker is directly in front of the listener. Then in a clockwise rotation, the right ear is 90°, directly behind the listener is 180°, and the left ear is 270°. This notation is illustrated in Figure 5-9, in which three loudspeakers (A, B, and C) are shown at 0°, 90°, and 270°, respectively.

A second notation useful in understanding the sound field environment is that of *near ear* and *far ear*. These designations simply indicate the ear nearer to or farther from the signal source. For example, from Figure 5-9, if loudspeaker B (a 90° azimuth position) was the signal source, then the right ear would be the near ear and the left ear would be the far ear. The right ear is in the direct path of the signal from loudspeaker B, whereas the head intervenes between the signal source (loudspeaker B) and the left ear. The left ear in this example is located farther from the signal source (by the width of the head) than is the right ear, and in the acoustic shadow that is cast by the head. This phenomenon, termed the *head shadow effect*, produces interaural temporal disparities and frequency-dependent amplitude reductions at the far ear in comparison to the near ear. For a comprehensive discussion of these characteristics in sound field, the reader is referred to Dirks, Stream, and Wilson (1972) and Dirks and Wilson (1980).

The influence of the loudspeaker azimuth position on the recognition threshold for spondaic words is shown in Figure 5-10 in which the thresholds are expressed in decibels regarding the threshold obtained at the 0° azimuth position. The thresholds were obtained from the left ear with the right ear occluded by an earplug and an earmuff, which in combination produced 25 to 45 dB of attenuation. The near and far ear conditions were created by changing the azimuth position of the loudspeaker that was located one meter from the center of the head. The data in Figure 5-10 indicate that the spondaic word thresholds are enhanced 3 to 4 dB in the near ear conditions with the lowest threshold obtained at the 300° azimuth position. In contrast, the far ear

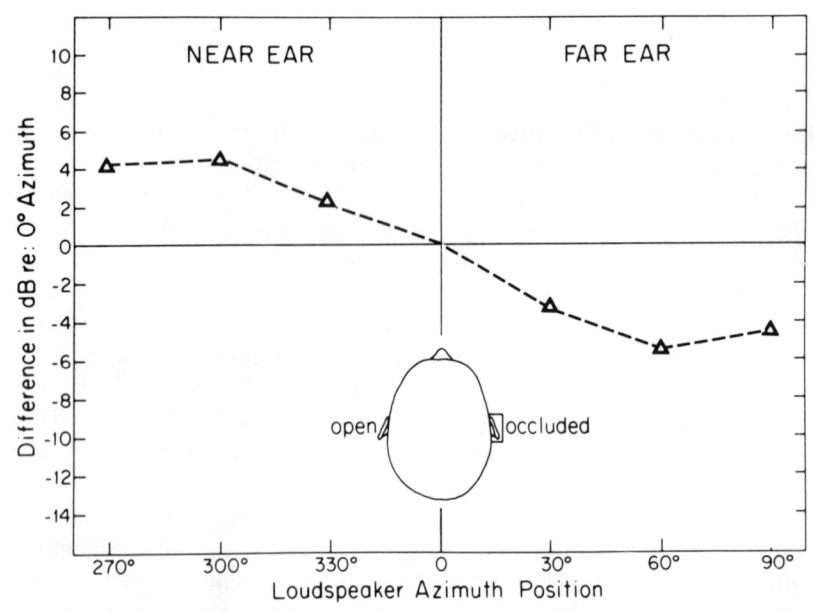

Figure 5-10. The spondaic word thresholds (in decibels with regard to the threshold at 0° azimuth) obtained on the left ears (open ear) of twelve listeners seated in an anechoic chamber.

Table 5-4. Comparison of MAP-MAF threshold differences (spondaic words) in decibels rounded to nearest 0.5 dB for four investigations

Investigation	Loudspeaker location				
	0°	30°	45°	60°	90°
Breakey and Davis, 1949	3.5				
Tillman, Johnson, and Olsen, 1966			7.5		
Dirks, Stream, and Wilson, 1972	3.5		7.5		
Stream and Dirks, 1974	3.0	5.0		7.0	5.0

conditions resulted in thresholds that are depressed by 3 to 5 dB with reference to the threshold at the 0° azimuth position. The differences between the near ear and far ear conditions, therefore, range from 5 to 10 dB, depending on the azimuth positions involved.

The data just described indicate that loudspeaker location must be considered when the sound field environment is calibrated for use with speech stimuli. In addition, the differences between speech thresholds obtained under earphones, that is, minimum audible pressure (MAP), and in sound field, minimum audible field (MAF), must be considered. Although the MAP-MAF differences are not specified currently in an ANSI standard, several investigations (Breakey and Davis, 1949; Dirks, Stream and Wilson, 1972; Stream and Dirks, 1974; and Tillman, Johnson, and Olsen, 1966) have documented the disparities between the two listening conditions. The data in Table 5-4 represent the differences, in decibels, between the speech recognition thresholds obtained through earphones and the thresholds obtained with a loudspeaker located at five azimuth positions in sound field. First, the data in the table again demonstrate that the intensity level required to establish the threshold for speech varies as a function of the azimuth position. Second, in all conditions, the threshold for speech in sound field is attained at a lower sound pressure level than is the threshold for speech established through an earphone. The appropriate sound pressure level for speech in sound field can be determined from the data in Table 5-4 by subtracting the MAP-MAF threshold difference (at a given azimuth) from the standard earphone sound pressure level for speech. For example, with a 20-dB SPL earphone reference for speech, the sound field should be calibrated to 16.5 dB SPL (0° azimuth) or 12.5 dB SPL (45° azimuth). Further details for sound field calibration are given by Dirks et al. (1972).

COMMENT

In most audiology centers the speech recognition threshold measurement is entrenched securely in the test battery routinely employed for the clinical evaluation of auditory function. The rationale for the clinical use of this measurement is based on the following considerations:

1. Validity. Because communicative disability was the major concern of clinicians involved in the development of hearing tests, it seemed desirable to obtain a sensitivity measurement using speech stimuli. The speech recognition threshold was thought to relate in some valid way to the communication process.
2. Check on Pure Tone Thresholds. The speech recognition threshold offers a method for checking the accuracy of pure tone thresholds. Disparities between thresholds for pure tone and speech stimuli are sometimes interpreted as evidence of pseudohypacusis, nerve VIII disease, or poor measurement technique.
3. Reference Level for Other Tests. The speech recognition threshold is often used as a reference level for the presentation of stimuli used for other tests, such as suprathreshold word recognition measurements.
4. Reliability with Difficult-to-Test Patients. Patients who are very young and/or mentally retarded may respond reliably to speech but cannot be conditioned to respond to tonal stimuli.

On closer examination the foregoing arguments suggest that the speech recognition threshold may be useful under some circumstances, but the procedure probably does not deserve its current high standing among auditory tests. The following reconsideration of the rationale for this measurement is offered by the authors.

1. Validity. Although the use of speech stimuli for threshold estimation has a certain face validity, that validity is more apparent than real. The materials most commonly used for the speech recognition threshold, spondaic words, were selected because they are among the most easily recognized speech materials. It commonly is observed that patients with severe communicative handicaps are able to recognize spondaic words. In other words, the ability to recognize spondaic words has little to do with communicative function. For the purpose of estimating the sensitivity of the auditory system, speech stimuli suffer from two important disadvantages: stimulus intensity is difficult to specify, and speech stimuli lack frequency selectivity. Pure tone stimuli are free of these problems. The validity of the speech recognition threshold is questionable on grounds that 1) the stimulus materials are not representative of speech used for communicative purposes; 2) the ability to recognize spondaic words is not highly correlated with

communicative function; 3) the stimuli cannot be specified precisely; and therefore, 4) standardization of the stimuli across clinics is poor.
2. Check on Pure Tone Thresholds. Although the speech recognition threshold can be helpful as a check on pure tone threshold measurements, this alone is not a convincing argument for its routine use. Many patients seen in audiology clinics have been seen on previous visits so that their reliability often is well established. For patients who have not been evaluated previously, a more appropriate check on the repeatability of pure tone thresholds would be to repeat the pure tone threshold measurements. Conversely, comparison of the speech recognition threshold with averaged pure tone threshold data provides some indication of the overall compatability or agreement between these two different auditory measurements. For patients who are suspected of pseudohypacusis, the speech recognition threshold should be included in the battery of tests designed to evaluate that possibility. Student clinicians would be well advised to perform both pure tone threshold measurements and speech recognition thresholds in order to acquire the necessary experience with both procedures and so that the agreement between the two measurements can be observed.
3. Reference Level for Other Tests. It is conventional to present stimuli for suprathreshold speech recognition testing at a level relative to the speech recognition threshold. The level at which word recognition test materials are presented commonly is specified as the *sensation level*, that is, the intensity level above the recognition threshold. The term sensation level is not appropriate in this context because different stimuli typically are used for the two measurements. Just as 40 dB sensation level for a 4000-Hz tone is referenced to the threshold for the 4000-Hz tone, not to the threshold at some other frequency, the sensation level for speech stimuli should be referenced to the threshold for the same stimulus. Furthermore, the threshold that serves as a reference for *sensation level* should be a detection threshold, not a recognition threshold. It is not necessary, however, to reference the presentation level for speech recognition testing to a threshold for speech. A perfectly legitimate procedure would be to select the presentation level with reference to the sensitivity for pure tones. Procedures for averaging pure tone thresholds were discussed in a previous section. This practice would obviate the need for the speech recognition threshold measurement, conserving the valuable time of the patient and clinician, while providing an adequate means of deciding what level to employ for the presentation of speech recognition test materials.

4. Reliability with Difficult-to-Test Patients. For patients that cannot be conditioned to respond to tonal stimuli, the clinician is obliged to employ any reasonable means for evaluating auditory function. Certainly, speech stimuli can be helpful under these circumstances.

In summary, the speech recognition threshold measurement is one of the clinician's tools that can be helpful in the auditory evaluation of patients. It is useful under certain circumstances, but its limitations should be kept in mind. The role of all auditory tests should be evaluated carefully in the framework of the audiologic evaluation. No single measurement procedure should be accepted as indispensable without a thoughtful and thorough development of the rationale for the test. If patients are expected to spend their time and money in the audiology clinic, then they deserve the benefit of an ongoing critical evaluation of clinical procedures.

REFERENCES

American National Standards Institute. 1954. American National Standard Practice for Volume Measurements of Electrical Speech and Program Waves, ANSI C16.5-1954. American National Standards Institute, Inc., New York.

American National Standards Institute. 1969. American National Standards Specifications for Audiometers, ANSI S3.6-1969. American National Standards Institute, Inc., New York.

American National Standards Institute. 1973. American National Standard Psychoacoustical Terminology, ANSI S3.20-1973. American National Standards Institute, Inc., New York.

American Speech-Language-Hearing Association Subcommittee on Speech Audiometry. 1979. Guidelines for determining the threshold level for speech. Asha 21:353–356.

Beattie, R. C., B. J. Edgerton, and D. V. Svihovec. 1975. An investigation of Auditec of St. Louis recordings of Central Institute for the Deaf spondees. J. Am. Audiol. Soc. 1:97–101.

Beattie, R. C., D. V. Svihovec, and B. J. Edgerton. 1975. Relative intelligibility of the CID spondees as presented via monitored live voice. J. Speech Hear. Disord. 40:84–91.

Bilger, R. C., and M. D. Wang. 1976. Consonant confusions in patients with sensorineural hearing loss. J. Speech Hear. Res. 19:718–748.

Bowling, L. S., and B. S. Elpern. 1961. Relative intelligibility of items on CID Auditory Test W-1. J. Aud. Res. 1:152–157.

Breakey, M. R., and H. Davis. 1949. Comparisons of thresholds for speech; word and sentence tests; receiver versus field and monaural versus binaural listening. Laryngoscope 59:236–250.

Bryant, W. S. 1904. A phonographic acoumeter. Arch. Otolaryngol. 33:438–443.

Carhart, R. 1946. Speech reception in relation to pattern of pure tone loss. J. Speech Hear. Disord. 11:97–108.

Carhart, R., and L. S. Porter. 1971. Audiometric configuration and prediction of threshold for spondees. J. Speech Hear. Res. 14:486–495.

Carr, R. R. 1979. Unpublished data. V. A. Medical Center, Long Beach, Ca.

Chaiklin, J. B. 1959. The relation among three selected auditory speech thresholds. J. Speech Hear. Res. 2:237–243.

Chaiklin, J. B., J. Font, and R. F. Dixon. 1967. Spondee thresholds measured in ascending 5 dB steps. J. Speech Hear. Res. 10:141–145.

Chaiklin, J. B., and I. M. Ventry. 1964. Spondee threshold measurement: A comparison of 2- and 5-dB methods. J. Speech Hear. Disord. 29:47–59.

Cherry, C. 1966. On Human Communication. M.I.T. Press, Cambridge, Mass.

Conn, M., J. Dancer, and I. M. Ventry. 1975. A spondee list for determining speech reception threshold without prior familiarization. J. Speech Hear. Disord. 40:388–396.

Cramer, K. D., and N. P. Erber. 1974. A spondee recognition test for young hearing-impaired children. J. Speech Hear. Disord. 39:304–311.

Curry, E. T., and B. P. Cox. 1966. The relative intelligibility of spondees. J. Aud. Res. 6:419–424.

Davis, H. 1970. Audiometry. In H. Davis and S. R. Silverman (eds.), Hearing and Deafness. Holt, Rinehart, & Winston, Inc., New York.

Dirks, D. D., C. Kamm, D. Bower, and A. Bettsworth. 1977. Use of performance intensity functions for diagnosis. J. Speech Hear. Disord. 42:408–415.

Dirks, D. D., R. W. Stream, and R. H. Wilson. 1972. Speech audiometry: Earphone and sound field. J. Speech Hear. Disord. 37:162–176.

Dirks, D. D., and R. H. Wilson. 1980. Binaural hearing in sound field. In E. Libby (ed.), Binaural Hearing and Amplification. Vol. I. Zenetron Hearing Instruments, Inc., Chicago.

Eisenberg, R. B. 1976. Auditory competence in early life: The roots of communicative behavior. University Park Press, Baltimore.

Erber, N. P. 1969. Interaction of audition and vision in the recognition of oral speech stimuli. J. Speech Hear. Disord. 12:423–425.

Erber, N. P. 1971. Auditory detection of spondaic words in wide band noise by adults with normal hearing and by children with profound hearing losses. J. Speech Hear. Res. 14:373–381.

Erber, N. P. 1974. Pure-tone thresholds and word-recognition abilities of hearing-impaired children. J. Speech Hear. Res. 17:194–202.

Feldmann, H. 1960. A history of audiology: A comprehensive report and bibliography from the earliest beginnings to the present. (Transl. by J. Tonndorf from: Die geschichtliche Entwicklung der Horprufungsmethoden, kuze Darstellung und Bibliographie von der Anfongen bis zue Gegenwart, in Zwanglose Abhandungen aus dem Gebeit der Hals- Nasen- Ohren- Heilkunde. H. Leicher, R. Mittermaiser, and G. Theissing (eds.). Georg Thieme Verlag, Stuttgart, 1960.) Transl. Beltone Inst. Hear. Res. 22:1–111.

Finney, D. J. 1952. Statistical Method in Biological Assay. C. Griffen, London.

Fletcher, H. 1929. Speech and Hearing. Van Nostrand, New York.

Fletcher, H. 1940. Auditory patterns. Rev. Mod. Physics 12:47–65.

Fletcher, H. 1950. A method of calculating hearing loss for speech from an audiogram. J. Acoust. Soc. Am. 22:1–5.

Fletcher, H., and W. Munson. 1937. Relation between loudness and masking. J. Acoust. Soc. Am. 9:1–10.

Fletcher, H., and J. C. Steinberg. 1929. Articulation testing methods. Bell Systems Tech. J. 7:806–854.

Flower, R. M., and R. Viehweg. 1961. Review of audiologic findings among patients with cerebellopontine angle tumors. Laryngoscope 71:1105–1126.

Fowler, E. P. 1941. Hearing standards for acceptance, disability rating, and discharge in the military and in industry. Laryngoscope 51:937–956.

French, N. R., and J. C. Steinberg. 1947. Factors governing the intelligibility of speech sounds. J. Acoust. Soc. Am. 19:90–119.

Graham, J. T. 1960. Evaluation of methods for predicting speech reception threshold. Arch. Otolaryngol. 72:347–350.

Green, D. M., and J. A. Swets. 1966. Signal Detection Theory and Psychophysics. John Wiley & Sons, Inc., New York.

Gruber, J. 1891. A Text-Book of the Diseases of the Ear. (Translated by E. Law and C. Jewell from the second German edition). D. Appleton and Company, New York.

Harris, J. D., H. L. Haines, and C. K. Myers. 1956. A new formula for using the audiogram to predict speech hearing loss. Arch. Otolaryngol. 63:158–176.

Hawkins, J. E., and S. S. Stevens. 1950. Masking of pure tones and of speech by white noise. J. Acoust. Soc. Am. 22:6–13.

Hawley, M. E. 1977. On the application of the new Edison phonograph to general hearing measurement. In M. E. Hawley (ed.), Speech Intelligibility and Speaker Recognition, pp. 247–252. Dowden, Hutchinson and Ross, Inc., Stroudsburg, Pa.

Hirsh, I. J. 1947. Clinical application of two Harvard auditory tests. J. Speech Hear. Disord. 12:151–158.

Hirsh, I. J. 1952. The Measurement of Hearing. McGraw-Hill Book Company, Inc. New York.

Hirsh, I. J., and W. D. Bowman. 1953. Masking of speech by bands of noise. J. Acoust. Soc. Am. 25:1175–1180.

Hirsh, I. J., H. Davis, S. R. Silverman, E. G. Reynolds, E. Eldert, and R. W. Benson. 1952. Development of materials for speech audiometry. J. Speech Hear. Disord. 17:321–337.

Hudgins, C. V., J. E. Hawkins, Jr., J. E. Karlin, and S. S. Stevens. 1947. The development of recorded auditory tests for measuring hearing loss for speech. Laryngoscope 57:57–89.

Hughson, W., and E. A. Thompson. 1942. Correlation of hearing acuity for speech with discrete frequency audiograms. Arch. Otolaryngol. 36:526–540.

Jerger, J. F., R. Carhart, T. W. Tillman, and J. L. Peterson. 1959. Some relations between normal hearing for pure tones and for speech. J. Speech Hear. Res. 2:126–140.

Jerger, J., and S. Jerger. 1971. Diagnostic significance of PB word functions. Arch. Otolarynol. 93:573–580.

Johnson, E. 1968. Auditory findings in 200 cases of acoustic neurinomas. Arch. Otolaryngol. 88:598–603.

Jones, J. H., and V. O. Knudsen. 1924. Functional tests of hearing. Laryngoscope 39:1–16.

Kärber, G. 1931. Beitrag zue kollektiven behandlung pharmakologischer reihenversuche. Arch. Exp. Path. Pharm. 4:480–483.

Kiang, N. Y. S., and E. C. Moxon. 1974. Tails of tuning curves of auditory-nerve fibers. J. Acoust. Soc. Am. 55:620–630.

Kruel, E. J., D. W. Bell, and J. C. Nixon. 1969. Factors affecting speech discrimination test difficulty. J. Speech Hear. Res. 12:281–287.

Kryter, K. D., C. Williams, and D. M. Green. 1962. Auditory acuity and the perception of speech. J. Acoust. Soc. Am. 34:1217–1223.

Levitt, A., and B. Voroba. 1974. Binaural hearing. In S. Gerber (ed.), Introductory Hearing Science. W.B. Saunders Company, Philadelphia.
Levitt, H., and L. R. Rabiner. 1967a. Binaural release from masking for speech and gain in intelligibility. J. Acoust. Soc. Am. 42:601–608.
Levitt, H., and L. R. Rabiner. 1967b. Predicting binaural gain in intelligibility and release from masking in speech. J. Acoust. Soc. Am. 42:820–829.
Lichwitz, L. 1889. Über die Anwendung des neuen Edison's chen Phonographen als allgemeinen Hörmesser. (On the application of the new Edison Phonograph to general hearing measurement.) Prager med. Wochenschr. 14:547–549.
Licklider, J. C. R., and G. A. Miller. 1951. The perception of speech. In S. S. Stevens (ed.), Handbook of Experimental Psychology, pp. 1040–1074. John Wiley & Sons, Inc., New York.
Liden, G. 1954. Speech audiometry. Acta Otolaryngol., 114:1–45. (Suppl.)
Lindner, W. A. 1968. Recognition performance as a function of detection criterion in a simultaneous detection-recognition task. J. Acoust. Soc. Am. 44:204–211.
MacMillan, N. A. 1971. Detection and recognition of increments and decrements in auditory intensity. Percept. Psychophysics 10:233–238.
MacMillan, N. A. 1973. Detection and recognition of intensity changes in tone and noise: The detection-recognition disparity. Percept. Psychophysics 13:65–75.
Newby, H. A. 1958. Audiology: Principles and Practice. Appleton-Century-Crofts, New York.
Newby, H. A. 1979. Audiology. Prentice-Hall, Englewood Cliffs, New Jersey.
Northern, J. L., and M. P. Downs. 1978. Hearing in Children. Williams & Wilkins Company, Baltimore.
Novak, R. E. 1977. The use of the MLD to assess presbycusis. Doctoral dissertation. The University of Iowa, Iowa City.
Olsen, W. O., and N. D. Matkin. 1979. Speech audiometry. In W. F. Rintelmann (ed.), Hearing Assessment. University Park Press, Baltimore.
Owens, E., and E. D. Schubert. 1968. The development of constant items for speech discrimination testing. J. Speech Hear. Res. 11:656–667.
Parker, W., R. L. Decker, and W. H. Gardner. 1962. Auditory function and intracranial lesions. Arch. Otolaryngol. 76:425–435.
Pollack, I., H. Rubenstein, and L. Decker. 1959. Intelligibility of known and unknown message sets. J. Acoust. Soc. Am. 31:273–279.
Quiggle, R. R., A. Glorig, J. H. Delk, and A. B. Summerfield. 1957. Predicting hearing loss for speech from pure tone audiograms. Laryngoscope 67:1–15.
Rintelmann, W. F. 1979. Pseudohypacusis. In W. F. Rintelmann (ed.), Hearing Assessment. University Park Press, Baltimore.
Sanders, J. W., and W. F. Rintelmann. 1964. Masking in audiometry: A clinical evaluation of three methods. Arch. Otolaryngol. 80:541–556.
Schultz, M. C. 1972. A critique of speech recognition testing preliminary to hearing therapy. J. Speech Hear. Disord. 37:195–202.
Snyder, J. M. 1973. Interaural attenuation characteristics in audiometry. Laryngoscope 83:1847–1855.
Spearman, C. 1908. The method of "right and wrong cases" ("constant stimuli") without Gauss's formulae. Br. J. Psychol. 2:227–242.
Stream, R. W., and D. D. Dirks. 1974. Effect of loudspeaker position on differences between earphone and free-field thresholds (MAP and MAF). J. Speech Hear. Res. 17:549–567.

Swets, J. A. 1961. "Is there a sensory threshold?" Science 134:168–177.
Thurlow, W. R., S. R. Silverman, H. Davis, and T. E. Walsh. 1948. A statistical study of auditory tests in relation to the fenestration operation. Laryngoscope 58:43–66.
Tillman, T. W., and J. F. Jerger. 1959. Some factors affecting the spondee threshold in normal-hearing subjects. J. Speech Hear. Res. 2:141–146.
Tillman, T. W., R. M. Johnson, and W. O. Olsen. 1966. Earphone versus sound-field threshold sound pressure levels for spondee words. J. Acoust. Soc. Am. 39:125–133.
Tillman, T. W., and W. O. Olsen. 1973. Speech audiometry. In J. Jerger (ed.), Modern Developments in Audiology, pp. 37–74. 2nd Ed. Academic Press, Inc., New York.
Ventry, I. M., and J. B. Chaiklin (eds.). 1965. Multidiscipline study of functional hearing loss. J. Aud. Res. 5:179–272.
Wathen-Dunn, W., and D. W. Lipke. 1958. On the power gained by clipping speech in the audio band. J. Acoust. Soc. Am. 30:36–40.
Wilson, R. H., and J. K. Antablin. 1980. A picture identification task as an estimate of the word-recognition performance of non-verbal adults. J. Speech Hear. Disord. 45:223–238.
Wilson, R. H., D. E. Morgan, and D. D. Dirks. 1973. A proposed SRT procedure and its statistical precedent. J. Speech Hear. Disord. 38:184–191.
Wilson, R. H., R. W. Stream, and D. D. Dirks. 1973. Spread-of-masking effects on pure tones and several speech stimuli. J. Speech Hear. Res. 16:385–396.
Young, L., B. Dudley, and M. Gunter. Thresholds and psychometric functions of the individual spondaic words. J. Speech Hear. Res. In press.

CHAPTER 6

CLINICAL ASSESSMENT OF SPEECH RECOGNITION

Fred H. Bess

CONTENTS

SPEECH RECOGNITION MATERIALS FOR ADULTS	128
Nonsense Syllables	128
Monosyllabic Words: Open-Set Response	130
Monosyllabic Words: Closed-Set Response	135
Sentence Materials	140
SPEECH RECOGNITION MATERIALS FOR CHILDREN	144
Monosyllables and Spondees	144
Sentence Materials	152
Use of Adult Materials with Children	156
Nonconventional Materials	157
PROCEDURAL STRATEGIES IN SPEECH RECOGNITION	159
Mode of Presentation	159
Method of Response and Error Analysis	163
Abbreviated Recognition Tests	164
Adverse Listening Conditions	168
Speech Recognition by Bone Conduction	171
Special Considerations for Children	172
CLINICAL UTILIZATION OF SPEECH RECOGNITION TESTS	173
Estimating Social Efficiency	173
Diagnostic Implications	175
Hearing Aid Selection	187
Aural Rehabilitation	189
AFTERWORD	191
ACKNOWLEDGMENTS	191
REFERENCES	191

For more than four decades the assessment of speech recognition has served as an important measure for determining an individual's ability to identify phonetic nuances. Speech recognition is used routinely by the audiologist to qualitatively evaluate communicative efficiency, to aid in the selection and evaluation of appropriate amplification, to delineate site of lesion, and to assess specific rehabilitative needs. Depending on the purpose for measuring speech recognition, the audiologist must decide which is the best test material to use and what procedure should be employed to administer the test. This chapter reviews the current status concerned with the clinical measurement of speech recognition. Toward this end, the chapter focuses on three general areas: test materials for adults and children; procedures for administering the tests; and clinical utilization.

SPEECH RECOGNITION MATERIALS FOR ADULTS

Initial attempts to assess speech recognition can be traced to Campbell, who in 1910 was conducting research with Bell Telephone Laboratories (BTL) for the purpose of developing techniques to evaluate telephone circuits (Olsen and Matkin, 1979). Campbell's assessment technique consisted of a talker reading a list of nonsense syllables on one end of a telephone channel and a listener on the other end identifying the speech stimuli. The percentage of test items identified correctly was used to determine the speech intelligibility score (Levitt and Resnick, 1978).

Since 1910, numerous tests have been proffered for evaluating the speech recognition of both normal and hearing-impaired individuals. These tests have varied in terms of the type of speech material employed as well as the format used to measure speech intelligibility. In the past, those test materials most commonly employed in speech recognition assessment have been monosyllables and sentences. These materials may be subcategorized further on the basis of whether the items are meaningful or nonmeaningful. Nonsense syllables, for example, are nonmeaningful monosyllabic materials sometimes used as a test for speech recognition. Furthermore, speech stimulus items may appear in an open-set response format or in a closed-set response paradigm. An open-set response implies that a listener may select any possible number of alternatives within the confines of the individual's receptive vocabulary. In contrast, a closed-set mode restricts the available choices to a given set of stimulus items. This section reviews some of the more common auditory tests used in the measurement of speech recognition for adults. Because many of the traditional materials have received comprehensive coverage from several other sources (Bess, 1982; Davis and Silverman, 1978; Olsen and Matkin, 1979) the discussion here will provide greater focus on the more recent tests which are perhaps less well known.

Nonsense Syllables

Nonsense syllables were one of the earliest materials used in the assessment of speech recognition. These early tests were designed primarily for assessing communication systems rather than measuring the recognition abilities of the hearing impaired. The original lists developed by BTL consisted of a sequential series of consonant-vowels (CV), vowel-consonants (VC) or consonant-vowel-consonants (CVC). The research conducted by BTL (Campbell, 1910; Fletcher, 1922; Fletcher and Steinberg, 1929) served as a model for future nonsense syllable tests. During these early years, the Psycho-Acoustic Laboratories at Harvard (PAL) also became involved in the development of nonsense materials for evaluating communication systems. The Harvard group developed lists that consisted of isolated vowels, CV, and VC syllables.

It was not until the 1970s, however, that nonsense syllable tests were considered seriously for clinical use with the hearing-impaired population. The major limitations that apparently discouraged clinical audiologists from using these materials were: the fact that material was nonmeaningful and hence not representative of everyday speech; inherent difficulties in eliciting an appropriate response from the listener; and problems associated with scoring the response. Edgerton and Danhauer (1979), however, emphasized that there is no documented evidence to support the latter two limitations and then highlighted the many advantages offered by using nonsense stimulus items. These advantages include: increased analytic accuracy; minimal contamination by memory and word familiarity effects; sample test construction; and increased diagnostic efficiency.

A promising nonsense syllable test has been developed by Resnick for use in hearing aid evaluations (Levitt and Resnick, 1978; Resnick et al., 1976). Termed the *nonsense syllable test* (NST), it is comprised of seven subtests, each of which contains seven to nine nonsense syllables of the CV or VC type. The nonsense syllables used in the various subtests contain all of the major consonant sounds and three vowels which are in the extreme positions of the vowel triangle. In the selection of the seven subtests greater emphasis was given to those sounds that are known to give difficulty to hearing-impaired adults. The seven subtests which comprise the NST are shown in Figure 6-1. It can be seen that the subtests differ in the class of consonants represented (voiced or voiceless), the position of the consonants and the vowel context. Each subtest employs a closed-set response format and the response foils are essentially all of the remaining syllables within the subtest. It should also be noted that the test was designed so that the response foils correspond with the most frequent perceptual confusions of both normal hearers and hearing-impaired individuals. The complete NST contains 62 stimulus items including one repeat item in each subtest. There are 16 randomized forms available. Test time varies from 8 to 15 minutes depending on the age and astuteness of the listener.

Sound field performance intensity functions of normal hearers for the NST in quiet and under two different noise conditions are shown in Figure 6-2. These data, taken from Levitt and Resnick (1978), were obtained with the stimuli presented from a loudspeaker located at 0° azimuth and with one ear of the listener covered with an ear protector. The percent correct scores represent average data for seven subtests

<u>1</u>	<u>2</u>	<u>3</u>	<u>4</u>	<u>5</u>	<u>6</u>	<u>7</u>
ɑf	uθ	iʃ	ɑb	fɑ	lɑ	nɑ
ɑʃ	up	if	ɑdʒ	tɑ	bɑ	vɑ
ɑt	us	it	ɑd	pɑ	dɑ	mɑ
ɑk	uk	ik	ɑm	hɑ	gɑ	zɑ
ɑs	ut	is	ɑz	θɑ	rɑ	gɑ
ɑp	uf	iθ	ɑg	tʃɑ	jɑ	bɑ
ɑθ	uʃ	ip	ɑn	sɑ	dʒɑ	ðɑ
			ɑŋ	ʃɑ	wɑ	dɑ
			ɑv	kɑ		

Figure 6-1. Test items comprising the NST. Each column represents a subtest of the NST. (From Resnick et al.; 1976, reproduced with permission.)

taken from male and female talkers. It can be seen that in the quiet condition the function is gradual, increasing at a rate of about 3 percent/dB. As the listening condition becomes less favorable, the growth of the function decreases and at a signal-to-noise (S/N) ratio of 0 the slope is only 0.75 percent/dB.

Monosyllabic Words: Open-Set Response

A major contribution to the clinical measurement of speech recognition was the development of phonetically balanced (PB) monosyllabic word lists by researchers at the Harvard Psycho-Acoustic Laboratories (Egan, 1948). Known as the PAL PB-50 lists, these materials were constructed using the following basic criteria outlined by Egan: monosyllabic structure; equal average difficulty; equal range of difficulty; equal composition of phonetic classes; composition representative of English speech; and the words in common usage. Egan postulated that in order for a speech intelligibility test to be valid it was desirable that each list have an equal representation of speech sounds. That is, whenever possible, the frequency of occurrence of basic speech sounds should be reflected in each test list. Toward this end, the phonetic composition of the PAL PB-50 lists were based on Dewey's (1923) frequency count from a sample of 100,000 English words found in newsprint. This frequency count of each phonetic class in the initial, medial, and final positions was determined and an attempt was made to approximate this speech sound composition into each list. The work by Egan at the Psycho-Acoustic Laboratories resulted in a total of 20 lists of 50 monosyllables each.

During World War II, the PB-50 lists were commonly used in those military programs that provided aural rehabilitation. Two specific limitations of this test, however, seemed to preclude its widespread clinical acceptance. First, clinical experience revealed that the lists had a sufficient number of unfamiliar words to influence the performance scores of those patients with limited receptive vocabularies. In addition, one of the first clinically available recordings (made by Rush Hughes) of some of these lists had certain acoustical features which made the test even more difficult. These recordings also failed to include a carrier phrase.

In an effort to eliminate some of the problems associated with the PAL PB-50 test, a research team from the Central Institute for the Deaf

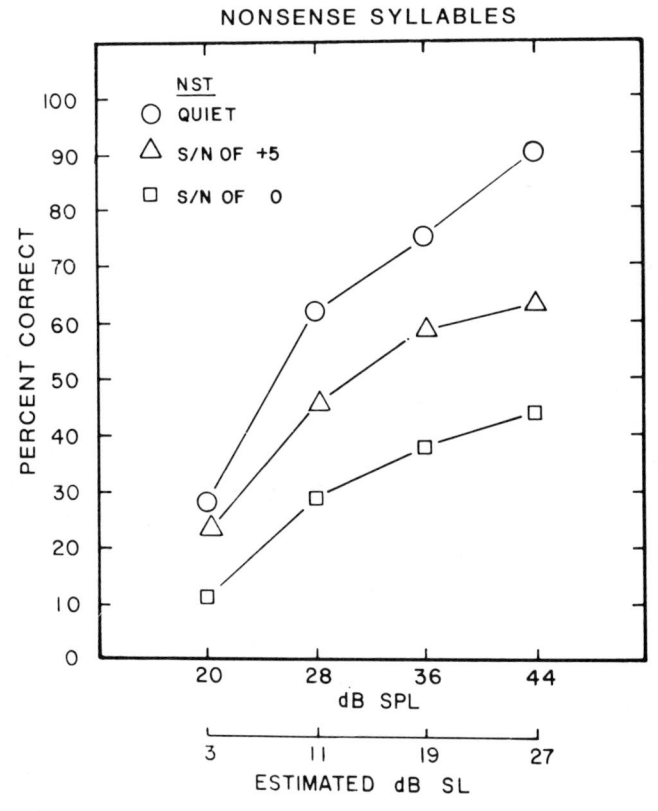

Figure 6-2. Performance intensity functions obtained with the NST in normal hearers under quiet and two noise conditions. S/N, signal to noise ratio. (Adapted from Levitt and Resnick, 1978)

(CID) developed a modified version of the PAL lists that incorporated a simpler vocabulary, an improved phonetic balance, and standardized, commercially available recordings (Hirsh et al., 1952). To improve the phonetic composition of this new test a criterion of spoken rather than written English was used—thus offering greater face validity. The two sources used to satisfy the phonetic criterion were Dewey's (1923) study of phonetic composition and the BTL study of business telephone calls in New York City. These revised lists are recognized as the CID W-22s and are comprised of 200 words categorized into four lists of 50 words each. The CID W-22s are the most widely used clinical tool in speech audiometry (Martin and Forbis, 1978).

After reviewing some of the limitations inherent in the PAL PB-50s and the CID W-22 materials, Tillman, Carhart, and Wilber (1963) developed a new monosyllabic word test of the consonant-nucleus-consonant (CNC) variety. This test, based on the original work of Lehiste and Peterson (1959), was developed using a criterion of phonemic rather than phonetic balancing. Lehiste and Peterson differentiated between phonetics and phonemics in the following manner (p. 281):

> As the term phonetics is normally used in American linguistics, it concerns the physiological and acoustical properties of speech. Auditory phonetics might refer to the mechanical analysis of speech by the ear, but a listener's own linguistic background will strongly influence his judgements about any speech which he hears. Essentially perceptual phonetics is phonemics and phonetics is the study of the physiological and physical properties of speech sounds.

Hence, Lehiste and Peterson argued that there are limitations to phonetic balancing because speech elements in a word are directly influenced by contiguous sounds.

The test items developed by Lehiste and Peterson were selected on the basis of a high degree of familiarity, carefully controlled phonemic balance, and use of consonant-nucleus-consonant words. Phonemic balancing was established by determining the frequency of occurrence for each initial, medial, and final phoneme in a corpus of familiar words ($N = 1263$; Thorndike and Lorge, 1952), and then ensuring that the phonemic composition for each 50-word list was proportional to the original 1263 words. Tillman and coworkers (1963) developed two new lists known as the Northwestern University auditory test No. 4 (NU #4) using the pool of words generated by Lehiste and Peterson. In order to provide greater flexibility for research and clinical use, the original two lists of the NU #4 were later expanded to four 50-word lists and called the Northwestern University auditory test No. 6 (NU #6) (Tillman and Carhart, 1966). Four scramblings of each list of the NU #6 are available, providing a total of 16 lists. Normative data have been reported for the NU #6 on list equivalency, effect of presentation level in normals and sensorineural impaired ears, the use of half-lists, effects of counterbalancing vs. randomization, and finally, the effects of listener dialect (Beattie, Edgerton, and Svihovec, 1977; Rintelmann et al., 1974; Tillman and Olsen, 1973; Wilson et al., 1975).

Boothroyd (1968) developed "isophonemic" word lists that are comprised of 15 lists of 10 words. All words are of the CNC variety. The phonemes selected were those that occurred most frequently in the CNC pool. Boothroyd advocated scoring each phoneme rather than simply scoring the word as correct or incorrect. Thus, each list was comprised of 30 phonemes. The reported advantages of this speech recognition test are that it affords a means of phonemic analysis and the test may be administered in a short period of time (Olsen and Matkin, 1979).

With the exception of the NST, the monosyllabic materials described thus far contain materials that do not take into account the discriminative difficulties encountered by hearing-impaired individuals. In the opinion of Jerger (1980), a more adequate assessment of speech recognition for the hearing impaired is a test that contains materials that reflect the speech understanding problems encountered by persons with hearing loss. One such test is the "high-frequency" list developed by Pascoe (1975). This test is comprised of 50 monosyllabic words that focus on sound elements that are known to cause difficulty for the hearing impaired. The stimulus items contain only three vocalic nuclei and 63 percent of the consonant sounds are voiceless fricatives and voiceless plosives. No attempt was made to incorporate a phonetic balance because for every word selected as a test item, six or more similar sounding words were included to reduce learning effects with repeated presentations of the same list. In the original description of this list, Pascoe (1975) carefully familiarized the subject with the words and offered a period of pretest practice. Pascoe suggested that this familiarization and practice makes the test more of a closed-set than an open-set paradigm. This test, however, does seem to approximate more closely the format used by other open-set word lists already described in this section. Although the high-frequency lists appear to have potential, there is a paucity of information on the clinical applicability of this test. Published normative data for normal-hearing and hearing-impaired listeners are needed in such areas as effect of presentation level, learning effects, variability, and effect of 10-word presentation versus 50-word presentation before these lists can be used in the clinical setting with any degree of confidence.

Some preliminary research has been conducted on the *Pascoe high frequency* (PHF) word list by Gravel and coworkers (1981). The general purpose of this study was to establish performance intensity functions for the PHF list in both normal and hearing-impaired listeners. Male and female recordings were generated and each of these master lists were randomized six times to make twelve forms of the test. A multitalker babble was used for presenting the lists in competition. In addition to presentation level, data were reported on male versus female recordings, test-retest reliability, and the effects of competition. Thus far, the preliminary data suggest that the list does have clinical usefulness. In particular, the test appears to be sensitive to the word recognition difficulties experienced by individuals with high-frequency sensorineural hearing loss.

Representative performance intensity functions in normal hearers for several of the open-set monosyllable materials are shown in Figure 6-3A. These functions reflect the performance data of the original recordings for each of the test materials except the PHF word list. In addition, a function representative of a second recording of the CID W-22 lists is provided because of their widespread acceptance in clinical settings (Martin and Forbis, 1978). It is seen readily that differences exist among the various materials. The most difficult monosyllabic

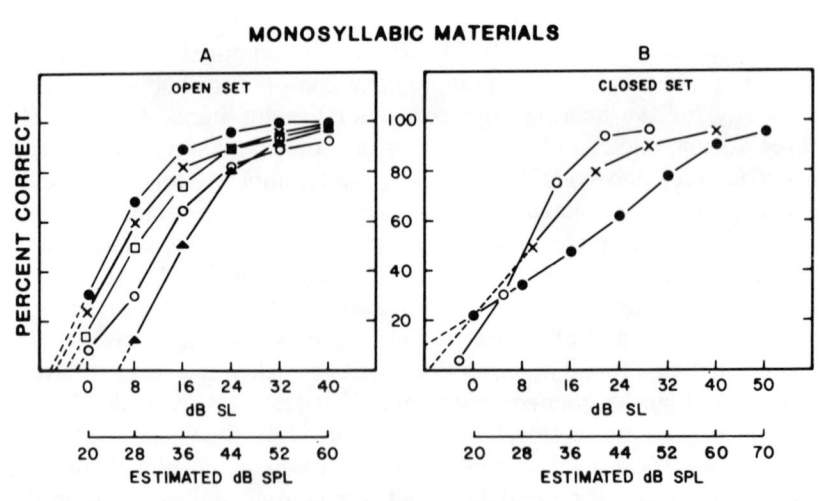

Figure 6-3. Performance intensity functions obtained in normal hearers with various monosyllabic word lists. Lists using an open-set response format (A) are ●──●, CID W-22; ×──×, NU #6; ○──○, PAL (Rush Hughes recording) PB-50; □──□, PHF (male talker version); ▲──▲, CID W-22 (Auditec recording). Lists using a closed-set response format (B) are: ○──○, picture identification task (PIT); ×──×, modified rhyme hearing test (MRHT) (96 percent correct performance level); ●──●, California consonant test (CCT); SL, sensation level; SPL, sound pressure level.

tests are the Harvard PAL PB-50s (Rush Hughes recordings) and the PHF word list (male talker) as evidenced by the gradualness of their slopes. On the most linear portion of the functions (between 20 and 80 percent) recognition increases at a rate of 2.4 percent/dB for the Harvard PAL PB-50s and 3.4 percent/dB for the PHF word list. It is seen also that the functions for the original NU #6 and CID W-22 recordings are quite similar and these recordings are somewhat easier than both the PHF word lists and the PAL PB-50s. The steepness of the functions for these two sets of materials are 5.6 percent/dB for the NU #6 and 5.0 percent/dB for the CID W-22.

Note the differences that exist in the functions of the two recordings of the CID W-22 materials. The function for the more recent recording of the CID W-22 (Beattie et al., 1977) is displaced to higher sensation levels and the slope of the curve is not as steep as for the original recordings. Indeed, such data illustrate clearly that two different recordings of the same material can yield distinctively different performance functions.

Monosyllabic Words: Closed-Set Response

Despite the widespread clinical use of 50-word open-set monosyllabic lists, many have emphasized the limitations of these materials and searched for alternative test formats. Among the major criticisms of the traditional open-set word lists were failure to differentiate between normal and sensorineural-impaired listeners, inability to analyze phonemic errors, and failure to differentiate between the performance of hearing aids. A closed-set multiple-choice format seemed to be a viable alternative for several reasons; this paradigm is not influenced significantly by word familiarity or word frequency, the potential for learning effects and auditor bias is minimal, pattern-error analysis is possible, and, finally, this format is easy to administer and simple to score.

Schultz and Schubert (1969) developed a closed message response set called the multiple choice discrimination test (MCDT) using the 200 stimulus items from the CID W-22 lists. For each stimulus word four response foils were generated using the following basic guidelines: word familiarity of the response foils should be the same as that of the stimulus word; all possible phoneme substitutions should have an equal probability of occurrence; and response foils should differ from the stimulus item by a single consonant phoneme substitution. Using these criteria, four lists of 50 stimulus items (5-word ensembles) were constructed. Further, each list was scrambled four times to produce a total of 16 available lists. Schultz and Schubert demonstrated in normal hearers that the slope of the function for the MCDT was considerably steeper than that of the traditional CID W-22 when each was administered under a comparable background of white noise. There is only limited information available, however, on the use of this test with hearing-impaired listeners.

Perhaps the most popular multiple-choice test used in the clinical setting is the *modified rhyme hearing test* (MRHT) developed by Kruel and coworkers (1968) at the Stanford Research Institute. The MRHT might be considered an outgrowth of the rhyme test introduced by Fairbanks (1958) 10 years earlier. The *rhyme test* was designed to study phonemic differentiation and was comprised of 250 common monosyllabic words grouped into 50 ensembles of five rhyming words. Subjects were presented a response form that contained the word stems and the listener's task was to complete the test word by writing in the appropriate consonant (i.e., _____ ot, _____ ay, _____ op). Hence, the response format may be classified as a semi-closed set. The stimulus items contained 18 consonants which approximated 90 percent of all consonants in the English language. When the rhyme test was administered at one intensity over various S/N ratios (+15 to −6 dB) a slope of about 3 percent/dB was established.

The rhyme test provided the impetus for the modified rhyme test (MRT) developed by House and colleagues (1965) for evaluating speech communications systems. The MRT incorporated a closed message set format and was comprised of 50 ensembles of six rhyming consonant-vowel-consonant test items. In one-half of the 50 ensembles the only difference among the words in the set was the initial consonant; whereas, in the other half the final consonant was the only phoneme varied. The subject was instructed to circle or draw a line through the stimulus item perceived. The lists were administered at six different S/N ratios and the performance intensity function was reported to be 5 percent/dB over the linear portion of the function.

The next modification of the rhyme test was the introduction of Griffiths (1967) rhyming minimal contrasts test. Based on research by House and coworkers (1965), this test used a closed message set consisting of 50 ensembles of five words each. More than half of the stimuli for this test were taken from the MRT. Griffiths classified phonemes on the basis of place (position in the mouth), manner (release of vocal air stream), and voicing (voiced, voiceless, nasal). The test consonants within each ensemble were varied unidimensionally or multidimensionally to allow for minimal contrast comparisons among phoneme classifications (place, manner, voicing). Similar to the MRT, the task involved initial consonant identification for 25 ensembles; whereas, 25 sets required final consonant recognition.

The MRHT (Kruel et al., 1968) is considered the clinical version of the MRT and it uses essentially the same vocabulary. A small number of the original test items were changed to avoid repetition or because some of the words were considered objectionable. The MRHT is composed of six 50-word lists, with each list comprised of 50 six-word ensembles. Each ensemble of words varied relative to initial consonant or final consonant position, while the stem of the word was held constant. The original recordings included a background of noise that had been adjusted so that the average normal hearing adult achieved 96, 83, or 75 percent correct performance. It was recommended that the test be administered at a most comfortable loudness (MCL) level. A sample of some of the test ensembles for both the initial and final consonant variation is shown in Table 6-1.

Pederson and Studebaker (1972) described a minimal contrasts closed-set monosyllabic word test known as *The University of Oklahoma closed response speech test* (UOCRST) which contained three subtests: initial and final consonant subtests and a median vowel subtest. The following criteria were employed in the selection of the stimulus items that comprise this test: meaningful words were used wherever possible; consonant-vowel-consonant materials were used; test items within a set were varied in one phoneme position; and test items were selected on the basis of familiarity. Two additional criteria employed for the consonant subtests were that the phoneme vowel within each set varied only in the place of articulation (when possible) and identical sets of phonemes were employed for both subtests. The consonant subtests were comprised of five ensembles of four stimulus items for a total of 20 stimulus words per subtest. Each stimulus word was used four times, thus producing 80 items on each consonant subtest. An example of some of the words used in the consonant subtests is shown in Table 6-2. The vowel subtest is comprised of one ensemble of eight monosyllabic words (see Table 6-2). Each stimulus word is used eight times thus producing a total of 64 items in this subtest.

The items for all three subtests were recorded on tape by a male talker and then rerecorded for equal intensity. The subtests were

Table 6-1. Sample ensembles from the modified rhyme hearing test (MRHT)

Initial consonant variation		Final consonant variation	
mark	bark	bath	back
park	hark	bun	bad
lark	dark	bass	bat
peel	keel	peach	peas
feel	eel	peal	peak
reel	heel	peat	peace

Table 6-2. Sample ensembles from the consonant subtests and the entire median vowel subtest from the UOCRT

Initial-consonant subtest		Final-consonant subtest		Median-vowel subtest	
pair	care	pop	pock	beat	bait
tear	air	pot	pa	bit	boat
				bet	bat
bale	gale	robe	rogue	bat	boot
dale	ale	rode	row		

administered monaurally to normal hearers at five different S/N ratios. Performance S/N functions revealed a steep slope for the vowel subtests (6.4 percent/dB) and gradually rising slopes for the two consonant subtests (initial-consonant, 2.4 percent/dB; final-consonant, 2.3 percent/dB).

Wilson and Antablin (1980) developed a *picture identification task* (PIT) for the purpose of assessing the word recognition abilities of adults unable to provide a verbal response, such as expressive aphasics. The test was designed to approximate the recognition performance obtained with conventional monosyllabic materials. Monosyllabic materials of the consonant-nucleus-consonant variety that could be readily pictoralized and which satisfied Lehiste and Peterson's (1959) criteria for phonemic balance were selected from Thorndike and Lorge (1944). The test is comprised of four equivalent lists of 50 words each. Each stimulus item is accompanied by three rhyming alternatives pictoralized on a response plate in a quadrant formation. Of the 200 stimulus items, 183 have alternative words that rhyme in the initial position, whereas the remainder have alternatives that rhyme in the initial position. The authors recommended that the test be administered at two intensity levels, 50 and 70 dB hearing level (HL) using half-lists for each presentation. Wilson and Antablin (1980) reported that the picture identification task provides a good estimate of word recognition and recommended its use with nonverbal adult populations.

In 1977, Owens and Schubert introduced a multiple-choice consonant identification test known as the *California consonant test* (CCT). This test of consonant recognition was developed because of the authors' firm belief that a need existed for a test which provided for phoneme variation in only one position in any given item; used an easily manageable number of foils, and contained a test format and standardization based on the results of a clinical population for whom the test was intended. Furthermore, because Owens and Schubert were concerned with the phonemic confusions of hearing-impaired listeners, it would be of value to "select items by a process of elimination, from a wide variety of test items, rather than to amass data on a particular available test" (page 464).

Historically, the CCT was based on earlier research on consonant identification of hearing-impaired listeners (Owens, Benedict, and Schubert, 1972; Owens and Schubert, 1968; Schubert and Owens, 1971). Several experimental forms were developed using a corpus of multiple-choice stimulus items, in order to obtain a better understanding of the phonemic errors made by hearing-impaired listeners. The final modification of these forms (form 7) represents the clinical version of this test known as the CCT. In its present form, the CCT is comprised of two different scramblings of 100 test items, each of which is arranged within an ensemble of four CVC monosyllabic words. For each item the words are assembled so that either the initial two phonemes are the same with the final one or two phonemes varying, or the final two phonemes are the same with the initial one or two phonemes varying (Table 6-3). Of the 100 test items, 36 assess consonant identification in the initial position and 64 assess recognition in the final position (Schwartz and Surr, 1979). Previous research had shown that hearing-impaired subjects experience more difficulty with consonant identification in the final position.

The clinical application of this test appears to have considerable potential. The reliability of the CCT is reportedly high and it does differentiate among hearing-impaired patients with varying degrees of speech recognition problems. Consequently, this test may have value in the hearing aid selection process as well as assisting the audiologist in the determination of appropriate rehabilitation procedures. Schwartz and Surr (1979) have conducted three basic experiments on the clinical utility of the CCT. First, performance intensity functions were obtained on both normal and hearing-impaired listeners; second, word recog-

Table 6-3. Sample ensembles from the CCT

Phonemes vary in initial position	Phonemes vary in final position
thin ___	cash ___
tin ___	cat ___
sin ___	cap ___
shin ___	catch ___
tore ___	rode ___
core ___	robe ___
pore ___	rove ___
chore ___	rose ___

nition scores from the CCT in a group of 60 sensorineural hearing-impaired subjects were compared to their performance scores on the NU #6; and third, the CCT was examined for split-half reliability. The performance scores obtained with the CCT for hearing-impaired subjects were considerably poorer overall when compared to the data obtained with the NU #6. It was also reported that the wide variability between half-list scores precluded the use of half-list testing.

Representative performance intensity functions for three of the closed-set monosyllabic materials are shown in Figure 6-3B. The function for the MRHT represents the S/N condition that approximates a 96 percent correct performance level in normal hearers. The most difficult of these materials, as evidenced by the steepness of the slopes, is the CCT, followed by the MRHT and the PIT. The slope for the CCT test is 1.6 percent/dB; whereas, the slopes for the MRHT and PIT are 3.0 and 5.2 percent/dB, respectively.

Sentence Materials

Several attempts have been made to use sentences as a means of assessing speech recognition on the basis that such materials offer a more "realistic" listening condition for everyday communication and thus provide for improved face validity. Other more specific desirable features inherent in sentential stimuli are: they include a temporal domain that adds to the discriminatory task (Jerger, 1970); they impart thoughts and concepts that require discriminatory processing (Jerger and Jerger, 1979); and they afford greater diagnostic flexibility than other types of stimuli in that they provide a measure of both central and peripheral function, especially when used in association with a competing message (Jerger and Jerger, 1979). Given these stated advantages it is somewhat surprising to find so few sentence tests available.

One of the first sentence tests to receive some clinical acceptance was the everyday speech sentence test developed and recorded at the Central Institute for the Deaf (Silverman and Hirsh, 1955; Davis and Silverman, 1978). This sentence test was constructed using a set of criteria for representing everyday speech that was outlined by a working group of the Armed Forces—National Research Council Committee on Hearing and Bioacoustics (CHABA). Some of the more important criteria used in the development of these sentences included an appropriate adult vocabulary, representative length and form of sentences, a low level of abstraction, a high degree of redundancy, a variation in grammatic structure, and no phonetic loading. The CID sentence test uses an open-set response format and is comprised of 100 sentences divided into 10 sets of 10 sentences each. The sentence length varies from two to 12 words and there are 50 key words within each set of sentences. The lists are homogeneous in their level of difficulty and the key 50 words within each list are representative of the phoneme content of everyday English. The listener's response may be written or spoken and the scoring is based on the percentage of key words correctly perceived.

Because the sentence length varied considerably, Harris and coworkers (1961) revised the lists so that each sentence contained six to nine words while retaining the 50 key words of the original test. Additional sets of sentences were also constructed using the original words from the original CID version. Giolas and Duffy (1973) found that the equivalency of the CID and the revised CID sentence (R-CID) tests was suspect when the materials were distorted (low-pass filtering at 420 Hz). At the present time, however, there are no commercial recordings of either version of these sentences and their clinical application has therefore been somewhat limited. A sample performance intensity function of the R-CID in normal hearers, taken from data produced by Elkins and Causey (1973), is shown in Figure 6-4A. The steepness of the linear portion of this function is quite sharp, rising at

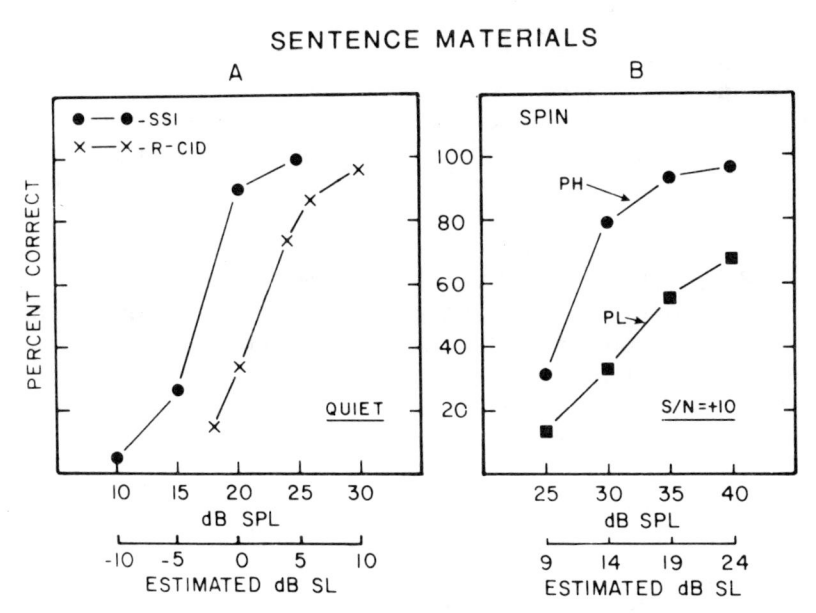

Figure 6-4. Performance intensity functions obtained in normal hearers with three different types of sentence materials; the synthetic sentence identification (SSI) test, the revised CID (R-CID) test and the speech perception in noise (SPIN) test (B, Modified from Hutcherson, Dirks, and Morgan, 1979).

a rate of almost 11 percent/dB, and thus illustrates that these materials are easier to identify than nonsense syllables or monosyllabic stimuli.

A more recent sentence recognition test that also employs an open-set response format is the speech perception in noise test (SPIN) proffered by Kalikow, Stevens, and Elliott (1977). The SPIN is somewhat different from other speech recognition tests because an attempt is made to assess not only the acoustic-phonetic components of speech but also the linguistic-situational information. That is, in addition to testing for acoustic-phonetic data, the SPIN was designed to examine the utilization of such important variables as memory and the lexical, semantic, and syntactic cues of speech. The test is comprised of eight forms of 50 sentences each. The sentences are generally five to eight words in length and the last word of each sentence serves as the stimulus item. The recordings of these sentences also contain a background of babble-type competition which is comprised of 12 talkers reading continuously. It is thus possible for the examiner to manipulate any desired speech-to-babble (S/B) ratio. Twenty-five of the sentences within a test form contain a final stimulus item, always a monosyllabic noun, which is rated as having "high predictability" (PH). This means that the listener is aided in the identification process by the surrounding contextual cues in the sentence including the syntactic, semantic, and prosodic information. Another 25 sentences within a test form are rated as having "low predictability" (PL) on the basis that the listener receives only minimal contextual cues and must therefore identify the word from its acoustical properties as well as the lexical information. The response task involves simply repeating back or writing the final word of each sentence. Examples of key stimulus items which appear in sentences with high and low predictability are shown in Table 6-4.

In an attempt to learn more about the SPIN, Hutcherson, Dirks, and Morgan (1979) studied the effects of presentation level and S/B ratio on a group of normal-hearing listeners. Predictably, the subjects scored much poorer on the PL sentences than they did on PH sentences and general overall performance was affected significantly by the presentation level. An example of a performance intensity function at a S/B ratio of +10 obtained by Hutcherson and colleagues is shown in

Table 6-4. Examples of sentences from the SPIN test showing high predictability and low predictability

Sentence	Context
The watchdog gave a warning growl.	High
I had not thought about the growl.	Low
Cut the bacon into strips.	High
Bob heard Paul called about the strips.	Low

Figure 6-4B. The PH curve increases at a rate of 9 percent/dB whereas the PL function rises at a rate of only 4 percent/dB.

Perhaps the most common sentence test presently employed in the clinical setting is the *synthetic sentence identification* (SSI) test developed by Speaks and Jerger (1965). These materials are called synthetic sentences because they are not "actual" sentences, but rather approximate actual sentences in the sense that the succession of words is based on conditional probabilities of word sequences (Jerger, 1970). That is, with the exception of the initial word, each new word within a sentence is dependent or "conditional" on the preceding word or words. Under such circumstances it is possible to construct sentences with a specified length and with varying approximations to real sentences. Examples of typical synthetic sentences with different levels of approximation are shown in Table 6-5. First-order synthetic sentences are constructed by selecting each word at random from Thorndike and Lorge's (1944) pool of 1000 most common words to develop a sentence of specified length. Hence, the succession of words have no meaningful relationship to one another. Second-order approximation sentences may be constructed by selecting a word at random from the word pool, and then asking an individual to select a second word that would logically and syntactically follow the first word. Without having knowledge of the first word another individual selects a third word from the pool that could ostensibly follow the second word. Third-order approximations may be developed by randomly selecting a word pair from the second-order sentences and then adding a third word from the pool that would reasonably be expected to follow the word pair. The first word would then be discarded and another individual would be asked to choose an appropriate word to complete the triplet.

With this construction procedure a group of 24 10-sentence ensembles representing four different levels of sentential approximation were constructed by Speaks and Jerger (1965). The test procedure involves presenting a closed set of 10 sentences and asking the subject to identify the sentence that was perceived. A sample performance-intensity function for the SSI under quiet conditions is shown in Figure

Table 6-5. Examples of sentences from the Synthetic Sentence Identification (SSI) test showing different levels of approximation to actual sentences

Sentence	Approximation level
Due his fit along sick near nearly	First
Three came home on any woman can	Second
Agree with him only to find out	Third

6-4A. The steepness of the function is similar to that of the R-CID material, rising at an approximate rate of 12 percent/dB. To increase the difficulty of this material a competing speech message was mixed with the sentences. A message-to-competition ratio (MCR) of 0 dB is comparable to the performance of normal hearers on monosyllabic materials in quiet.

SPEECH RECOGNITION MATERIALS FOR CHILDREN

Assessment of speech recognition among children is a difficult task and there is a need for the audiologist to give more careful consideration to this component of hearing assessment. The major modification required in the evaluation of children is to ensure that the speech material is within the receptive vocabulary of the child under test. It is important to rule out the possibility of difficult material as a potential variable in producing a poor speech recognition score. The limited research currently available on speech recognition assessment with children is a direct reflection of the problems associated with this clinical procedure. Indeed, if speech audiometry is to afford the audiologist any information of value in this population, attentive thoughtfulness must be given to such important variables as the kind of information sought; the selection of an appropriate test material; the type of response task the test requires; and finally, the need for a reinforcement paradigm (Olsen and Matkin, 1979).

The intent of this portion of the chapter is to review some of the various speech materials commonly used in speech recognition assessment of children. Similar to the section on adults, this discussion will be divided into a review of the types of materials most commonly used for children. A general guide of some of the more common tests used with children is summarized in Table 6-6.

Monosyllables and Spondees

The traditional speech recognition materials are comprised primarily of monosyllabic word lists with either open or closed response formats. Perhaps one of the earliest efforts to develop a speech recognition test using a vocabulary appropriate for children was made by Hudgins in 1944. Four monosyllabic word lists, referred to as the *phonetically balanced familiar* (PBF) lists, were constructed by selecting words that appeared in the PAL PB-50 lists as well as the list of 10,000 words used most frequently in children's literature (Thorndike and Lorge, 1944). These lists required an open-set response and were reported useful in the speech assessment of children at Clarke School for the Deaf.

Another popular open-response monosyllabic word test used for children is comprised of the lists developed by Haskins (1949). Using essentially the same design that was used in the development of the PAL PB-50s, Haskins selected words from the PAL PB-50 lists that also appeared in the International Kindergarten Vocabulary list. Hence, a pool of 425 monosyllabic words considered appropriate for young children was categorized into four lists of 50 words each. Because the lists were developed using a pattern of phonetic composition similar to that used in the PAL PB-50s the lists were referred to as phonetic balanced kindergarten 50s (PBK-50s). These word lists, standardized on a group of 22 normal-hearing adults, were analyzed to determine their relative difficulty and reliability. Haskins reported that lists 1, 3, and 4 were essentially equivalent to a list on the PAL PB-50 test; however, list 2 was noted to be considerably easier. The reliability of the PBK-50 test did not appear to differ significantly from the PAL PB-50s. Interestingly, Haskins did not assess the performance of normal-hearing or hearing-impaired children with this test.

For many younger children the open-response design is a complicated task and subsequently causes difficulty in the administration and scoring of the test. A child with a speech problem, for example, is difficult to evaluate because responses may not represent what the child actually perceived. In addition, children sometimes lose interest in the task because of the tedium associated with this type of format. Many children's lists have incorporated a closed-set response format as a means of minimizing some of the above problems.

One of the earlier multiple-choice speech recognition tests for preschool children was described by Sortini and Flake (1953). Using an object pointing method a child was asked to identify small toys that represented either spondee or phonetically balanced words. With this technique estimates could be made of a child's ability to hear and recognize speech. The test was reported to have several favorable attributes including subject cooperation and relatively short administration time.

In the same year, Pronovost and Dumbleton (1954) constructed a picture-pointing speech recognition task that was based on a pictorialized test developed by Mansur (1950). This test was comprised of 36 picture word pairs that contrasted vowels, semi-vowels, and consonants. Three sets of word pairs were represented on a test page, one pair that were "unlike" (cat-bat) and two "like" pairings (bat-bat and cat-cat). The subject was instructed to identify the appropriate response from one dissimilar and two similar word pairings. When the test was administered to 437 first grade children it was found that about

Table 6-6. Summary of common speech recognition materials used with children

Test name	Investigator(s)	Material	Number of lists	Items per list	Response format	Response task	Age range	Commercially available?
Children's lists								
1. PBK-50	Haskins (1949)	Monosyllables	4	50	Open set	Verbal	6–9 years	No
2. Discrimination by Identification of Pictures (DIP)	Siegenthaler and Haspiel (1966)	Monosyllables	3	48	Closed set (2 picture matrix)	Psychomotor	2 years, 10 months 8 years, 3 months	Yes
3. Word Intelligibility by Picture Identification (WIPI)	Ross and Lerman (1970)	Monosyllables	4	25	Closed set (6 picture matrix)	Psychomotor	3–6 years	Yes
4. Goldman-Fristoe-Woodstock Test of Auditory Discrimination (GFW)	Goldman, Fristoe, and Woodcock (1970)	Monosyllables	1	30	Closed set (4 picture matrix)	Psychomotor	≥ 4 years	Yes
5. Sound Effects Recognition Test (SERT)	Finitzo-Hieber et al. (1980)	Environmental Sounds	3	10	Closed set (4 picture matrix)	Psychomotor	≥ 3 years	Yes
6. Spondee Recogni-	Erber (1974)	Spondees	1	25	Closed set	Written	8–16 years	No

7.	WIPI Sentences		Sentences	4	Closed set (6 picture matrix)	Psychomotor	3–6 years	No
8.	Five Sound Test	Weber and Redell (1976)	Vowels /u/, /a/, /i/, /ʃ/, /s/	1	Open set	Psychomotor	Infant/ children	No
9.	Perception of Words and Word Patterns	Ling (1978)	Monosyllables, spondees and trochees	3	Closed set	Psychomotor and verbal	9–13 years	No
10.	Childrens Perception of Speech (CHIPS)	Erber and Witt (1977)	Monosyllables	4[a]	50	Psychomotor	≥ 3 years	No
11.	Synthetic Sentence Identification of Children (SSIC)	Katz and Elliott (1978)	Synthetic sentences	10[a]	10	Verbal	≥ 7 years	No
12.	BKB Sentences	Wilson (1978)	Sentences	21 / 11	16 / 16	Open set / Verbal	8–15 years	No
13.	Auditory Numbers Test (ANT)	Bench, Koval, and Bamford (1979)	Numbers	1	5	Closed set / Psychomotor	3–8 years	No
14.	Pediatric Speech Intelligibility Test	Erber (1980)	Monosyllables Sentences	1 / 2	20 / 10	Closed set / Verbal	3–10 years	No
		Jerger et al. (1980)						

Speech Recognition 147

148   Bess

Table 6-6. (Continued)

Test name	Investigator(s)	Material	Number of lists	Items per list	Response format	Response task	Age range	Commercially available?
Adult lists								
1. Northwestern University Auditory Test No. 6 (NU-6)	Tillman and Carhart (1966)	Monosyllables	4	50	Open set	Verbal/written	$\geqslant$ 9 years	Yes
2. Central Institute for the Deaf W-22 (CID W-22)	Hirsh et al. (1952)	Monosyllables	20	50	Open set	Verbal/written		Yes
3. Oklahoma University Closed Response Test (OUCRT)	Jones and Studebaker (1974)	Monosyllables Words	4	20	Closed set	Written	$\geqslant$ 9 years	No
4. Nonsense Syllable Test (NST)	Levitt and Resnick (1978)	Syllables	16[b]	62	Closed set	Written	$\geqslant$ 6 years	No
5. Speech Perception in Noise (SPIN)	Elliott (1979)	Sentences	1	50	Open set	Verbal	15 years	No

[a] Randomizations
[b] Seven subtests within a list

10 percent experienced difficulty with speech sound recognition. Although this test was reported to have good reliability and validity, some difficulty with pictorializing certain phonetic contrasts was noted.

In 1963, Myatt and Landes developed a pictorialized speech recognition test for young children that was comprised of 80 pictures representing monosyllabic words judged to be within the vocabulary of preschool-age children. The pictures were categorized into twenty plates of four words each. The Myatt and Landes test was then administered to several different groups of children. The findings showed that the information obtained from this test was the same as that of the phonetically balanced list employed with adults. This test, however, did not undergo any type of standardization.

Realizing the potential of the picture format concept comprised by Myatt and Landes (1963), Lerman, Ross, and McLaughlin (1965) administered the test to a group of hearing-impaired children using professionally drawn pictures. The test was found to have good reliability for assessing the speech recognition skills of hearing-impaired children. In a follow-up investigation, Ross and Lerman (1970) noted limitations associated with the Myatt and Landes pictures that prompted them to incorporate modifications in the test. Some of the reported problems were too difficult a vocabulary, inadequate pictorialization of some of the words, and the potential for high chance scores. The Ross and Lerman (1970) revision essentially eliminated most of the aforementioned shortcomings and it soon became commonly recognized as the *word intelligibility by picture identification* (WIPI) test. In its final form there were four lists of stimulus words and these test items were arranged into 25 plates of six pictures each. Each of the four lists were equal in their level of difficulty and the lists contained both gross and fine discrimination tasks. After field testing the WIPI on a group of children with moderate to severe hearing losses (5 to 6 years of age) it was concluded that the test was clinically useful. Schwartz (1971) examined the usefulness of the WIPI with normal-hearing preschool children and found that the test (lists 1 and 2) could also be used reliably with children as young as 2½ years.

Katz and Elliott (1978) developed a picture-pointing speech recognition test for very young children known as the *Northwestern University—children's perception of speech* (NU-CHIPS) test. This instrument was designed so that monosyllabic nouns would be within the receptive vocabulary of 3-year-old inner city children. The test consists of four randomizations of a 50-word list. A picture of each stimulus word appears on a plate with three other foil items. Male talker recordings were made of each randomization and a preliminary field analysis on normal hearers (adults and children) revealed that the test is reliable, easy to administer, and appropriate for children as young as 3 years of age.

It is important to note at this point that recognition performance for children's tests varies as a function of age; or, more appropriately, receptive vocabulary. To illustrate, Sanderson-Leepa and Rintelmann (1976) compared the performance of a group of normal hearing children using three common types of speech materials: the WIPI, the PBK-50; and the NU #6. Sixty normal hearers were categorized into the following age groups: 3½, 5½, 7½, 9½, and 11½ years. After obtaining performance intensity functions with the different materials, the following pertinent conclusions were drawn: the WIPI appeared to be the most suitable instrument for the assessment of speech recognition in the 3½-year-old group; for the 5½-year-old group both the WIPI and the PBK-50 tests seemed appropriate, but the WIPI was preferable because it is not limited by speech and language dissimilarities, it is a more interesting task, and it is a shorter test; and for those age groups 7½ and above, the NU #6 was noted to be more difficult than the PBK-50 test.

In a sequence of three studies, Erber (1974, 1977, 1980) proffered several auditory tests that can be used in the assessment of speech recognition abilities of hearing-impaired children. These auditory tests were developed for delineating among those children who could respond to the spectral components of the acoustic signal and those who perceived only intensity or stress patterns. Erber (1974) first reported on a spondee recognition test that was comprised of 25 bisyllabic words representing a wide variety of speech sounds. The words were considered to be within the receptive reading and lipreading vocabularies of hearing-impaired children between the ages of 8 and 16 years. The stimuli were recorded on tape and presented monaurally (TDH-49 earphones) to 72 hearing-impaired children at a preferred listening level. The spondee recognition scores were plotted as a function of average pure tone threshold level (500, 1000, 2000 Hz). The findings revealed that children with hearing levels better than 85 dB scored well on the test (70 to 100 percent); whereas, spondee recognition was poor (0 to 30 percent) for those whose average hearing levels were greater than 100 dB. Interestingly, there was a wide range of scores that occurred in the hearing level range of 85 to 100 dB.

In another study, Erber and Witt (1977) outlined an auditory test that was designed to assess the speech perception abilities of children with moderate-to-severe and profound hearing loss. The test was developed in an attempt to establish the stimulus intensity at which a child perceives speech most effectively. The stimuli for this test were comprised of 10 monosyllables, 10 trochees, and 10 spondees. The two syllables for the trochees and spondees were separated by a stop consonant so that the two syllables could be perceived easily. No attempt was made to balance the words phonetically. The test items were presented monaurally through a miniature hearing aid receiver that was coupled to the subject's hearing aid. The 30 words were presented in blocks of six at various intensities ranging from detection to discomfort. Children were required to identify both the stress pattern and the specific word. When these words were administered to the children with profound hearing loss it was found that word recognition was very poor and failed to exhibit much improvement with increasing intensity. Conversely, scores for word categorization were much better and showed considerable improvement as the stimulus intensity was raised above speech detection threshold.

In a follow-up investigation, Erber (1980) developed a simpler test of speech perception for children with severe to profound hearing loss who did not possess the vocabulary required for responding to traditional word recognition tests. This instrument, known as the *auditory numbers test* (ANT) requires only that the child be able to count from one to five and to apply these number labels to blocks of from one to five items. As with the previous auditory tests, the ANT was designed to delineate children who actually perceive the spectral characteristics of speech from those who respond only to the patterns of the acoustic stimulus. First, the child's detection and preferred listening levels are determined. Next, five colored cards depicting groups of one to five ANTs and corresponding numerals are placed before the child. After a preliminary practice session the mouth of the clinician is covered and a single number (i.e., "five") is presented. The child is then required to point to the appropriate card. This same procedure is continued with all of the remaining numbers. The ANT was administered monaurally (auditory trainer or speech audiometer) to 39 hearing-impaired children. A sample of the information that can be obtained from this auditory test is shown in Figure 6-5. These data represent the identification scores (1 to 5) of each ear as a function of hearing threshold level (HTL). Scores are high for those children with hearing losses 98 dB HTL or better and low for those with impairments that exceed 118 dB HTL. Similar to the data described earlier, there was a great deal of overlap obtained between the average threshold levels of 100 to 113 dB. A high score (i.e., 3 to 5) suggests that a child is capable of perceiving the spectral characteristics of speech; whereas a low score (i.e., 1) means that a child should be classified as profoundly deaf. If a child responds only to intensity patterns, a remediation pro-

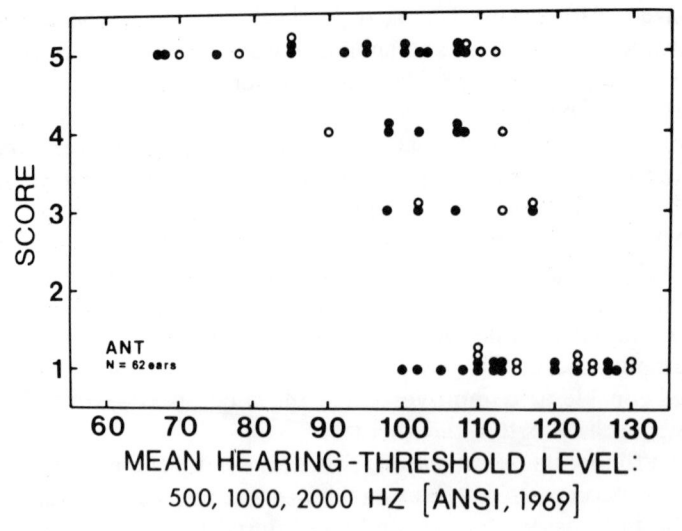

Figure 6-5. Monaural scores on the ANT plotted as a function of average pure tone hearing threshold level (500, 1000, 2000 Hz) for a group of hearing-impaired children. Open circles represent the ANT scores of children whose audiometric data were judged as questionable. (From Erber, 1980; reproduced with permission.)

gram should be established that focuses on improving the ability to recognize certain aspects of sound patterns such as pause, duration, and rate.

Sentence Materials

Several attempts have been made to develop children's speech recognition tests using sentence materials. Weber and Redell (1976) observed that the traditional WIPI test underestimated hearing-impaired children's speech recognition abilities. When the stimulus word was placed into a sentence context, however, the hearing-impaired children seemed to score at a level more consistent with their educational performance. Consequently, Weber and Redell constructed sentences from stimulus words of the WIPI. Normal-hearing and hearing-impaired children were shown a picture from the WIPI test booklet and asked to comment on what they saw. Sentences were then developed by using the most frequently solicited words from each stimulus item. For example, with the stimulus word *clown*, the most frequently elicited responses were *funny* and *circus*. Hence, the sentence that resulted from this information was "We laughed at the funny *clown* in the circus." The sentences were constructed so that the stimulus item was always centrally located. The child's task was to point to the picture on the WIPI plate that best represented the sentence.

Four 25-sentence lists were generated. When this modified version of the WIPI was administered to a clinical population it was found that the obtained recognition scores were more compatible with the teacher's observations of speech recognition ability.

Wilson (1978) developed a less difficult synthetic sentence identification test judged to be more suitable for young children than the conventional SSI. Wilson constructed 10 third-order synthetic sentences containing five words each using the general procedures outlined by Speaks and Jerger (1965). The most frequently occurring words spoken by 5-year-old children (Wepman and Hass, 1969) served as the vocabulary pool for the construction of the *synthetic sentence identification for children* (SSIC) test. The third-order sentences were generated by a group of normal-hearing 9- to 10-year-old children. A male talker tape recorded the sentences and a 5-minute segment of a passage from *Charlotte's Web* (White, 1952) was used as a competing message. An example of a simplified synthetic sentence is: "Story is good because they." Performance on the SSIC was compared with the SSI and the NU #6 tests in 60 normal-hearing children ranging in age from 7 years to 11 years, 11 months. The tests were also administered to hearing-impaired children in the moderate-to-severe, and severe-to-profound hearing loss range. The results of this study showed that the performance of the SSIC in normal hearers was similar to the SSI in terms of intertest homogeneity and performance intensity function. Further, the synthetic sentence tests at a MCR of O dB was comparable in level of difficulty to the NU #6 test in quiet.

The findings obtained with the hearing-impaired subjects, however, showed that the SSIC was considerably less difficult for both the moderate-to-severe and the severe-to-profound hearing loss categories—particularly under the more adverse listening conditions. The hearing-impaired subject's performance for the two synthetic sentence tests at various MCR ratios is shown in Figure 6-6. For the moderate-to-severe hearing loss group it is noted that the function for the SSIC is much steeper than for the SSI, especially at the three most difficult listening conditions. The mean scores for the SSIC at these test conditions were 5 to 23 percent better than for the SSI. Under the more favorable listening conditions, however, the findings were comparable. The differences in performance between the two tests are even greater in the group of subjects with severe-to-profound hearing loss. Interestingly, these children were unable to respond to the NU #6 test because of the difficulty of the listening task. These findings would suggest that the SSIC is a simpler and a more appropriate sentence test for hearing-impaired children—especially those with severe-to-profound hearing loss.

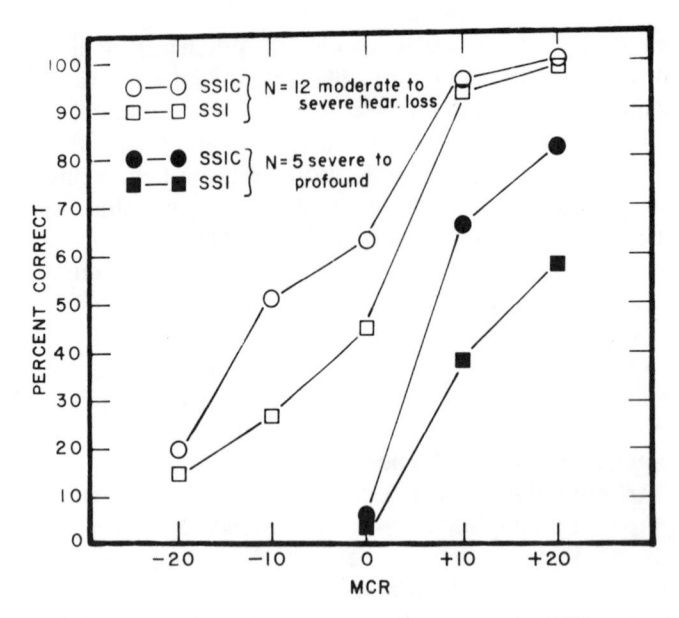

Figure 6-6. Comparison of mean percent correct scores on the SSIC test and the SSI test as a function of message-to-competition ratio for a group of children with moderate-to-severe hearing losses and a group of children in the severe-to-profound hearing loss category (Modified from Wilson, 1978)

Bench, Koval, and Bamford (1979) also developed a sentence speech recognition test for hearing-impaired children (BKB). The BKB used an open-set response and was developed as a test that would reflect better the natural language usage of hearing-impaired children. Language samples were elicited from hearing-impaired children (ages 8 to 15 years) who were asked to describe pictures which illustrated activities from play and home settings. The recordings made of each language sample were transcribed and subjected to a grammatical analysis and vocabulary count. The construction of the BKB sentences thus reflected the most common spoken usage of both vocabulary and grammar. In addition, sentence length was limited to seven syllables. Examples of these sentences are: "An old woman was at home": and "They broke all the eggs." The scoring consists merely of computing the percentage of key words (underlined) repeated correctly. The standard BKB sentence test (BKB-ST) is presently comprised of 21 lists of 16 sentences each of which contains 50 stimulus words. A more simplified version of this test, known as the *picture-related BKB sentence lists for children* (BKB-PR), incorporates corresponding drawings to depict the key words. This modified version contains 11 lists of 16 sentences and 50 stimulus words.

Preliminary analysis of the standard sentence materials revealed that the test was appropriate for the speech recognition assessment of children under natural listening conditions. In a follow-up investigation, Bench et al. (1979) compared the BKB-ST to a number of alternative speech recognition tests in a group of hearing-impaired children. They concluded that the BKB-ST is more appropriate linguistically for hearing-impaired children than other available tests designed primarily for an older population.

Jerger and coworkers (Jerger et al., 1980; Jerger, 1981) described a pediatric speech intelligibility test that is comprised of both word and sentence messages. This test was developed incorporating both types of materials because a comparison of performances between words and sentences can be of value in the identification of central auditory dysfunction. There were several stages involved in the generation of these materials. First, children's responses were obtained for 60 stimulus pictures, 30 of which represented monosyllabic words and 30 of which depicted action scenes that could be easily described in sentence form (i.e., a picture of a bear brushing his teeth). The illustrated nouns and action verbs were selected on the basis of previous research on normal language development in children. All of the children's responses were tape recorded and later transcribed. Next, the elicited sentences were categorized into four different construction patterns and these data were then examined in relation to chronological age, vocabulary, and receptive language skills. The results of this comparison showed that differences in vocabulary and receptive language were evident among the various construction patterns. Specifically, the most sophisticated construction patterns were composed by older children with more advanced language skills. It was reasoned that these sentences may be too difficult for children with poorer language skills and consequently two different sentences formats were employed— one that used a simpler sentence construction ("Show me a bear brushing his teeth"), and one that used a more sophisticated adult-like construction pattern ("A bear is brushing his teeth").

The number of sentences were reduced from 30 to 10. The selection of the final 10 sentences was accomplished by carefully examining the children's responses for the sentences in terms of the syntactic and semantic contents. That is, Jerger and coworkers were interested in establishing for each stimulus card what percentage of children responded with the target sentence or its equivalence in terms of syntactic and semantic properties. Ten cards were then selected that seemed to yield the most consistent responses among the children.

Unlike sentence materials, the children's responses for word cards were not found to differ as functions of age, vocabulary, or language skills. For test purposes, 20 cards were selected which yielded the highest percentage target responses.

Normative studies on this pediatric speech intelligibility test are still in the data collection stages. Nevertheless, this test appears to have potential as a clinical tool in the assessment of speech recognition abilities of young children.

Use of Adult Materials with Children

Some of the adult lists, especially the open-set response monosyllabic materials, have been shown to be useful with children. Larson, Peterson, and Jacquot (1974) demonstrated with the NU #6 in quiet that 5- and 6-year-old children performed essentially the same as adults. In a background of noise, however, word recognition scores for the children were significantly poorer than for adults at comparable listening conditions. Sanderson-Leepa and Rintelmann (1976) also demonstrated that the NU #6 test could be used with children. A group of 7½- and a group of 9½-year-old children achieved mean percent correct scores of 92.8 and 93.5, respectively; whereas 11½-year-old children obtained a mean score of 96.5 percent correct. Brooks and Goetzinger (1966) compared word recognition scores in three groups of children (grades 2, 4, and 6) using the Rush Hughes recording PB-50 (list 7) and the CID W-22. Although significant differences were reported between materials at each grade level, differences among grades were not found for either of these tests. Brooks and Goetzinger noted that by grade 6, children are able to perform similar to an adult population. Others have also reported on the usefulness of adult monosyllabic materials with young children (McNamee, 1960; Nielson, 1960; Wilson, 1978).

Jones and Studebaker (1974) compared the word recognition scores of hearing-impaired children on the University of Oklahoma Closed Response Speech Test and the CID W-22 test. The children ranged in age from 9 to 16 years. The subjects scored considerably poorer on the W-22s than they did with the UOCRT. Significantly, only nine subjects in this study were able to score above 0 percent on the CID W-22 test. Hence, the results showed that the UOCRT was a more appropriate and valid test for this population.

Studies also have examined the usefulness of adult sentence materials with a younger population. Wilson (1978), for example, demonstrated that the SSI was sufficiently easy to be used in testing both normal-hearing and hearing-impaired children. Elliott (1979) reported on the performance of children aged 9 to 17 years on the SPIN. Children 15 years of age and above scored similar to normal-hearing adults; whereas younger children exhibited significantly poorer scores, especially with the high predictability sentences in the presence of a competing babble.

Finally, it should be noted that the nonsense syllable test also can be used with younger children. At Vanderbilt University, for example, the NST has been found useful for the evaluation of syllable recognition skills of children between the ages of 7 and 13 years (Bess and Gibler, 1981). In general, these children achieve performance scores that are slightly lower and somewhat more variable than for adults.

The foregoing review thus indicates that certain adult lists can be used with some success in the evaluation of children. It must be recognized, however, that the selection of speech materials for children should be made on the basis of the level of a child's speech and language competence.

Nonconventional Materials

The children's speech recognition tests that have been discussed thus far presume at least some development of language skills. Unfortunately, however, the clinician often is faced with a child who has severely limited language ability, thus precluding the use of conventional word recognition materials. Under this circumstance it is desirable to have available a simple tool for obtaining an estimate of a child's perceptual abilities.

Ling (1978) has developed a rather simple speech recognition test for hearing-impaired children. The *five sound test* was developed as a means of measuring the effectiveness of a child's hearing aid. The five speech sounds employed in the test are /u/, /a/, /i/, /ʃ/, and /s/. These stimuli encompass the frequency range of all phonemes and the voiced sounds contain sufficient harmonics to convey suprasegmental information. The child is asked to indicate if the sound is perceived through the amplification system when the stimuli are presented at a conversational loudness level. According to Ling (1978), children with residual hearing through 1000 Hz are able to hear the three vowel sounds. Children with measurable hearing through 2000 Hz will be able to hear also the /ʃ/ sound and those who have auditory sensitivity up to 4000 Hz can perceive the /s/. Furthermore, by incorporating a competing noise signal it is possible to determine whether an upward spread of masking occurs—that is, the high consonants may not be perceived as well in the noise condition as they are in quiet. As noted, the five sound test is used as a means of measuring the effectiveness of a hearing aid. For example, if a hearing-impaired child is unable to hear the /ʃ/ sound while using amplification it would imply either insufficient residual hearing or hearing aid gain in the frequency region 2000 to 2500 Hz. Carrying this concept one step further, if the test indicates that /a/ is audible to a child with hearing up to 3000 Hz and /i/ is not, it would suggest that the gain at 2000 to 3000 Hz needs to be increased relative to the gain at 1000 to 1500 Hz.

Eilers, Wilson, and Moore (1977) developed a visually reinforced infant speech discrimination (VRISD) paradigm for assessing discriminative skills in young infants. The VRISD is simply a modification of the operant procedures used for assessing the hearing sensitivity of young infants (Wilson, Moore, and Thompson, 1976). With this technique, infants are conditioned to respond (head turn) to a signal state change and then reinforced for providing a correct response. The following speech contrasts were used as the stimuli: /sa/ versus /va/, /sa/ versus /a/, /sa/ versus /za/, /as/ versus /a:z/, /a:s/ versus /a:z/, /at/ versus /a:d/, /a:t/ versus /a:d/, /at/ versus /a:t/, /fa/ versus /θa/, and /fi/ versus /θi/. The first stimulus from a given paired set was presented via sound field at a rate of one syllable per second at 50 dB sound pressure level (SPL). When the attention of the infant is obtained (with the child's head at midline) the signal is changed to the second stimulus for 4 seconds at 65 dB SPL. Once the infant is conditioned to make an appropriate response at 65 dB SPL the stimuli are administered at equal intensities. A correct response is reinforced with the activation of an animated toy. The VRISD procedure has been used successfully with most infants between 6 and 14 months of age. The technique reportedly is useful in assessing the discriminative function of young infants thought to be delayed developmentally, in determining the developmental level for discrimination, and in assessing amplification systems (Moore and Wilson, 1978).

Finitzo-Hieber and coworkers (1980) developed a nonlinguistic test referred to as the *sound effects recognition test* (SERT). The 30 environmental sounds (plus one practice item) used in the test were selected on the basis of ease in sound recognition, ease in pictorialization, fidelity of the recording, and spectral content of the stimuli. Another important criterion for selection of a stimulus was the "... frequency that the name or synonym of the stimulus occurred in a spontaneous speech sample of kindergarten children" (Finitzo-Hieber et al., 1980, p. 272). It was reasoned that if the label of a sound was part of a kindergartener's spontaneous language then it would enhance the probability of young children being able to identify the stimulus. The 30 environmental sounds are divided into three sets of 10 items each. Each item appears on a response plate along with three foil pictures. The tape-recorded stimuli may be administered via earphones or through a loudspeaker. The stimuli are presented at 25 to 40 dB sensation level (SL) regarding the speech awareness threshold. The child's task is merely to point to the picture corresponding to the sound.

The authors emphasized that although the SERT should not be used as a substitute for speech recognition assessment the test can offer valuable information relative to a child's ability to recognize sounds.

PROCEDURAL STRATEGIES IN SPEECH RECOGNITION

Mode of Presentation

A number of procedural alternatives are available to the clinician for presenting speech recognition materials. Some of the fundamental issues that need consideration are: the use of a carrier phrase; the use of recorded materials or monitored live voice (MLV); the appropriate intensity level or levels for administering the speech test; and the use of adaptive methodologies.

Use of the Carrier Phrase For most speech recognition tests it is common practice to preface each stimulus item with a carrier phrase such as "Say the word _____ ," "You will say _____ ," or "Write the word _____ ." (Martin and Pennington, 1971; Martin and Forbis, 1978). The carrier phrase has been used in speech recognition assessment because it prepares the listener for the upcoming stimulus item and because it assists the clinician in monitoring the intensity presentation of the signal. Traditionally, the clinician monitors the carrier phrase on a V.U. meter at a predetermined intensity level and allows the stimulus item to be delivered naturally.

A number of researchers have questioned whether a carrier phrase is needed (Martin, Hawkins, and Bailey, 1962; McClennan and Knox, 1975). Martin and coworkers (1962) reported no differences in speech recognition scores with or without a carrier phrase, but observed that subjects with sensorineural hearing loss specified a preference for the carrier phrase. McClennan and Knox (1975) proposed a procedure that allowed the subject to control the delivery of the speech signal. This free operant system did not employ the carrier phrase because the self-initiating delivery was thought to be sufficient for preparing the subject for the stimulus item. When this technique was compared to traditional test presentation procedures that incorporate a carrier phrase, it was found that no differences in word recognition scores were obtained. In addition, many of the listeners expressed a preference for the free operant procedure. Conversely, Gladstone and Siegenthaler (1971) reported that scores were poorer when a carrier phrase was not used. Hence, although the use of a carrier phrase is common in the clinical setting, the majority of evidence suggests that it does not influence the outcome of the test.

Recorded Materials Versus Monitored Live Voice The clinician must also determine whether to use monitored live voice or a recorded version of the speech recognition test. The advantage of a monitored live voice presentation is that it affords the clinician greater clinical flexibility, and at least one investigator has suggested that acceptable test-retest reliability exists when using this technique (Resnick, 1962). There is far more convincing evidence, however, to support the use of a recorded presentation. Brandy (1966) demonstrated that recognition scores differed among normal hearers when the recorded materials were made by a single talker on 3 separate days; these differences were not found, however, with a single recording that was dubbed three times and then reordered. Brandy concluded that "recorded presentations which are equivalent in acoustic output provide more reliable listener performance than do live presentations which are unequivalent in acoustic output" (page 474). Penrod (1979) reported marked variability in word recognition scores among 30 subjects with hearing impairment when listening to the recordings of four different talkers (audiologists) who were accustomed to the monitored live voice technique. For 26 of the 30 subjects, the difference between the best and worst scores was 8 percent or greater. Penrod also observed that the variability of performance increased as scores decreased and thus questioned the validity of monitored live voice when used with persons having problems in speech understanding. Variability between talkers is also evident when speech is presented in a background of noise (Gengel and Kupperman, 1980).

In recognition of these talker differences Kruel et al. (1968) stated that "only the actual recording of the spoken lists of words can be considered to be the test materials" (page 281). More recently, Hood and Poole (1980) demonstrated that individual talkers play the prominent role in determining word difficulty for a particular list of words. That is, word difficulty with a list is, to a large extent, a function of the individual talker. The speaker, then, appears to be a most important variable affecting speech recognition.

An example of how different talkers can influence the performance intensity function of the same test material is shown in Figure 6-7. The differences among these functions for the NU #6 test using four separate recordings and talkers clearly show that the word lists themselves should not be considered as the test materials.

Presentation Level The speech stimulus should be presented at an intensity level that will offer the listener the best opportunity to understand clearly. This maximum value is often referred to as the *PB-max* when monosyllabic materials are employed. It is recognized, however, that the only true way that an individual can obtain a maximum

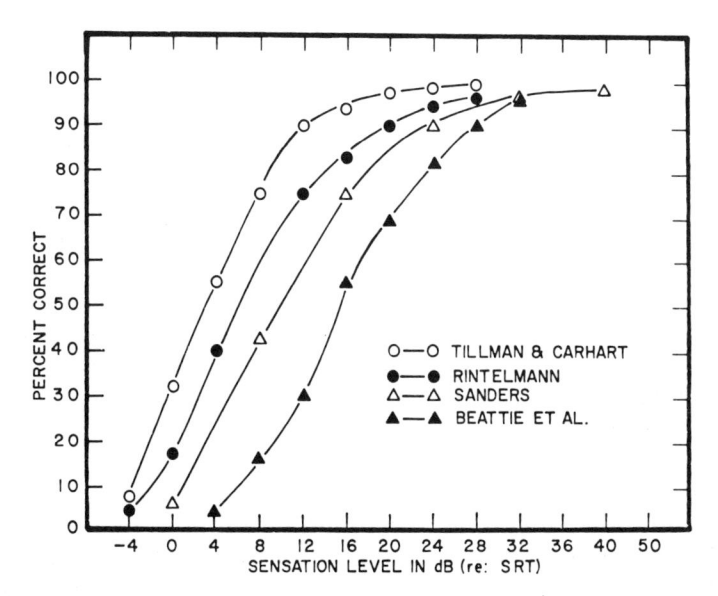

Figure 6-7. Comparison of performance intensity functions for four different recordings of the Northwestern University Auditory Test No. 6 (NU #6) [Beattie et al., 1977, Rintelmann et al., 1974 (Rintelmann Recording); Tillman and Carhart, 1966; Roe, 1965 (Sanders Recording)]. SRT, speech reception threshold.

speech recognition score is to obtain a performance intensity function. Because such a procedure is time consuming, clinicians usually attempt to estimate speech recognition ability by administering the test at only one or two intensity levels. The intensity needed to yield a maximum speech recognition score varies, depending upon such variables as the recording, type of test material, and the test format or response. Most speech recognition tests are presented at intensity levels ranging between 25 and 50 dB SL.

Some audiologists favor a most comfortable loudness level for presenting the speech recognition materials. Kruel and coworkers (1968), for example, suggested a most comfortable loudness level for administering the MRHT. A MCL presentation, however, will not necessarily yield a maximum speech recognition score among hearing-impaired listeners. Clemis and Carver (1967) have reported that a comfortable loudness setting failed to yield a maximum recognition score in a group of patients diagnosed as having Meniere's disease. Clevenger (1972) also observed in two cases of elderly subjects that the maximum score was not obtained at the most comfortable loudness presentation. Ullrich and Grimm (1976) noted that only three of ten listeners with hearing impairment achieved a maximum recognition at the MCL level. The remaining subjects yielded speech recognition scores that were 16 to 28 percent poorer than scores achieved at higher intensity level presentations.

Despite the time involved, some clinicians favor obtaining a complete performance intensity function—that is, speech recognition is assessed across a range of several intensity levels. The use of this approach is especially valuable for differentiating between cochlear and retrocochlear lesions (Jerger and Hayes, 1977; Jerger and Jerger, 1971). The clinical application of the performance intensity function is detailed later in this chapter. At a minimum, it is recommended that a speech recognition test be presented at two or three successively higher intensity levels. Olsen and Matkin (1979) suggested that a second word presentation of the stimulus items should be made at a hearing level that is several decibels above the pure tone threshold for 2000 Hz.

Adaptive Strategies An alternative method for measuring speech recognition is by adaptive testing, sometimes referred to as sequential or up-down transformed response testing (Bode and Carhart, 1973; Campbell and Lasky, 1968; Levitt, 1971, 1978). Several basic steps are common to these procedures (Bode and Carhart, 1972). The examiner first selects a specific percentage point on the performance intensity function and then determines the speech intensity required to achieve understanding at the selected percentage value. Next, the examiner chooses the adaptive method and criteria for the decision making that will lead to finding the desired percentage value. Finally, strategies are used that dictate decreasing the speech intensity when the examiner is above the selected percentage and increasing the intensity if below the desired percentage. Thus, a bracketing technique is used whereby the presentation level is varied above and below the target score. Let us say that we desire to find the S/N ratio needed to achieve a 50 percent word recognition score. The noise is kept at a fixed intensity and the examiner controls the intensity of the test items (signal). If the listener responds correctly to a test item the next word is decreased by a given step; conversely, if the listener responds incorrectly, the level of the next word is increased. The midpoints of several up-down sequences are then averaged to estimate the S/N ratio required for a 50 percent response level. Hence, adaptive methodology is not unlike the procedures commonly used to establish a pure tone threshold or speech reception threshold.

The use of this unique approach has been shown to be effective in estimating the recognition performance of both normal hearers and hearing-impaired listeners (Bode, 1978). A variation of this method can also be used for determining the optimum setting of a hearing aid

(Levitt, 1978). In addition, adaptive test procedures offer several advantages over the traditional test protocol for measuring speech recognition. The procedure is rapid, efficient, affords excellent test-retest reliability (in quiet or noise), and allows performance estimation at any desired preselected point on the performance-intensity function. Application of adaptive procedures are not restricted to speech recognition measures, but can also be used for assessing other speech audiometric phenomena. (See Chapter 7 for a discussion of this technique with MCL and LDL measurements.) A comprehensive review of adaptive methodology is proffered by Levitt (1978).

Method of Response and Error Analysis

The typical procedure for scoring the speech recognition test is for the subject to respond to each item verbally with the clinician judging whether the response was correct or incorrect (Martin and Pennington, 1971). Despite its common usage, there are known limitations to this approach. Merrell and Atkinson (1965) examined the differences between the verbal and written responses of a hearing-impaired subject using a 25-member panel of normal hearers. When using verbal responses, the recognition scores perceived by the panel members ranged from 14 to 21 percent, whereas scores for the written responses ranged only from 0 to 2 percent. Merrell and Atkinson also noted a tendency for the panel members to err in favor of accepting incorrect verbal responses. These investigators thus concluded that a written response would render a more reliable speech recognition score.

Additional evidence in support of the Merrell and Atkinson (1965) study has been reported by others (Lovrinic, Burgi, and Curry, 1968; Nelson and Chaiklin, 1970). Disarno and McGinnis (1977) also reported numerous examiner errors when sound field speech recognition testing was conducted in a background of noise.

Several factors are thought to contribute to examiner error when a verbal response is used. First, the limited bandwidth of the monitoring system may affect the clinician's perception of high frequency elements within the speech signal. Another factor is the poor S/N ratio usually achieved in the examiner room when testing under adverse listening conditions. Other variables include the absence of visual cues and the examiner's perception of the correct response, sometimes referred to as auditor bias.

As noted earlier an advantage of the closed-set response paradigm is that it affords the clinician a more accurate means to analyze specific errors made by the subject. In a review of the literature concerned with the phoneme scoring from hearing-impaired listeners, Olsen and

Matkin (1979) observed the following general trends:

1. Consonant errors are more often substitutions than omissions
2. Omissions occur with greater frequency for the final consonant
3. Voicing errors seldom occur; however, there are errors based on place and manner of articulation
4. Vowel errors occur for open-set materials, although fewer errors are noted in closed-set messages
5. A general relationship exists between errors and audiometric pattern
6. Errors made by the hearing impaired are not consistent from one occasion to the next

As noted in Chapter 11 of this text, such information can be helpful in planning the rehabilitative strategies for a hearing-impaired patient.

The performance score will differ, depending on the scoring method used. Markides (1978) examined the effect of whole word versus phoneme scoring on the word recognition performance of normal hearers and hearing-impaired listeners. In general, phoneme scoring yielded higher percentage scores with the average differences varying from 20 to 25 percent. These findings led Markides to conclude that clinicians should report the scoring method employed in the evaluation.

Abbreviated Recognition Tests

In an effort to reduce the test time and decrease patient and examiner fatigue, attempts have been made to abbreviate the speech recognition tests by presenting half lists rather than whole lists. According to a survey on audiometric practice (Martin and Forbis, 1978), many clinicians use only 25 words in the hearing evaluation and hearing aid selection process.

There is some literature that suggests that half-list testing can be used reliably for the measurement of speech recognition in normal hearers (Burke, Shutts, and King, 1965; Elpern, 1961; Manning et al., 1975; Resnick, 1962; Rintelmann et al., 1974; Shutts, Burke, and Creston, 1964) and sensorineural-impaired listeners (Campanelli, 1962; Rintelmann et al., 1974). Split-half testing has been opposed on the basis that erroneously high correlations occur because the subtest is part of the whole list score (Grubb, 1963a, b). The validity of using half-list speech recognition tests in the audiologic assessment has been challenged by several investigators. For example, Jirsa, Hodgson, and Goetzinger (1975) examined split-half reliability for the CID W-22 and NU #6 word recognition tests in both normal listeners and sensorineural-impaired subjects and noted that the results did not support the use of 25 word lists. Schwartz, Bess, and Larson (1977) also examined the use of half-list testing in normal listeners for the NU #6 and the MRHT at several different signal-to-noise ratios. The large individual variability among subjects did not support the use of half list measures when testing in a background of noise—at least for normal hearers. Over one-third of the speech recognition scores obtained between the first and second half lists exceeded 10 percent. Finally, Edgerton, Klodd, and Beattie (1978) examined the usefulness of half lists in the hearing aid selection process and concluded that such practice was not justified.

Alternative methods have been proffered for the purpose of decreasing the overall test time. In 1974, Rose developed a 10-word speech recognition test that could be used as a screening tool. Ten words from the CID W-22 list were selected on the basis of the most frequent errors made by a large group of sensorineural hearing-impaired subjects. If a subject failed to miss the first 10 (most frequently missed) words, there was not need to continue the remaining words. If one or more of the 10 words were missed, however, the examiner would continue with the complete list. Experience with NU #6 materials suggests that a 10-word presentation similar to that described by Rose has merit as a clinical screening tool.

Another approach to shortening the test procedure was suggested by Lynn (1962). In a pilot study, Lynn proposed pairing the words from the entire 50 words in the lists, thus administering two words after each carrier phrase (i.e., Say the words ball, tree). Using 10 normal hearers and 10 subjects with sensorineural hearing loss, Lynn found that paired word presentation produced scores that were essentially equivalent to a 50-word carrier phrase presentation. Stach (1979) also investigated the usefulness of paired word presentation in 10 normal hearers and 20 listeners with sensorineural hearing loss. Stach reported that the average differences between the paired word presentation and a whole list presentation were minimal and only one subject exhibited a difference between scores greater than 10 percent. Furthermore, the amount of hearing loss was unrelated to paired word versus whole list differences, the ear tested, the age of the subject, or the order of list presentation. Thus, Stach concluded that paired word testing had potential as a valid and reliable alternative to the standard procedure of speech recognition assessment.

The use of abbreviated tests has generally been criticized on two basic counts. It has been argued that reducing the number of stimulus items in the test disturbs the phonetic balance structure of the list.

Criticism has also been made on the basis of the binomial distribution in speech recognition testing.

Phonemic or Phonetic Balance Recall that Egan (1948) first pursued the possibility of using 25-word lists but concluded that lists shorter than 50 items failed to satisfy the criterion of phonemic balance. Many have since criticized the use of 25-word lists on the basis that it disturbs the phonemic balance originally created in 50-word lists (Carhart, 1965; Goetzinger, 1978; Grubb, 1963b).

There are those, however, that question the clinical value of phonemic balancing. Tobias (1964), for instance, commented that there is ". . . overwhelming clinical and experimental experience that indicates phonetic balance to be an interesting but unnecessary component of one of our current audiometric tests" (page 99). Carhart (1970) has also noted that "precise phonetic balance does not seem to be of major importance from the clinical point of view" (page 229). Further, clinical studies have shown that many tests containing differences in phonetic structure yield similar recognition scores (High, Fairbanks, and Glorig, 1964; Kopra, Blosser, and Waldron, 1968; Northern and Hattler, 1974). More recently, Aspinall (1973) developed four different lists of words with varying degrees of phonemic balance: a well-balanced list; a poorly balanced list comprised of "least commonly expected" phonemes; a poorly balanced list comprised of "most commonly expected" phonemes; and a list of words selected at random. When these four lists were administered to a group of subjects with sensorineural hearing loss, the scores did not differ significantly.

Binomial Characteristics of Speech Recognition An important element of any speech recognition test is that it yield good test-retest reliability. The reliability of a speech recognition score is influenced by two significant variables, the subject's performance level and the number of test items. As early as 1948, Egan noted that the reliability of a given test score is dependent, in part, on the subject's performance score. Egan observed that variability is greatest in the middle range of test scores and lowest in the regions of the two extremes of the percentage scale. Egan also recognized that variability is influenced by the length of the test list. Hence, as the number of test items increases, the variability decreases. Thornton and Raffin (1978) developed a probalistic model to describe the inherent variability of word recognition tests. This model is appropriate for those recognition tests in which the items are scored as correct or incorrect and the total score is expressed in terms of percentage of items perceived correctly. Speech recognition test scores may thus be described by a binomial distribution and the standard deviation (SD) of this distribution is expressed with the following formula:

$$SD = \sqrt{\frac{\text{probability of a single binary event} \times \text{probability of a complementary binary event}}{N \text{ of sample}}}$$

When this formula is applied to test scores obtained with traditional word recognition tests of different length, it can be demonstrated that the standard deviations will vary as functions of sample size and the probability of a binary event. The largest standard deviations occur with small sample sizes and scores that approach the middle range of the percentage scale.

Once the standard deviation of the distribution is known, it is possible to estimate the critical differences for different length tests at various levels of confidence. That is, given a subject's initial word recognition score, one can predict with a high degree of confidence (e.g., 0.05) the range of scores expected on a second test form. If the second test score is outside the predicted range, the two scores may be considered significantly different. An example of some of the critical differences at the 95 percent confidence level developed by Thornton and Raffin (1978) for different sample sizes is shown in Table 6-7. It is seen that when a subject scored 50 percent on a 50-item test there is a 95 percent probability that the retest score will fall within a range of 32 to 68 percent (± 18). For a 10-item list, the expected retest score would range between 10 and 90 percent (± 40).

The clinician should consider these factors when selecting the length of the test and when determining what constitutes a significant difference. In clinical practice, the audiologist should report not only the word recognition score but also the sample size and critical differences for a selected confidence level. Tables of critical differences have been constructed for comparing scores from word lists of both

Table 6-7. Extreme scores (%) not exceeding the critical difference ($P > 0.05$) as a function of test sample size

Initial test score (%)	100 Items (range)	50 Items (range)	25 Items[a] (range)	10 Items (range)
50	37–63	32–68	28–76	10–90
70	57–81	52–86	48–92	30–90
90	81–96	76–98	72–100	50–100

From Thornton and Raffin (1978).

[a] Critical differences calculated to the next highest 2 percent.

equal and unequal length by Raffin and Thornton (1980; Thornton and Raffin, 1978). To summarize, it is clear that a reduction in the number of test items will result in increased variability unless the scores occur at the upper or lower extremes of the percentage scale. The clinical implications of using only a 10-item list seem obvious. Thornton and Raffin (1978) state that "although it is tempting to try to devise a test with fewer items that will have the same variability across forms as a larger test, it is unlikely that this can be done without substantial changes in construction and scoring to eliminate the binomial characteristics" (page 517). Those who wish further detail on the binomial characteristics of speech recognition tests are referred to several sources (Hagerman, 1976; Olsen and Matkin, 1979; Raffin and Thornton, 1980; Thornton and Raffin, 1978).

Adverse Listening Conditions

Word recognition scores obtained in quiet conditions are not truly representative of what individuals typically encounter under everyday listening situations. Thus, many audiologists have begun to assess speech recognition using a background of noise or competing speech in an attempt to increase the face validity of the listening condition. Testing speech in the presence of noise increases the difficulty of the listening task by reducing the redundant cues in the speech signal. Under such adverse conditions, it is possible to identify communicative difficulties that are not readily seen under quiet conditions. Carhart (1968) emphasized the importance of assessing speech recognition under a typical noise environment and stated ". . . once we have developed good methods for measuring a patient's capacity to understand speech under adverse listening conditions, we will possess the audiological tools for dealing much more insightfully with his everyday listening problems" (page 715). In recognition of the importance of simulating a typical noise environment, many of the more recent speech recognition tests described previously have incorporated a background noise or competing speech on the test tape (i.e., MRHT, NST, MCDT, UOCRT, SPIN, R-CID). Despite the apparent widespread acceptance of speech recognition testing under adverse conditions, however, there does not exist presently a standardized procedure for its clinical implementation (Bess, 1982).

The evaluation of speech recognition under adverse conditions has been conducted using several types of background competition such as continuous broadband noise, continuous speech spectrum noise, modulated broadband noise, single talkers, multitalkers, and cafeteria noise. The amount of masking that these stimuli produce is dependent on the intensity, spectrum, and temporal patterns of both the speech stimulus and the masker. The dominant factor in masking, however, is the S/N ratio at those frequencies important in speech (Miller, 1947).

Perhaps the most common type of competition for testing speech reception is broadband noise because it is readily available on most clinical audiometers. There is a plethora of literature dealing with the effects of broadband noise on speech recognition (Egan, 1948; Humes, Bess, and Schwartz, 1978; Keith and Talis, 1970, 1972; Miller, 1947; Olsen, Noffsinger, and Kurdziel, 1975; Pollack, 1958; Rupp and Phillips, 1969; Sambataro and Pestalozza, 1952; Sever, 1973; Shapiro, Melnick, and VerMeulen, 1972; Schwartz, Bess, and Larson, 1977). The results from a representative group of these studies are shown in Table 6-8. Large differences in mean word recognition scores are noted between studies and are due, at least in part, to possible procedural differences as well as the inherent variability of the test measure. The large measures of dispersion demonstrate the marked variability that can occur when testing speech recognition in a noise background.

Research concerned with the effects of repeated measures on speech recognition in noise also demonstrates the large variability seen with this test procedure. Several investigators observed a practice effect associated with testing speech recognition in noise (Jerger, Malmquist, and Speaks, 1966; Sever, 1973; Shore, Bilger, and Hirsh, 1960; Tobias, 1973). As part of a larger study, Sever (1973) measured the word recognition scores in 16 normal hearers for several different S/N ratios (0, +4, +8). Examination of the data at a S/N of +8 reveals that 11 of the 16 subjects showed improvement from test to retest conditions. It should be noted, however, that some investigators have failed to observe a learning effect (Beattie and Edgerton, 1976; Gengel and Miller, 1976). Even if there is no learning effect, test-retest variability remains a problem. To demonstrate more clearly the variability

Table 6-8. Mean word recognition scores and dispersion measurements in normal hearers obtained in the presence of a broadband noise (S/N = 0) for several representative studies

Investigator(s)	Material	Mean word recognition (%)	SD	Range
Rupp and Phillips (1969)	CID W-22	72	—	36–92
Keith and Talis (1972)	CID W-22	82	—	10
Sever (1973)	NU #6	48	11	30–66
Olsen, Noffsinger, and Kurdziel (1975)	NU #6	74	—	56–94
Schwartz, Bess, and Larson (1977)	NU #6	63	21	—
Humes, Bess, and Schwartz (1978)	NU #6	68	21	—

obtained in noise, Sever's test-retest differences for the +8 S/N condition were plotted as a cumulative frequency distribution and shown in Figure 6-8. These data show that the test-retest reliability for the quiet condition was reasonably good—in fact, all of the subjects were within ±6 percent from the test to retest conditions and slightly more than 90 percent of the subjects were within ±4 percent. In a background of noise, however, only about 37 percent of the subjects were within ±6 percent from test to retest. If all subjects are included, some individual test-retest differences of 20 percent or more can be expected.

Some audiologists have criticized the use of a continuous noise on the basis that typical everyday backgrounds are fluctuating and usually contain several talkers. Although far less research has been conducted using fluctuating types of background competition, the available evidence suggests that variability continues to exist under these conditions (Cooper and Cutts, 1971; Danhauer and Leppler, 1979; Shapiro et al., 1972; Surr and Schwartz, 1980). Such wide variability represents an obvious limitation for using this approach in the clinical setting with any degree of confidence. Although this variability was obtained in normal hearers there is no reason to suspect that senso-

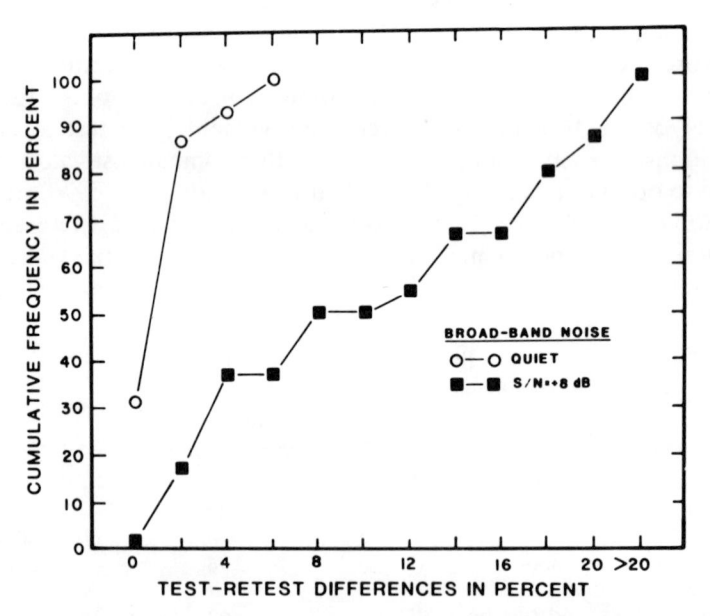

Figure 6-8. Cumulative frequency distribution of test-retest differences in normal hearers for the Northwestern University Auditory Test No. 6 (NU #6) (Rintelmann et al., 1974) presented in quiet and in a background of broad band noise (S/N = +8 dB). (Modified from Sever, 1973)

rineural-impaired listeners perform differently; some would even suggest that the hearing-impaired exhibit greater variability. Nevertheless, there is ample evidence to indicate that hearing-impaired subjects experience far greater difficulty coping with a background of noise or competing speech than do normal hearers. Consequently, it still seems advisable to measure speech recognition in the presence of a typical noise environment if one desires an estimate of the handicap imposed by the hearing impairment.

The clinical implications of such variability seem obvious, especially for hearing aid evaluations. When comparing speech performance among hearing aids, one must be able to determine with assurance that any demonstrated improvement in speech recognition is due to the hearing aid itself and not chance variation related to the speech recognition task per se. Based on the binomial characteristics of speech recognition tests one would expect a noise background to lower the true scores toward the middle range of the performance scale and thus increase the variability. It is therefore essential to use a table of critical differences for judging whether differences between scores are significant (Raffin and Thornton, 1980; Thornton and Raffin, 1978).

To summarize, the basis for assessing speech recognition in a background of noise does have merit and within certain limitations can afford the audiologist valuable information. Presently, however, no accepted standardized procedure exists for conducting this test measure. Hence, there is an urgent need to develop a clinical procedure for assessing speech performance in the presence of competition specifying the test material, noise type, S/N ratio, and general test procedure (Bess, 1982).

Speech Recognition by Bone Conduction

Several investigators have examined the feasibility of conducting speech audiometry with the stimuli transduced by a bone vibrator (Goetzinger and Proud, 1955; Hahlbrock, 1962; Hoople and Bradley, 1964; Kasden and Robinson, 1973; Robinson and Kasden, 1970). This technique can serve as a reliability check for bone conduction pure tone thresholds, offer valuable information in the assessment of young children or other difficult-to-test patients, and predict cochlear reserve in cases of chronic middle ear disease or in postoperative patients of middle ear surgery. A major limitation to bone conduction speech audiometry is the maximum output available in the more commonly used vibrators. Barry and Gaddis (1978) reported a maximum vibrator (Radioear B-70-A) output of 65 to 70 dB HL. Furthermore, Barry and Gaddis observed that the output level should not exceed 55 dB HL in order to keep harmonic distortion below 10 percent.

Special Considerations for Children

Many of the variables known to affect speech recognition for adults are also applicable to the pediatric population. Some procedural strategies for children, however, warrant special consideration. One such area is the intensity level at which the materials should be administered. Unlike adult lists, performance intensity functions are not available on many of the children's materials, thereby making it difficult to estimate the appropriate presentation level needed to approximate maximum achievement. Sanderson-Leepa and Rintelmann (1976) recommended 32 dB SL for normal-hearing children when using monosyllabic materials. Olsen and Matkin (1979) reported that sensation levels of 36 to 40 dB yield high speech recognition scores in children with mild to moderate hearing losses. These authors caution the clinician, however, about individuals with precipitous high frequency hearing losses, noting that the hearing level at 2000 Hz should be considered in determining the presentation level. Children with severe to profound hearing losses have been found to exhibit maximum recognition scores at intensity levels somewhat lower than the traditional 30 to 40 dB SL (Erber and Witt, 1977; Olsen and Matkin, 1979). Thus, in order to select the most appropriate presentation level for a given test it seems advisable for the clinician to develop performance intensity functions in normal-hearing children and children with varying degrees of hearing loss. Again, the importance of selecting a material within the receptive vocabulary of the child under test cannot be overemphasized.

Children in the severe-to-profound hearing loss category often lack the language skills needed to take many of the traditional speech recognition tests. Thus, Erber (1977) has proposed the following test battery approach for evaluating the speech perceptive skills of these children:

1. Determine the child's speech awareness, speech comfort, and speech discomfort levels for connected speech
2. Use a spondee recognition test or auditory numbers test to delineate children who perceive the spectral components of speech from those who receive only the time and intensity patterns of the signal
3. Distinguish children who can recognize words, children who can identify only stress patterns, and children who are unable to identify either
4. Evaluate the child's ability to understand connected speech with a hearing aid using videotaped sentences
5. Assess auditory and visual recognition of videotaped sentences differing in length and syntactic form. Such information can aid

the clinician in selecting which sensory system should be emphasized as well as in establishing appropriate classroom placement
6. Assess auditory and visual recognition of vowels and consonants in small closed set response formats using a videotaped syllable recognition test. Such a test can help identify perceptual problems with specific features within the speech signal

Finally, Olsen and Matkin (1979) emphasized that a reinforcement paradigm commonly used in testing the thresholds of young children, may also be employed effectively for evaluating speech recognition. They also noted that a reinforcer is appropriate when the listening task is difficult.

Hence, it can be seen that the audiologist is faced with numerous decisions relative to selecting the appropriate clinical strategies for assessing speech recognition. Many of these procedural variables have a significant influence on the performance score and must be considered in the test selection and interpretation of speech recognition findings.

CLINICAL UTILIZATION OF SPEECH RECOGNITION TESTS

Estimating Social Efficiency

An early application of speech audiometry was the prediction of an individual's efficiency under everyday listening conditions. In 1948, Silverman and coworkers described a social adequacy index (SAI) that used speech reception threshold and word recognition data to predict a hearing-impaired listener's ability to understand everyday speech. Essentially, the SAI expressed a relationship between sensitivity and maximum word recognition. The index value was based on word recognition data administered at soft, moderate, and conversational intensity levels using the Rush Hughes recordings of the PAL PB-50s. Difficulty with everyday listening situations reportedly began at a SAI of 67. At this point about two-thirds of the test items were perceived correctly when averaged across all three listening conditions (mentioned above). This performance score was found to occur between a speech reception threshold (SRT) of 28 dB (American National Standards Institute, 1970) if the speech recognition was perfect and a recognition score of 70 percent if the SRT was 2 dB (ANSI, 1970) or better. The threshold of social adequacy, or the point at which the subject was just "getting by," was 33. This occurred between a SRT of 46 dB (ANSI, 1970) if recognition was perfect and a SAI and 35 if the SRT was 2 dB (ANSI, 1970) or better. This concept, although interesting, failed to predict adequately the word recognition capabilities of hearing-impaired individuals. The limited standardization of the Rush Hughes PAL PB-50 recordings and failure to include a typical noise background were possibilities offered for the failure to predict communicative efficiency. Another measure, referred to as the social hearing index (SHI) has been proposed by Niemeyer (1965). This approach is similar to the SAI except sentence materials are used instead of monosyllables (Olsen and Matkin, 1979). To date, the SHI has not received clinical acceptance.

It is of interest to note that audiology programs within the Veterans Administration (VA) use speech audiometry as a means to estimate hearing handicap. The VA system defines normal hearing as a speech threshold of less than 26 dB (ANSI, 1970), a word recognition score of 92 percent or better, and pure tone thresholds better than 25 dB at four of the five octave frequencies 250 through 4000 Hz while not exceeding 40 dB at the remaining frequency (VA, 1976).

Several attempts have been made to estimate the hearing handicap by measuring speech recognition in the presence of a noise background (Anianssen, 1973; Elkins, 1971; Ross et al., 1965; Suter, 1978). These studies have all observed the importance of good hearing at frequencies 2000 Hz and above in order to cope effectively with competing backgrounds. Suter (1978) reported that many subjects with average hearing levels (500, 1000, 2000 Hz) of 26 dB (ANSI, 1970) or better, and thus classified as normal, experienced considerable difficulty understanding in a background of noise. Suter also noted that frequencies above 2000 Hz are better predictors of speech recognition than the traditional frequencies of 500, 1000, 2000 Hz.

Jerger and Jerger (1979) described an innovative audiovisual test procedure for quantification of the auditory handicap (QUAH). The QUAH is comprised of 25 questions or commands that require a psychomotor response. The test contains both simple and more difficult sentences that are mixed with a competing message. An example of a simple sentence is "Draw another circle." The task for the listener is merely to carry out the command of the sentence on the answer sheet provided. A block of sentences are presented first auditorially and then visually via a TV monitor. There are a total of 10 practice items and 40 test items. The QUAH was administered to a group of 53 normal hearers under several different MCRs. The authors observed that although the subjects had no difficulty with the task, the clinical application of this test seemed somewhat limited. The amount of test time and the level of intellectual skill were two variables that precluded the clinical utility of the QUAH.

Another approach to the quantification of a hearing handicap has been through the use of questionnaires. There are numerous questionnaires or scales that have been devised for this purpose. These procedures have been criticized, however, for the following reasons: results are related primarily to hearing loss; outcomes vary as functions of age and occupation; and results are confounded by the site of auditory lesion (Jerger and Jerger, 1979). Those who wish to review some of the efforts to develop handicap scales are referred elsewhere (Chapter 11 of this text; Dirks and Carhart, 1962; Ewertson and Birk-Nielsen, 1973; High et al., 1964; Giolas et al., 1979; Noble and Atherley, 1970).

Diagnostic Implications

A common misconception among many audiologists is that speech recognition tests can yield informative diagnostic data regarding the location of auditory pathology. The literature is replete with references to the limited diagnostic value of speech audiometry—especially when a recognition test is administered at only one intensity level (Bess, 1982; Carhart, 1965; Dirks, 1978; Johnson, 1977; Olsen and Matkin, 1979; Sanders, Josey, and Glasscock, 1974). The major drawback of these tests is the wide dispersion of performance scores commonly seen within the various auditory disorders. Because of this wide overlap in performance, it simply is not possible to obtain an expected score or even a range of scores for a given etiologic category. Despite the diagnostic limitations of speech recognition tests, they continue to be used as part of the basic audiometric evaluation for assessing the communicative efficiency among various types of hearing impairments. This portion of the chapter is designed to review and discuss speech audiometric findings among various types of hearing impairment. Specifically, this discussion will be confined to disorders of the middle ear, cochlea, and nerve VIII. The use of speech audiometry in the assessment of cases of central auditory dysfunction is covered in Chapter 8.

Disorders of the Middle Ear and Cochlea Individuals with conductive hearing loss experience only minimal problems understanding speech when the intensity of the signal is sufficiently loud. The mean word recognition scores for three groups of conductive hearing loss and several categories of sensorineural hearing loss are shown in Table 6-9. It is readily apparent that word recognition is quite good by comparison for the conductive groups and that the range of performance scores does not appear to be excessive. The greatest dispersion of scores among the middle ear disorders is seen in the glomus tumor group, and is probably due to the known presence of mild sensorineural involvement in this population (Bratt et al., 1979). Examples of per-

Table 6-9. Mean word recognition scores (NU #6) obtained from various etiologic groups

Diagnosis	N	Ears (%)	Mean word recognition (%)	SD	Range (%)
Conductive					
Otitis media	50	62	96	6.8	80–100
Glomus tumor	32	32	93	9.0	60–96
Otosclerosis	25	25	91	6.0	82–100
Sensorineural					
Sudden deafness	19	19	32	32.0	0–100
Meniere's disease	112	136	78	26.0	8–100
Presbycusis	139	208	93	10.0	56–100
Cochlear otosclerosis	9	9	74	9.5	62–88
Acoustic neuroma	105	105	54	34.0	0–100

formance intensity functions for a normal hearer (1), a conductive loss (2), and three different types of sensorineural hearing loss (3–5) are shown in Figure 6-9. For the normal hearer it is seen that as the intensity of the speech signal is increased above threshold, word recognition improves dramatically, reaching an asymptote at 100 percent correct. The performance intensity function for the conductive hearing loss is essentially the same as that for the normal hearer, except that it is displaced to the right by the amount of hearing loss. When the speech intensity is sufficient to overcome the conductive hearing loss, word identification increases at a rate similar to that of the normal listener and also asymptotes at 100 percent correct. Hence, individuals with a conductive hearing loss generally experience little difficulty in speech understanding, usually exhibiting performance scores in the vicinity of 90 percent or better when obtained at moderate sensation levels unless there is also some sensorineural involvement. According to Hood and Poole (1971), subjects with conductive loss experience less trouble understanding speech than one might even predict from the loss in hearing sensitivity.

In contrast to conductive hearing loss, persons with cochlear impairment exhibit varying degrees of difficulty understanding speech. Referring again to Table 6-9, the mean word recognition scores for the different types of sensorineural hearing loss are seen to be significantly poorer than the groups with middle ear problems. Although mean differences between groups exist, note the large values for the measures of dispersion. For some categories the entire range of possible scores (0 to 100 percent) was obtained. Given such large variability in scores, it is no wonder that speech recognition tests have limited diagnostic value.

Examples of performance intensity functions for subjects with cochlear involvement are shown in Figure 6-9. Curve 3 represents the performance intensity function for a subject with a mild-to-moderate cochlear loss. First, it is noted that the function is displaced to the right by the amount of hearing loss similar to that of the subject with conductive involvement. The maximum performance score achieved, however, is significantly poorer than in the normal or conductively impaired listener. Some subjects with cochlear involvement actually exhibit a slight decrease in word recognition with increasing intensity once the maximum performance score has been achieved. An example of such a function is depicted by curve 4 in Figure 6-9.

Disorders of Nerve VIII Because acoustic tumors constitute a sizable proportion of nerve VIII disorders, many clinicians develop the misconception that all nerve VIII complications are a consequence of such tumors (Jerger, 1973). It should be emphasized, however, that there are a number of pathologic conditions that can produce an au-

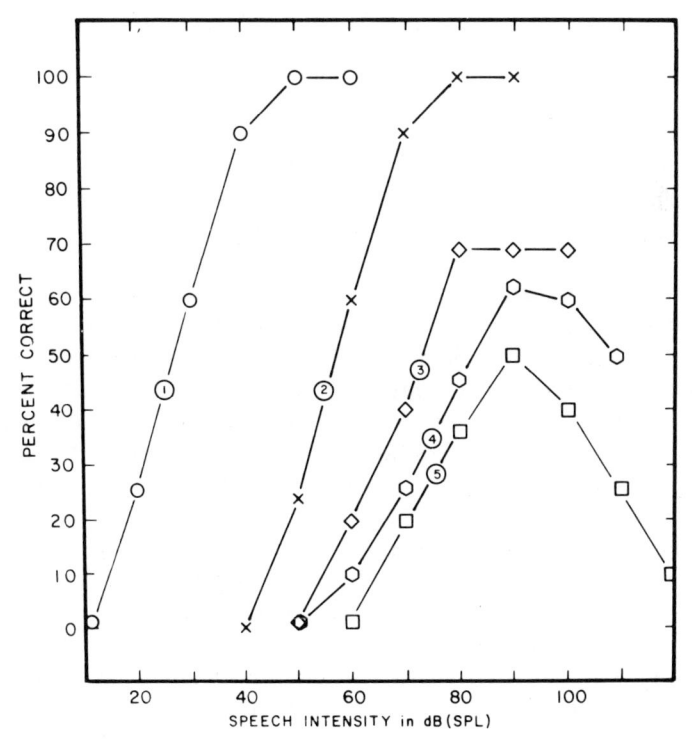

Figure 6-9. Examples of performance intensity functions for monosyllabic materials seen in normal hearers (1), conductive hearing losses (2), sensorineural impairments (3 and 4), and retrocochlear lesions (5).

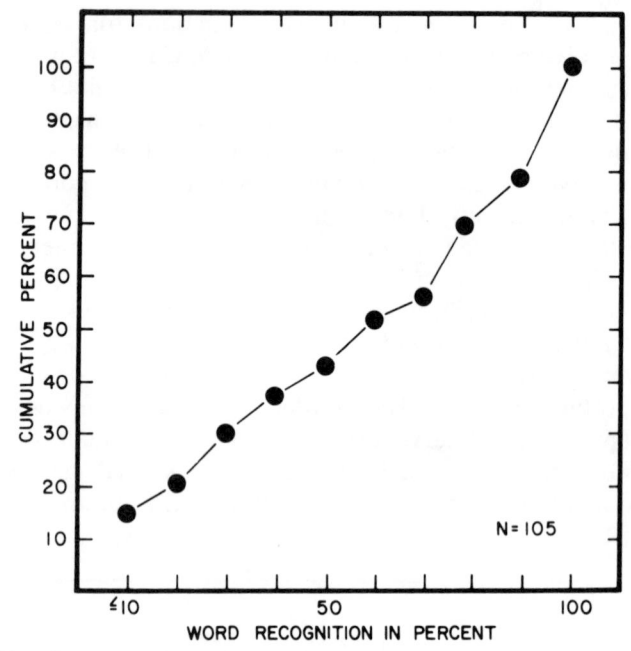

Figure 6-10. Cumulative frequency distribution of word recognition scores (NU #6) obtained in 105 ears with nerve VIII pathology

ditory disorder of nerve VIII including acoustic tumors, viral infections, vascular insult, trauma, neural atrophy associated with presbycusis, and multiple sclerosis.

It is generally recognized that subjects with nerve VIII lesions yield low performance scores for speech understanding. A maximum speech recognition score of 0 to 30 percent has long been considered a strong indication of a retrocochlear lesion. Unfortunately, however, the wide range in scores makes it almost impossible to use such data diagnostically with any degree of confidence. This is exemplified by the data in Table 6-9 for the 105 subjects with surgically confirmed nerve VIII tumors that reveal a mean speech recognition score of 54 percent with a standard deviation of 33.8 percent and a range of 100 percent.

A more striking illustration of the rather wide distribution of scores seen among subjects with nerve VIII tumors when only one presentation intensity level is used is shown in Figure 6-10.[1] This figure represents a cumulative frequency distribution for the word recognition scores of the same 105 subjects shown in Table 6-9. Note that whereas

---

[1] The data reported in Table 6-9 and Figures 6-10 to 6-14 were compiled by the author and taken from the patient files of the Bill Wilkerson Hearing and Speech Center and The Otology Group, Nashville, Tennessee.

about 30 percent of the subjects exhibited word recognition scores of 30 percent or less, slightly more than 50 percent of the subjects scored 60 percent or better. Thus, although a recognition score of ≤30 percent continues to be a good indication of a retrocochlear lesion, it is obvious that a large percentage of subjects with nerve VIII disorders will exhibit speech recognition scores higher than 30 percent.

In an effort to delineate better those variables that contribute to the wide dispersion of scores, the speech recognition data from 105 subjects with acoustic tumors were analyzed in terms of the degree of hearing loss and tumor size. The effect of sensitivity loss on speech understanding in shown in Figure 6-11. This figure depicts the mean word recognition scores and their respective standard deviations as a function of average hearing loss. It may be seen that the variable of hearing loss has a definite influence on speech perception, especially as hearing loss increases. In the normal-to-mild hearing loss categories the effect is minimal. As the sensitivity loss becomes moderate-to-

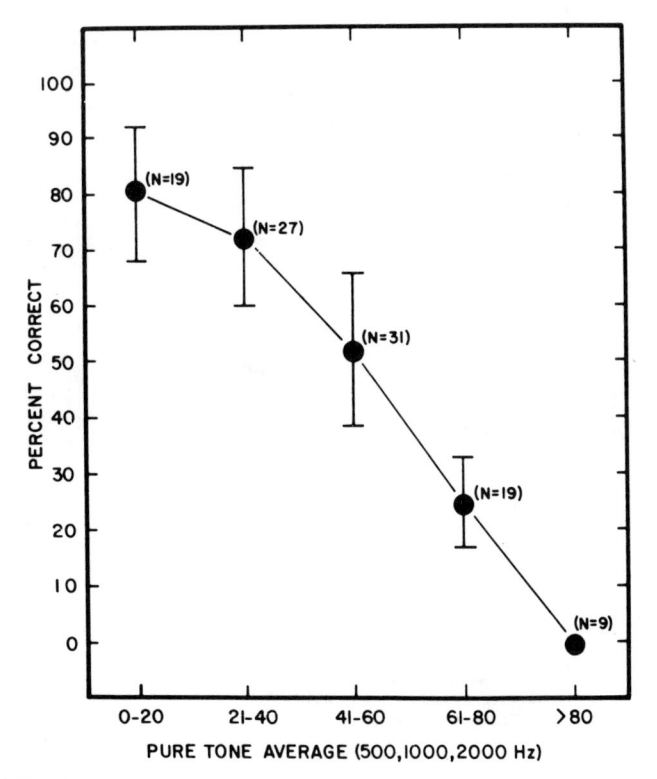

Figure 6-11. Mean word recognition scores (NU #6) and standard deviations plotted as a function of hearing levels in 105 ears with nerve VIII pathology

severe, however, the debasement of speech recognition is quite pronounced. The data in the most severe hearing loss category (>80 dB) should be interpreted with some degree of caution because it was occasionally necessary to present the speech intensity at a reduced sensation level.

The effect of tumor size on speech recognition is shown in Figure 6-12. This figure represents mean word recognition scores and standard deviations as a function of tumor size while controlling for differing degrees of hearing loss. Tumor size is seen to have no effect on speech perception. Rather, the degree of hearing loss seems to be the predominant factor.

Factors that Contribute to Problems in Speech Understanding   There are several reasons why individuals with hearing impairment experience difficulty understanding speech. As previously noted, persons with conductive hearing loss exhibit only minor problems, if any, with speech recognition. Whatever difficulties they do experience are most

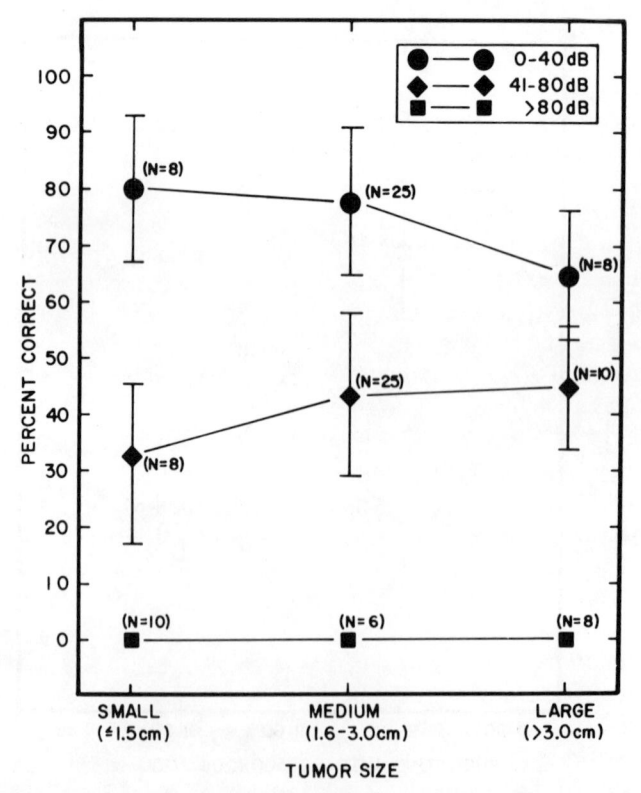

Figure 6-12. Mean word recognition scores (NU #6) and standard deviations plotted as a function of tumor size and controlling for degree of hearing loss.

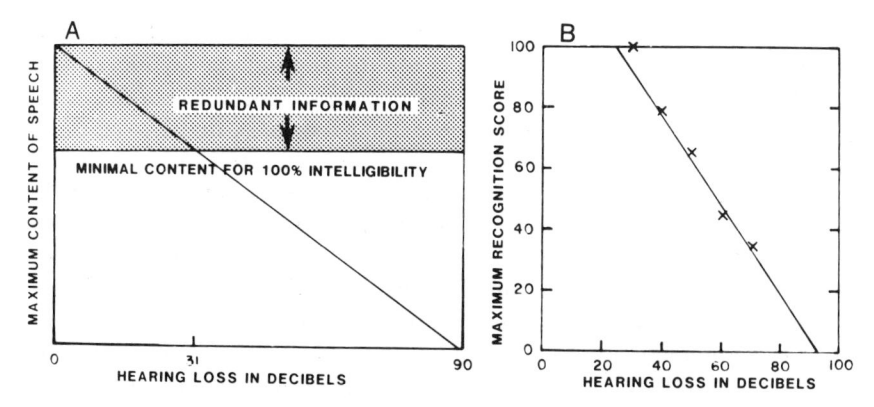

Figure 6-13. A, Model demonstrating the manner in which degree of hearing loss affects speech recognition. The shaded area represents the redundant information present in speech and the unshaded portion depicts the minimal information necessary for 100 percent recognition. The diagonal line shows how content information is progressively reduced with increasing hearing loss and associated recruitment. B, Demonstration of how the model works in a group of Meniere's cases. (Modified from Hood and Poole, 1971)

likely due to a decrease in the loudness of the signal as well as the possible filtering effects produced by the shape of the hearing loss causing differential sensitivity to various frequencies. With regard to cochlear-impaired subjects, however, the explanation for a breakdown in speech recognition is not as simple. With this group, a number of speculated factors are thought to interact in a rather complicated way to produce a breakdown in the reception of speech. Some of the factors mentioned most frequently are amount of hearing loss, shape of the hearing loss, and masking.

Amount of Hearing Loss It is generally recognized that speech understanding deteriorates progressively as the amount of hearing loss increases. Hood and Poole (1971) suggested that both the magnitude of the hearing impairment and associated recruitment (abnormally rapid growth in loudness) interact in some unknown manner to produce poor speech understanding, at least for those individuals who exhibit hearing levels greater than 31 dB. In a group of 43 cases of Meniere's disease, Hood and Poole demonstrated systematically that the maximum recognition score, as well as the shape of the performance intensity function, was directly related to the degree of hearing loss and subsequently the amount of recruitment. Hood and Poole noted that the progressive debasement of speech intelligibility as hearing loss increases is due to the reduction of redundant cues present in normal speech sounds. An example of this concept is illustrated in Figure 6-13. The shaded area (A) represents the redundant information normally present in speech; whereas the unshaded area below depicts the minimal information content necessary for 100 percent intelligibility. The diagonal line demonstrates how critical information content is systematically reduced as a consequence of increasing hearing loss and associated recruitment. Note that the diagonal line crosses the minimal content line at 31 dB, implying that discrimination will not be seriously affected for hearing levels below this point. Once a hearing level of 90 dB has been reached, however, all informational content needed for understanding has been essentially eliminated. One can see from Figure 6-13B that such a model is indeed appropriate, at least for cases of Meniere's disease. This figure depicts maximum recognition scores for a group of Meniere's cases falling into different hearing loss categories. Beyond a hearing loss of 31 dB, speech understanding is seen to deteriorate in a progressive manner until a hearing loss of 90 dB is reached—a hearing level at which understanding has been reduced to zero. It is important to mention, however, that these data represent only average scores and that the variability of recognition performance and recruitment among hearing-impaired listeners is considerable.

Shape of Hearing Loss Although the amount of hearing loss is thought to be a prominent variable in the perception of speech, it is generally conceded that other factors interplay in some complicated manner to produce a deterioration in recognition ability. Certainly, the audiometric configuration must be considered an important variable in speech understanding.

Early studies on filtered speech have shown that as high frequencies are eliminated, consonant identification is affected more adversely than vowel identification. Conversely, when the low frequencies are filtered, vowels are affected more than consonants. It is not surprising, then, to note that an individual with a high frequency loss will no doubt experience problems perceiving the high frequency consonant information in the speech signal. Stated otherwise, much of the energy in consonant sounds is concentrated in the higher frequencies and this energy is attenuated by the amount of high-frequency hearing loss. In support of this concept, the literature is replete with references dealing with the deterioration of speech understanding in normal hearers as more frequencies are eliminated or filtered from the signal (Egan and Wiener, 1946; French and Steinberg, 1947; Kiukaanniemi, 1979; Liden, 1954; Pederson, 1970; Pollack, 1948). Findings from studies on hearing-impaired listeners have also shown progressive debasement of speech as the extent of the high frequency loss increases beyond 2000 Hz. For example, Liden (1967) compared the maximum word recognition scores for subjects with varying degrees of high frequency hearing losses. The average performance scores for different groups of subjects with cutoff frequencies at 3000, 2000, 1500, 1000, and 500 Hz were 96, 93, 83, 70, and 50 percent, respectively. Kiukaanniemi (1980) also observed increasingly poorer speech recognition in hearing-impaired subjects (without recruitment) showing mild, moderate, and severe high frequency losses. Interestingly, however, the group with a moderate hearing impairment exhibited poorer performance scores at the higher intensity levels (97 and 107 dB SPL) than did subjects with severe hearing loss. There is also evidence to suggest that better speech recognition occurs when the hearing loss is constant as a function of frequency. That is, subjects with flat audiometric configurations exhibit considerably less difficulty understanding speech than individuals with high frequency hearing loss (Bess and Townsend, 1977; Liden, 1967; Schuknecht, 1954; Thompson and Hoel, 1962). Hence, the "filtering effect" produced by a differential loss for frequency, especially with the falling configuration, must be considered a contributing factor in the deterioration of speech intelligibility.

Masking Another common explanation for poor speech recognition in subjects with high frequency sensorineural hearing loss is the upward spread of masking. At suprathreshold levels it has been suggested that increased energy in the low frequency region may serve to mask out the important high frequency cues needed for adequate speech perception (Martin and Pickett, 1970). Studies by Danaher, Osberger, and Pickett (1973) and Martin, Pickett, and Colten (1972) have shown that when the second formant (F2) of synthetic speech stimuli was presented alone, some differences in discriminative performance were observed between normal listeners and sensorineural hearing-impaired subjects. When the subjects listened to the F2 transitions in the presence of the first formant (F1), however, the differences in performance between the two groups became much greater, although considerable variability was evident. From these data, the authors concluded that the low frequency energy of F1 interferes with the discrimination of F2 transitions in sensorineural hearing-impaired subjects.

Consistent with the foregoing, there is a large amount of research on masking that has resulted in the conclusion that hearing-impaired listeners exhibit a greater upward spread of masking than do normal hearers (Clack and Bess, 1969; de Boer and Bouwmeester, 1974, 1975; Harbert and Young, 1965; Jerger, Tillman, and Peterson, 1960; Leshowitz, 1977; Leshowitz and Lindstrom, 1977; Rittmanic, 1962). A close examination of this topic, however, reveals that the upward spread of masking among hearing-impaired listeners appears to be no different than for normal hearers when measured at the same sound pressure level. Nevertheless, in order for speech to be perceived by hearing-impaired listeners, the signal must be presented at higher than normal sound levels, and under such conditions the ear of the hearing-impaired listener will most likely exhibit a greater upward spread of masking.

For reasons not altogether clear, subjects with nerve VIII involvement experience more difficulty in speech understanding than do cochlear-impaired listeners. In all probability, variables such as the amount and configuration of hearing loss will also affect the speech reception capabilities of this group. Indeed, we have seen that the effect of sensitivity loss is a most prominent factor (Figure 6-11).

No doubt other variables play important roles in the perception of speech variables for all hearing-impaired subjects which, to date, have received only incidental attention. Some of the physiopathologic variables of importance undoubtedly include etiology, duration of loss, present age, and age at onset. Some of the psychological factors that can affect performance outcome are memory, reaction time, power of concentration, and receptive vocabulary. Hence, speech recognition is dependent on both the integrity of the auditory system and the intelligence and education of the listener (Liden, 1967).

Differentiating between Cochlear and Nerve VIII Disorders As noted earlier, the overlap in performance scores between cochlear and nerve VIII disorders serves to limit the diagnostic value of the traditional speech recognition test. Furthermore, it has been shown that lesions from both anatomical sites exhibit a relationship between speech performance and hearing level such that word recognition decreases progressively with increasing hearing loss.

Measuring speech recognition in a background of noise reportedly improves the sensitivity of the test (Cohen and Keith, 1976; Liden, 1967). For example, it has been observed that a low pass filtered white noise was an effective tool for differentiating among hearing-impaired listeners. Olsen and coworkers (1975), however, examined the usefulness of testing speech understanding against a noise background with various types of auditory disorders. Although 62 percent of the subjects with retrocochlear lesions demonstrated a marked decrease in understanding, 38 percent did not. Considerable overlap in scores was reported among the different disorders. Consequently, introduction of a competing noise in speech recognition assessment does not appear to enhance the sensitivity of this measure to identify either cochlear or retrocochlear disorders.

During the early 1970s Jerger and Jerger (1971) proposed the use of performance intensity functions for phonetically balanced monosyllables (PI-PB) as a means of differentiating between cochlear and nerve VIII disorders. Briefly, the establishment of a complete performance intensity function involves the repeated presentation of lists of 25 monosyllabic words at successively higher intensities. Jerger and Jerger (1971) demonstrated that the PI-PB functions from ears with cochlear pathology exhibit a plateau or slight decrease in speech understanding as the intensity level presentation increases beyond maximum performance (see curves 3 and 4, Figure 6-9). Subjects with nerve VIII disorders, however, showed a significant breakdown in speech recognition with increases in intensity beyond maximum recognition. An example of a typical performance intensity function seen in subjects with nerve VIII disorders is shown in Figure 6-9 (curve 5). This progressive deterioration in word recognition with increasing speech intensity was referred to as the "rollover effect." By quantifying the amount of rollover, Jerger and Jerger were able to differentiate quite effectively cochlear from retrocochlear lesions. Other studies have since confirmed the diagnostic efficiency of the PI-PB function (Bess, Josey, and Humes, 1979; Dirks et al., 1977). Figure 6-14 demonstrates the effectiveness of PI-PB functions for delineating cochlear from retrocochlear lesions. The figure presents word recognition data for 15 subjects with Meniere's disease and 30 subjects with surgically confirmed nerve VIII tumors. The top portion of the figure (A) presents a scatterplot of maximum word recognition scores as a function of speech reception thresholds for each group. Predictably, when only one intensity presentation level is used, considerable overlap exists between the two sets of data. The lower left panel (B) presents the magnitude of the rollover (magnitude = PB max − PB min) as a function of the speech reception threshold for each group. It is quite apparent from this analysis that such a quantification of the rollover can serve to distinguish the nerve VIII tumor cases from those with Meniere's disease. The vast majority of the nerve VIII tumors exhibited rollover values of 25 percent or more; whereas, all of the Meniere's cases yielded rollover scores of 20 percent or less.

Jerger and Jerger (1971) observed that the rollover value has some dependence on the maximum recognition score, especially when that performance score is low. To correct for this "bias effect" they suggested that the magnitude of the rollover value be divided by the maximum recognition score. This value is known as the rollover index (RI) and it is essentially normalized to each subject's maximum recognition score. The RI data for the 15 Meniere's and 30 nerve VIII cases previously discussed are plotted in the lower right panel (C) of Figure 6-14. The RI provides good differentiation between the two groups of subjects. In this analysis a rollover index of 0.25 was found to be most effective; only three retrocochlear cases yielded index values below 0.25 and one subject with Meniere's disease had an index value that was above 0.25.

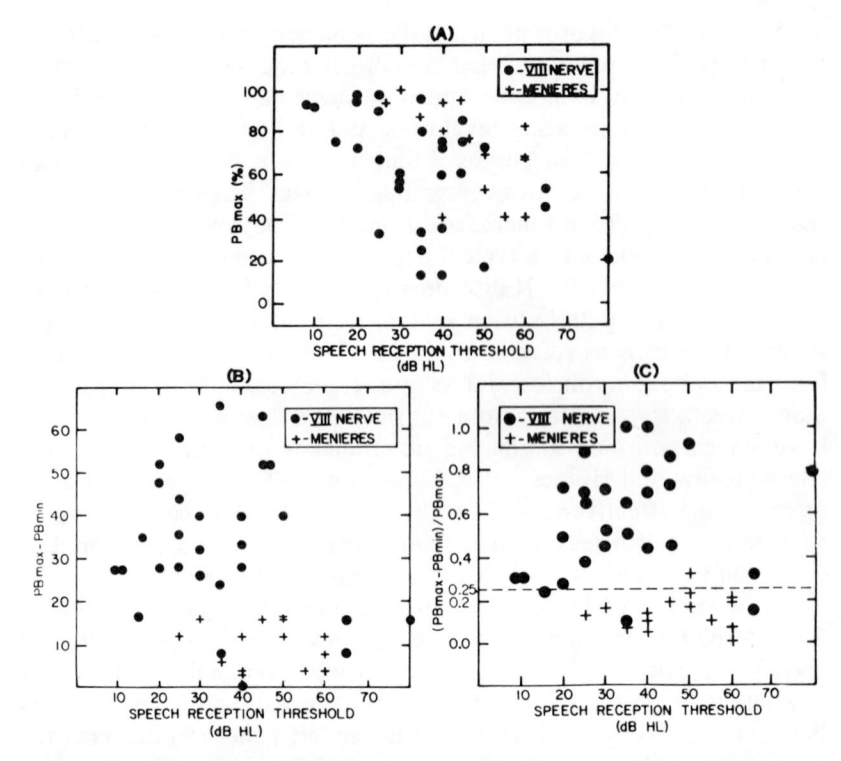

Figure 6-14. Word recognition data (NU #6) for 15 subjects with Meniere's disease and 30 subjects with surgically confirmed nerve VIII tumors. Scatterplots depict: maxium word recognition scores as a function of SRT(A); magnitude of rollover (PB max-PB min) as a function of SRT (B); and rollover index $\left(\dfrac{\text{PB max} - \text{PB min}}{\text{PB max}}\right)$ as a function of SRT (C).

The reader must be aware of several variables with regard to the use of the PI-PB function for differentiating cochlear from retrocochlear disorders. First, rollover indices can vary, depending on the speech materials used, talker differences, nature of the population studied, and other possible differences in test conditions. Jerger and Jerger (1971) as well as Dirks and coworkers (1977), for instance, reported an index value of 0.45 as the most effective cutoff level for distinguishing between cochlear and retrocochlear disorders. Thus, in keeping with the recommendation of Dirks and coworkers, each clinic should develop normative data and establish their own rollover index. A viable alternative to this procedure, however, would be the standardization of procedures and materials (tape recorded) that could be used across clinics.

It is also important to note that with some subjects it is not possible to obtain a PI-PB function either because of a very poor maximum recognition score (usually less than 30 percent) or because of a profound hearing impairment. In the former case, however, an initial score of ≤ 30 percent would seem to be sufficient to alert the clinician to the possibility of a retrocochlear lesion. Finally, the clinician should know that the degree of hearing loss in nerve VIII disorders can influence the index ratio such that the rollover is less pronounced for ears having either a mild or severe hearing loss for speech. In general, however, the use of the PI-PB function as a differential assessment tool is most impressive, especially when one considers the simple instrumentation and procedures required to administer the test.

According to Jerger and Hayes (1977), the diagnostic potential of the performance intensity function can be improved by comparing the results for two sets of materials, phonemically balanced words and synthetic sentences. In patients with cochlear disorders three distinctive patterns emerge based on the audiometric configuration. If the hearing loss is flat, the functions for both materials will be similar; if there is a high frequency hearing loss, the function for the words will fall below the function for sentences; and if there is a rising audiometric contour, the sentence function will fall below the word function. The comparison of PI-PB functions for these materials can be useful in the following ways:

1. If the relationship between materials is consistent with the audiometric configuration and no significant rollover is evident, cochlear involvement is the probable site of origin.
2. If the relationship between the two functions is out of proportion with the degree or shape of the hearing loss and rollover is evidenced in either function, the probable site is nerve VIII.
3. If the sentences fall below the words and this finding cannot be explained on the basis of audiometric pattern (i.e., rising audiometric pattern), a central deficit can be suspected.
4. The audiometric configuration and the direction and magnitude of difference between the words and sentences can offer the clinician a general indication of the amount of peripheral and central involvement.

Hearing Aid Selection

Another common application of speech recognition measures is concerned with the assessment of hearing aid performance. In 1946, Carhart described a comparative evaluation procedure that involved measuring speech recognition in quiet and noise with different hearing aids.

The Carhart approach, or more commonly some modification of this procedure, continues to be used in hearing aid evaluations and the majority of audiologists prefer to use monosyllabic materials in this hearing aid selection process. It has been argued, however, that such materials fail to differentiate effectively among amplification systems. Consequently, other types of speech stimuli have been advocated for hearing aid evaluations.

Jerger and Hayes (1976) described a procedure that uses synthetic sentences in the belief that these materials represent more appropriate, realistic stimuli to use in the evaluation of amplification. Different hearing aid arrangements can be evaluated with these sentence materials at varying MCRs. Orchik and Roddy (1980) compared the SSI and the NU #6 in the hearing aid evaluation using normal hearers and hearing-impaired listeners. Subject performance was assessed under three MCRs. The results failed to show a preference for one speech material over the other in the hearing aid evaluation. A similar result was reported by Gerber and Fisher (1979) when comparing the SSI and CID W-22 test materials. In another study, however, Madory (1978) examined the ability of the SSI to differentiate among four hearing aids with different frequency responses in a group of subjects with sensorineural hearing loss. The results of this study revealed that the Jerger and Hayes (1976) approach failed to demonstrate differences among the four hearing aids.

Pascoe (1975) and Skinner (1980) favored the use of high frequency lists (HF) in the hearing aid evaluation process. In a comparison between PB and the HF lists, Pascoe reported that the HF materials differentiated among hearing aids more effectively under quiet conditions. Levitt and coworkers (1978) demonstrated that the NST had distinct advantages over other speech materials in the hearing aid evaluation. Levitt et al. compared hearing aid performance with the NST, the CID W-22 word lists in quiet, the HF lists at a S/N ratio of +20 dB, and CHABA sentences at a S/N ratio of +5 or +10 dB in a group of subjects with sensorineural hearing loss. Greater performance score differences were found when using the NST. A significant factor that seemed to afford the NST an advantage in the hearing aid evaluation was its lower test-retest variability. Under actual clinical use the NST was found to be comparable to the minimum binomial error variance. This finding must be considered a distinct advantage for using nonsense materials, especially in the assessment of amplification.

Thus, it can be seen that an important research need in the hearing aid evaluation process is the development of speech materials that can help identify experimentally the most satisfactory hearing aid for an individual. According to Levitt and Resnick (1978), there is a need to develop two types of speech tests for the hearing aid evaluation. The first type should provide a realistic estimate of hearing aid performance; the second should offer specific information relative to which features of speech are giving the listener difficulty. Levitt noted that "the development of tests of the above type is not an extraordinarily difficult problem and would be a major addition to our armamentarium of tests for hearing-aid evaluation" (page 217). The use of speech recognition measures in the hearing aid evaluation is discussed in detail in Chapter 10.

Aural Rehabilitation

In addition to the assessment of amplification performance, speech recognition measures can be valuable for structuring aural rehabilitation strategies. Once the audiologist identifies the presence of a hearing impairment, it becomes equally important to determine the nature of the individual's handicap. This stage of the assessment process is generally referred to as the rehabilitation evaluation because it assists the clinician in developing a rehabilitation plan for the patient. In part, this evaluation may include assessment of auditory, visual, and auditory-visual speech recognition abilities. The CCT and similar tests of phonemic identification can provide the clinician with a good estimate of the consonant sounds that a hearing-impaired listener finds difficult to recognize (Owens, 1978). With such information auditory recognition of consonants can be improved through special training. In addition to evaluating identification of individual phonemes, it is also sometimes helpful to assess the perception of sentence material. This may offer information relative to a hearing-impaired listener's ability to use additional contextual information (Alpiner, 1978). Another application of speech recognition materials in the rehabilitation process is to assess the success of a particular strategy. In this context, the progress made by a patient in rehabilitative treatment is estimated by using a speech recognition test. Depending upon the results of such a measure, the specific strategy may be continued, discontinued, or perhaps modified to better reflect the patient's communicative needs. Unfortunately, there has been very little research conducted in these areas, and it is thus difficult to provide recommendations for specific uses of various materials. Nonetheless, aural rehabilitation is an important audiologic function and it appears that speech recognition measures can assist in both the planning and evaluation of rehabilitative strategies. A more detailed discussion of speech recognition assessment for rehabilitation is found in Chapter 11.

To summarize, a review of the clinical utilization of speech recognition tests demonstrates clearly that this assessment procedure has numerous applications. It is emphasized here that the type of speech material and test format to be used should vary depending on the purpose of the test. Some materials and response paradigms recommended for different clinical purposes are summarized in Table 6-10. If the clinician desires to assess the efficiency of hearing in everyday life, the use of handicap scales and/or sentence materials presented in a background of noise would seem appropriate. For diagnostic purposes, however, it is recommended that performance intensity functions be obtained for monosyllabic words or monosyllabic words and sentences in combination. In the hearing aid selection process it seems advisable to use nonsense syllables for subjects with high frequency sensorineural hearing losses and sentences for those cases with rising audiometric contours. Sentences would be more appropriate for rising configurations because this material is more dependent on low frequency information. An alternative approach for the hearing aid selection would be to use both nonsense syllables and sentences with all cases. The nonsense syllables could offer valuable data relative to the specific speech features the patient has difficulty perceiving. Thus, the clinician could modify the characteristics of the hearing aid to compensate for these difficulties. Sentence materials, on the other hand, could provide a measure of everyday listening efficiency. Finally, the speech materials to be used with aural rehabilitation should afford the clinician with information about phonemic errors and social efficiency. Accordingly, nonsense syllables or monosyllables in a closed-set response format and sentences would be generally recommended for this purpose. This test battery approach is certainly not a new concept in speech recognition assessment. As early as 1955, Silverman and Hirsh in their seminal publication on problems related to the use of speech in clinical audiometry highlighted the "need to think in terms of different tests for different purposes" (page 1243). Unfortunately, au-

Table 6-10. Speech recognition materials and response formats recommended for various clinical applications

Purpose	Speech recognition materials	Response format
Social adequacy	Handicap scales	
	Sentences	Open or closed set
Diagnosis	Meaningful monosyllables[a]	Open or closed set
	Sentences[a]	Open or closed set
Hearing aid selection	Nonsense syllables and sentences	Closed set
		Open or closed set
Aural rehabilitation	Nonsense syllables or monosyllables	Closed set
	Sentences	Open or closed set

[a] Administer at several intensities

diologists have been reticent to accept this advice and continue to use the same monosyllabic materials irrespective of the test purpose.

AFTERWORD

This chapter has focused on a review of many of the speech recognition materials currently available for both adults and children and discussed the more common procedural strategies and clinical applications of these tests. Special emphasis was placed on a coverage of children's materials since other textbooks have given this topic only incidental treatment. Because there are several clinical applications for speech recognition assessment, the criteria for selecting a material and response format should vary, depending on the clinician's purpose. Hence, the concept of a test battery approach is encouraged—that is, selecting test material and procedures that will best meet the audiologist's purpose for assessing speech recognition. It is somewhat distressing, however, to observe that audiologists continue to use traditional monosyllabic words no matter what the clinical use. As noted by Jerger (1980), "We are, at the moment, becalmed in a windless sea of monosyllables. We can sail further only on the fresh winds of imagination" (page 135).

ACKNOWLEDGMENTS

Some of the data reported herein were provided by the Bill Wilkerson Hearing and Speech Center, and Ms. Anne Forrest Josey and The Otology Group, Nashville, Tennessee. The author gratefully acknowledges Don Riggs for preparing the figures.

REFERENCES

Alpiner, J. G. (ed.). 1978. Handbook of Adult Rehabilitative Audiology. Williams & Wilkins Company, Baltimore.

American National Standards Institute. 1969. American National Standards Specifications for Audiometers, ANSI-S3.6-1969, American National Standards Institute, Inc., New York.

Anianssen, G. 1973. Binaural discrimination of "everyday" speech. Acta Otolaryngol. 75:334–336.

Aspinall, K. B. 1973. The effect of phonemic balance on discrimination for speech in subjects with sensorineural hearing loss. Doctoral dissertation. University of Colorado, Boulder, Colo.

Barry, S. J., and S. Gaddis. 1978. Physical and physiological constraints on the use of bone-conduction speech audiometry. J. Speech Hear. Disord. 43:220–226.

Beattie, R. C., and B. J. Edgerton. 1976. Reliability of monosyllabic discrimination tests in white noise for differentiating among hearing aids. J. Speech Hear. Disord. 41:464–476.

Beattie, R. C., B. J. Edgerton, and D. V. Svihovec. 1977. A comparison of the Auditec of St. Louis cassette recordings of NU-6 and CID W-22 on a normal hearing population. J. Speech Hear. Disord. 42:60–64.

Bench, J., J. M. Bamford, I. M. Wilson, and I. Clefft. 1979. A comparison of the BKB sentence lists for children with other speech audiometry tests. Austral. J. Audiol. 1:61–66.

Bench, J., A., Koval, J. Bamford. 1979. The BKB (Bamford-Koval-Bench) sentence lists for partially-hearing children. Br. J. Audiol. 13:108–112.

Bess, F. H. 1982. Basic hearing measurement. In N. J., Lass, L. V., McReynolds, J. L. Northern, and D. E. Yoder. (eds.), Speech, Language, and Hearing, pp. 913–943. W. B. Saunders Company, Philadelphia.

Bess, F. H. and A. Gibler. 1981. Syllable recognition skills of unilaterally hearing-impaired children. Paper presented at the convention of the American Speech-Language-Hearing Association, November 20–23, Los Angeles.

Bess, F. H., A. F. Josey, and L. E. Humes. 1979. Performance intensity functions in cochlear and eighth nerve disorders. Am. J. Otol. 1:27–31.

Bess, F. H., and T. H. Townsend. 1977. Word discrimination for listeners with flat sensorineural hearing losses. J. Speech Hear. Disord. 42:232–237.

Bode, D. L. 1978. Adaptive speech testing applied to hearing-impaired listeners. Paper presented at the convention of the American Speech-Language-Hearing Association, November 18–21.

Bode, D. L., and R. Carhart. 1972. Intelligibility and discrimination testing with adaptive methodology. Paper presented at the Conference on Speech Communication and Processing, Boston.

Bode, D. L., and R. Carhart. 1973. Measurement of articulation functions using adaptive test procedures. IEEE Trans. Audio Electroacoustics 21:196–201.

Boothroyd, A. 1968. Developments in speech audiometry. Sound 2:3–10.

Brandy, W. T. 1966. Reliability of voice tests of speech discrimination. J. Speech Hear. Res. 9:461–465.

Bratt, G. W., F. H. Bess, G. W. Miller, and M. E. Glasscock. 1979. Glomus tumor of the middle ear: Origin, symptomatology, and treatment. J. Speech Hear. Disord. 44:121–135.

Brooks, R., and C. P. Goetzinger. 1966. Vocabulary variables and language skills in the PB discrimination of children. J. Aud. Res. 6:357–370.

Burke, K. S., R. E. Shutts, and W. P. King. 1965. Range of difficulty of four Harvard phonetically balanced word lists. Laryngoscope 75:289–296.

Campanelli, P. A. 1962. A measure of intra-list stability of four PAL word lists. J. Aud. Res. 2:50–55.

Campbell, G. A. 1910. Telephonic intelligibility. Phil. Mag. 19:152–159.

Campbell, R. A., and E. Z. Lasky. 1968. Adaptive threshold procedures: BUDTIF. J. Acoust. Soc. Am. 44:537–541.

Carhart, R. 1946. Selection of hearing aids. Arch. Otolaryngol. 44:1–18.

Carhart, R. 1965. Problems in the measurement of speech discrimination. Arch. Otolaryngol. 82:253–260.

Carhart, R. 1968. Future horizons in audiological diagnosis. Ann. Otol. Rhinol. Laryngol. 77:706–716.

Carhart, R. 1970. Discussion, questions, answers, comments. In C. Røjskjer (ed.), Speech Audiometry, p. 229. Second Danavox Symposium, Andelsbogtrykkeriet i Odense, Denmark.

Clack. T., and F. H. Bess. 1969. Aural harmonics: The tone-on-tone masking versus the best-beat method in normal and abnormal listeners. Acta Otolaryngol. 67:399–412.
Clemis, J. D., and W. F. Carver. 1967. Discrimination scores for speech in Meniere's disease. Arch. Otolaryngol. 86:614–618.
Clevenger, J. P. 1972. The Modified Rhyme Test: A new clinical procedure for testing speech discrimination. Master's thesis. Central Michigan University, Mount Pleasant, Mich.
Cohen, R. L., and R. W. Keith. 1976. Use of low-pass noise in word recognition. J. Speech Hear. Res. 19:48–54.
Cooper, J. C., and B. P. Cutts. 1971. Speech discrimination in noise. J. Speech Hear. Res. 14:332–337.
Danaher, E. M., M. J. Osberger, and J. M. Pickett. 1973. Discrimination of formant frequency transitions in synthetic vowels. J. Speech Hear. Res. 16:439–451.
Danhauer, J. L. and J. G. Leppler. 1979. Effects of four noise competitors on the California Consonant Test. J. Speech Hear. Disord. 44:354–361.
Davis, H., and R. S. Silverman. 1978. Hearing and Deafness. 4th Ed. Holt, Rinehart & Winston, New York.
deBoer, E., and I. Bouwmeester. 1974. Critical bands and sensorineural hearing loss. Audiology 13:236–254.
deBoer, E. J., and I. Bouwmeester. 1975. Clinical psychophysics illustrated by the problem of auditory overload. Audiology 14:274–299.
Dewey, G. 1923. Relative Frequency of English Speech Sounds, Harvard University Press, Cambridge.
Dirks, D. 1978. Effects of hearing impairment on the auditory system. In E. C. Caterette and M. P. Friedman (eds.), Handbook of Perception, Vol. IV, pp. 567–608. Academic Press, New York.
Dirks, D., and R. Carhart. 1962. A survey of reactions from users of binaural and monaural hearing aids. J. Speech Hear. Disord. 27:311–322.
Dirks, D., C. Kamm, D. Bower, and A. Betsworth. 1977. Use of performance-intensity functions for diagnosis. J. Speech Hear. Disord. 42:408–415.
Disarno, N. J., and M. S. McGinnis. 1977. Variability of examiner error in speech discrimination testing in noise. Paper presented at the convention of the American Speech-Language-Hearing Association, November 2–5, Chicago.
Dubno, J. R., and D. D. Dirks. 1982. Evaluation of hearing-impaired listeners using a nonsense-syllable test. I. Test reliability. J. Speech Hear. Res. 25:135–141.
Dubno, J. R., D. D. Dirks, and L. R. Langhofer. 1982. Evaluation of hearing-impaired listeners using a nonsense-syllable test. II. Syllable recognition and consonant confusion patterns. J. Speech Hear. Res. 25:141–148.
Dubno, J. R., and H. Levitt. 1981. Predicting consonant confusions from acoustic analysis. J. Acoust. Soc. Am. 69:249–261.
Edgerton, B. J., and J. L. Danhauer. 1979. Clinical Implications of Speech Discrimination Testing Using Nonsense Stimuli. University Park Press, Baltimore.
Edgerton, B. J., D. A. Klodd, and R. C. Beattie. 1978. Half-list speech discrimination measures in hearing aid evaluations. Arch. Otolaryngol. 104:669–672.

Egan, J. 1948. Articulation testing methods. Laryngoscope 558:955–991.

Egan, J. P., and F. M. Wiener. 1946. On the intelligibility of bands of speech in noise. J. Acoust. Soc. Am. 18:435–441.

Eilers, R. E., W. R. Wilson, and J. M. Moore. 1977. Developmental changes in speech discrimination in infants. J. Speech Hear. Res. 20:766–780.

Elkins, E. 1971. Evaluation of Modified Rhyme Test results from impaired and normal-hearing listeners. J. Speech Hear. Res. 14:589–595.

Elkins, E., and G. D. Causey. 1973. Normal listener performance on the revised CID sentence lists. Paper presented at the convention of the American Speech-Language-Hearing Association, October 12–15, Detroit.

Elliott, L. L. 1979. Performance of children aged 9 to 17 years on a test of speech intelligibility in noise using sentence material with controlled word predictability. J. Acoust. Soc. Am. 66:651–662.

Elliott, L. L., S. Connors, E. Kille, S. Levin, K. Ball, and D. Katz. 1979. Children's understanding of monosyllabic nouns in quiet and in noise. J. Acoust. Soc. Am. 66:12–21.

Elpern, B. 1961. The relative stability of half list and full list discrimination tests. Laryngoscope 71:30–36.

Erber, N. P. 1974. Pure-tone thresholds and word-recognition abilities of hearing-impaired children. J. Speech Hear. Res. 17:194–202.

Erber, N. P. 1977. Evaluating speech-perception ability in hearing impaired children. In F. H. Bess (ed.), Childhood Deafness: Causation, Assessment and Management, pp. 173–181. Grune & Stratton, New York.

Erber, N. P. 1980. Use of the auditory numbers test to evaluate speech perception abilities of hearing-impaired children. J. Speech Hear. Disord. 45:527–532.

Erber, N. P., and L. H. Witt. 1977. Effects of stimulus intensity on speech perception by deaf children. J. Speech Hear. Disord. 42:271–278.

Ewertson, H. W., and Birk-Nielsen, H. 1973. Social hearing handicap index. Audiology 12:180–187.

Fairbanks, G. 1958. Test of phonemic differentiation: The Rhyme test. J. Acoust. Soc. Am. 30:596–600.

Finitzo-Hieber, T., I. J. Gerlin, N. D. Matkin, and E. Cherow-Skalka. 1980. A sound effects recognition test for the pediatric evaluation. Ear Hear. 1:271–276.

Fletcher, H. 1922. The nature of speech and its interpretation. J. Franklin Inst. 193:729–747.

Fletcher, H., and J. Steinberg. 1929. Articulation testing methods. Bell Systems Tech. J. 8:806–854.

French, N. R., and J. C. Steinberg. 1947. Factors governing the intelligibility of speech sounds. J. Acoust. Soc. Am. 19:90–119.

Gengel, R. W., and G. L. Kupperman. 1980. Word discrimination in noise: Effect of different speakers. Ear Hear. 1:156–160.

Gengel, R. W., and L. S. Miller. 1976. A clinical pass/fail criteria for word discrimination in noise. Paper presented at the convention of the American Speech-Language-Hearing Association, November 20–23, Houston.

Gerber, S. E., and L. B. Fisher. 1979. Prediction of hearing aid users satisfaction. J. Am. Aud. Soc. 5:35–40.

Giolas, T. G., and J. R. Duffy. 1973. Equivalency of CID and Revised CID Sentence Lists. J. Speech Hear. Res. 16:549–555.

Giolas, T. G., E. Owens, S. H. Lamb, and E. D. Schubert. 1979. Hearing performance inventory. J. Speech Hear. Disord. 44:169–195.

Gladstone, V. S., and B. M. Siegenthaler. 1971. Carrier phrase and speech intelligibility score. J. Aud. Res. 11:101–103.

Goetzinger, C. P. 1978. Word discrimination testing. In J. Katz (ed.), Handbook of Clinical Audiology, pp. 149–158. 2nd Ed. Williams & Wilkins Company, Baltimore.

Goetzinger, C. P., and G. O. Proud. 1955. Speech audiometry by bone conduction. Arch. Otolaryngol. 62:632–635.

Goldman, R., M. Fristoe, and R. Woodcock. 1970. Test of auditory discrimination. American Guidance Services, Inc., Circle Pines, Minn.

Gravel, J. S., M. G. Ochs, D. F. Konkle, and F. H. Bess. 1981. The Pascoe High Frequency word list: Performance of normal and hearing-impaired listeners. Paper presented at the convention of the American Speech-Language-Hearing Association, November 20–23, Los Angeles.

Griffiths, J. D. 1967. Rhyming minimal contrasts: A simplified diagnostic articulation test. J. Acoust. Soc. Am. 42:236–241.

Grubb, P. 1963a. A phonemic analysis of half-list speech discrimination tests. J. Speech Hear. Res. 6:271–276.

Grubb, P. 1963b. Some considerations in the use of half-list speech discrimination tests. J. Speech Hear. Res. 6:294–297.

Hagerman, B. 1976. Reliability in the determination of speech discrimination. Scand. Audiol. 5:219–228.

Hahlbrock, K. 1962. Bone conduction speech audiometry. J. Int. Audiol. 1:186–188.

Harbert, F., and I. M. Young. 1965. Spread of masking in ears showing abnormal adaptation and conductive deafness. Acta Oto-Laryngol. 60:49–58.

Harris, J. D., H. L. Haines, P. A. Kelsey, and T. D. Clack. 1961. The relation between speech intelligibility and the electroacoustic characteristics of low fidelity circuitry. J. Aud. Res. 1:357–381.

Haskins, H. A. 1949. A phonetically balanced test of speech discrimination for children. Master's thesis. Northwestern University, Evanston, Ill.

High, W. S., G. Fairbanks, and A. Glorig. 1964. Scale for self-assessment of hearing handicap. J. Speech Hear. Disord. 29:215–230.

Hirsh, I. J., H. Davis, S. R. Silverman, E. G. Reynolds, E. Eldert, and R. W. Bensen. 1952. Development of materials for speech audiometry. J. Speech Hear. Disord. 17:321–337.

Hood, J. D., and J. P. Poole. 1971. Speech audiometry in conductive and sensorineural hearing loss. Sound 5:30–38.

Hood, J. D., and J. P. Poole. 1980. Influence of the speaker and other factors affecting speech intelligibility. Audiology 19:434–455.

Hoople, G., and W. A. Bradley. 1964. A practical method for assessing cochlear reserve. Trans. Am. Acad. Opthalmol. Oto-laryngol. 68:70–73.

House, A. S., C. E. Williams, M. H. L. Hecker, and K. D. Kryter. 1965. Articulation testing methods. Consonantal differentiation in a closed-response set. J. Acoust. Soc. Am. 37:158–166.

Hudgins, C. V. 1944. A method of appraising the speech of the deaf. Volta Rev. 51:597–601.

Humes, L. E., F. H. Bess, and D. M. Schwartz. 1978. Thresholds of aural overload, word discrimination in noise, and the "fragile ear." J. Am. Aud. Soc. 3:253–257.

Hutcherson, R. W., D. D. Dirks, and D. E. Morgan. 1979. Evaluation of the speech perception in noise (SPIN) test. Otolaryngol. Head Neck Surg. 87:239–245.

Jerger, J. 1970. Development of synthetic sentence identification (SSI) as a tool for speech audiometry. In C. Røjskjer (ed.), Speech Audiometry, pp. 44–65. Second Danavox Symposium, Andelsbogtrykkeriet i Odense, Denmark.

Jerger, J. 1973. Diagnostic audiometry. In J. Jerger (ed.), Modern Developments in Audiology, pp. 75–115. 2nd Ed. Academic Press, New York.

Jerger, J. 1980. Research priorities in auditory science—The audiologist's view. Ann. Otol., Rhinol. Laryngol. 89(Suppl. 74, No. 5, Part 2):134–135.

Jerger, J., and D. Hayes. 1976. Hearing aid evaluation. Arch. Otolaryngol. 102:214–255.

Jerger, J., and D. Hayes. 1977. Diagnostic speech audiometry. Arch. Otolaryngol. 103:216–222.

Jerger, J., and S. Jerger. 1971. Diagnostic significance of PB word functions. Arch. Otolaryngol. 93:573–580.

Jerger, S. 1981. Evaluation of central auditory function in children. In R. Keith (Ed.), Central Auditory and Language Disorders in Children. College Hill Press, Houston.

Jerger, S., and J. Jerger. 1979. Quantifying auditory handicap—A new approach. Audiology 18:225–237.

Jerger, S., S. Lewis, J. Hawkins, and J. Jerger. 1980. Pediatric speech intelligibility test. I. Generation of test materials. Int. J. Ped. Otorhinolaryngol. 2:217–230.

Jerger, J., C. Malmquist, and C. Speaks. 1966. Comparisons of some speech intelligibility tests in the evaluation of hearing aid performance. J. Speech Hear. Res. 9:136–149.

Jerger, J. F., T. W. Tillman, and J. L. Peterson. 1960. Masking by octave bands of noise in normal and impaired ears. J. Acoust. Soc. Am. 32:385–390.

Jirsa, R. E., W. R. Hodgson, and C. P. Goetzinger. 1975. Unreliability of half-list discrimination tests. J. Am. Aud. Soc. 2:47–49.

Johnson, E. W. 1977. Auditory test results in 500 cases of acoustic neuroma. Arch. Otolaryngol. 103:152–158.

Jones, K. O., and G. A. Studebaker. 1974. Performance of severely hearing-impaired children on a closed-response auditory speech discrimination test. J. Speech Hear. Res. 17:531–540.

Kalikow, D. N., K. N. Stevens, and L. L. Elliott. 1977. Development of a test of speech intelligibility in noise using sentence materials with controlled word predictability. J. Acoust. Soc. Am. 61:1337–1351.

Kasden, S. D., and M. Robinson. 1973. Bone conduction speech discrimination in different pathologies. J. Aud. Res. 13:268–270.

Katz, D. R., and L. L. Elliott. 1978. Development of a new children's speech discrimination test. Paper presented at the convention of the American Speech-Language-Hearing Association, November 18–21, Chicago.

Keith, R. W., and H. P. Talis. 1970. The use of speech in noise in diagnostic audiometry. J. Aud. Res. 10:201–204.

Keith, R., and H. Talis. 1972. The effects of white noise on PB scores of normal and hearing impaired listeners. Audiology 11:177–186.

Kiukaanniemi, H. 1979. Simulation of high frequency hearing loss in a Finnish speech discrimination test. Acta Otolaryngol. 87:445–450.

Kiukaanniemi, H. 1980. Speech discrimination of patients with high frequency hearing loss. Acta Otolaryngol. 89:419–423.

Kopra, L. L., D. Blosser, and D. L. Waldron. 1968. Comparison of Fairbanks Rhyme Test and CID Auditory Test W-22 in normal and hearing-impaired listeners. J. Speech Hear. Res. 11:735–739.

Kruel, E. J., J. C. Nixon, K. D. Kryter, D. W. Bell, J. S. Lang, and E. D. Schubert. 1968. A proposed clinical test of speech discrimination. J. Speech Hear. Res. 11:536–552.

Larson, G. W., B. Peterson, and W. S. Jacquot. 1974. Use of Northwestern University No. 6 for speech discrimination testing with children. J. Aud. Res. 14:287–292.

Lehiste, I., and G. E. Peterson. 1959. Linguistic considerations in the study of speech intelligibility. J. Acoust. Soc. Am. 31:280–286.

Lerman, J. W., M. Ross, and R. M. McLaughlin. 1965. A picture identification test for hearing impaired children. J. Aud. Res. 5:273–278.

Leshowitz, B. 1977. Speech intelligibility in noise for listeners with sensorineural hearing damage. IPO Annual Progress Report, 11-23. Institute for Perception Research, Eindhoven, Holland.

Leshowitz, B., and R. Lindstrom. 1977. Measurement of nonlinearities in listeners with sensorineural hearing loss. In E. F. Evans and J. P. Wilson (eds.), Psychophysics and Physiology of Hearing, pp. 1–10. Academic Press, London.

Levitt, H. 1971. Transformed up-down methods in psychoacoustics. J. Acoust. Soc. Am. 49:467–477.

Levitt, H. 1978. Adaptive testing in audiology. Scand. Audiol. 6(Suppl.):241–291.

Levitt, H., M. J. Collins, J. R. Dubno, S. B. Resnick, and R. E. C. White. 1978. Development of a protocol for the prescriptive fitting of a wearable master hearing aid. Final Report of NINCDS Contract No. NIH-NO1-NS-4-2323.

Levitt, H., and S. B. Resnick. 1978. Speech reception by the hearing impaired: Methods of testing and the development of new tests. Scand. Audiol. 6(Suppl.):107–130.

Liden, G. 1954. Speech audiometry. Acta Otolaryngol. Suppl. 114.

Liden, G. 1967. Undistorted speech audiometry. In A. B. Graham (ed.), Sensorineural Hearing Processes and Disorders, pp. 339–357. Little, Brown & Company, Boston.

Ling, D. 1978. Auditory coding and reading—an analysis of training procedures for hearing-impaired children. In M. Ross and T. G. Giolas (eds.), Auditory Management of Hearing-Impaired Children, pp. 181–218. University Park Press, Baltimore.

Lovrinic, J. H., E. J. Burgi, and E. T. Curry. 1968. A comparative evaluation of five speech discrimination measures. J. Speech Hear. Res. 11:372–381.

Lynn, G. 1962. Paired PB-50 discrimination test. A preliminary report. J. Aud. Res. 2:34–36.

McLennan, R. O., Jr., and A. W. Knox. 1975. Patient controlled delivery of monosyllabic words in a test of auditory discrimination. J. Speech Hear. Disord. 40:538–543.

McNamee, J. 1960. An investigation of the use of the CID Auditory Test W-22 with children. Master's thesis. Ohio State University, Columbus, Ohio.

Madory, R. D. 1978. The test-retest reliability on the synthetic sentence identification hearing aid evaluation procedure. Master's thesis. Central Michigan University, Mount Pleasant, Mich.

Manning, W. H., C. K., Shaw, J. E., Maki, and D. S. Beasley. 1975. Analysis of half-list scores on the PBK-50 as a function of time compression and age. J. Am. Aud. Soc. 3:109–111.

Mansur, R. 1950. The construction of a picture test for speech sound discrimination. Master's thesis. Boston University, Boston, Mass.

Markides, A. 1978. Whole-word scoring versus phoneme scoring in speech audiometry. Br. J. Audiol. 12:40–46.

Martin, E. S., and J. M. Pickett. 1970 Sensorineural hearing loss and upward spread of masking. J. Speech Hear. Res. 13:426–437.

Martin, E. S., J. M. Pickett, and S. Colten. 1972. Discrimination of vowel formant and transition by listeners with severe sensorineural hearing loss. In G. Fant (ed.), Speech Communication Ability and Profound Deafness, pp. 81–98, A. G. Bell Association for the Deaf, Washington.

Martin, F. N., and N. K. Forbis. 1978. The present status of audiometric practice: A follow-up study. AsHA 20:531–541.

Martin, F. N., R. R. Hawkins, and H. A. T. Bailey. 1962. The non-essentiality of the carrier phrase in phonetically balanced (PB) word testing. J. Aud. Res. 2:319–322.

Martin, F. N., and C. D. Pennington. 1971. Current trends in audiometric practices. ASHA. 13:671–677.

Merrell, H. B., and C. J. Atkinson. 1965. The effect of selected variables upon discrimination scores. J. Aud. Res. 5:285–292.

Miller, G. A. 1947. The masking of speech. Psychol. Bull. 44:105–129.

Moore, J. M., and W. R. Wilson. 1978. Visual reinforcement audiometry (VRA) with infants. In S. E. Gerber and G. T. Mencher (eds.), Early Diagnosis of Hearing Loss, pp. 177–213. Grune & Stratton, New York.

Myatt, B., and B. Landes. 1963. Assessing discrimination loss in children. Arch. Otolaryngol. 77:359–362.

Nelson, D. A., and J. B. Chaiklin. 1970. Writedown versus talkback scoring and scoring bias in speech discrimination testing. J. Speech Hear. Res. 13:645–654.

Nielson, K. 1960. Speech sound discrimination of pre-school children as measured by the CID Auditory Test W-22. Master's thesis. Michigan State University, East Lansing, Mich.

Niemeyer, W. 1965. Speech audiometry with phonetically balanced sentences. Int. Audiol. 4:97–101.

Noble, W. G., and G. R. C. Atherly. 1970. The hearing measurement scale. J. Aud. Res. 10:229–250.

Northern, J. L., and K. W. Hattler. 1974. Evaluation of four speech discrimination test/procedures on hearing impaired patients. J. Aud. Res. 1(Suppl.):1–37.

Olsen, W., and N. D. Matkin. 1979. Speech audiometry. In W. F. Rintelmann (ed.), Hearing Assessment, pp. 133–206. University Park Press, Baltimore.

Olsen, W. O., D. Noffsinger, and S. Kurdziel. 1975. Speech discrimination in quiet and in white noise by patients with peripheral and central lesions. Acta Otolaryngol. 80:375–382.

Orchik, D. J., and N. Roddy. 1980. The SSI and NU-6 in clinical hearing aid evaluation. J. Speech Hear. Disord. 45:401–407.

Owens, E. 1978. Consonant errors and remediation in sensorineural hearing loss. J. Speech Hear. Disord. 43:331–347.

Owens, E., M. Benedict, and E. D. Schubert. 1972. Consonant phonemic errors associated with pure tone configurations and certain kinds of hearing impairment. J. Speech Hear. Res. 15:308–322.

Owens, E., and E. D. Schubert. 1968. The development of consonant items for speech discrimination testing. J. Speech. Hear. Res. 11:656–667.

Owens, E., and E. D. Schubert. 1977. Development of the California Consonant Test. J. Speech Hear. Res. 20:463–474.

Pascoe, D. P. 1975. Frequency responses of hearing aids and their effects on the speech perception of hearing-impaired subjects. Ann. Otol. Rhinol. Laryngol. 84(Suppl. 23, No. 5, Part 2):5–40.

Pederson, O. J. 1970. Some basic factors of importance for the intelligibility of speech. In C. Røjskjer (ed.), Speech Audiometry, pp. 12–27. Second Danavox Symposium, Andelsbogtrykkeriet i Odense, Denmark.

Pederson, O. T., and G. A. Studebaker. 1972. A new minimal contrasts closed-response-set speech test. J. Aud. Res. 12:187–195.

Penrod, J. P. 1979. Talker effects on word-discrimination scores of adults with sensorineural hearing impairment. J. Speech Hear. Disord. 44:340–349.

Pollack, I. 1948. Effects of high pass and low pass filtering on the intelligibility of speech in noise. J. Acoust. Soc. Am. 20:259–266.

Pollack, I. 1958. Speech intelligibility at high noise levels; effect of short term exposure. J. Acoust. Soc. Am. 30:282–285.

Pronovost, W., and C. Dumbleton. 1954. A picture-type speech sound discrimination test for children. J. Speech Hear. Res. 19:360–366.

Raffin, M. J. M., and A. R. Thornton. 1980. Confidence levels for differences between speech-discrimination scores—a research note. J. Speech Hear. Res. 23:5–18.

Resnick, D. M. 1962. Reliability of the twenty-five word phonetically balanced lists. J. Aud. Res. 2:5–12.

Resnick, S. B., J. R. Dubno, D. G. Howie, S. Hoffnung, L. Freeman, and R. M. Slosberg. 1976. Phoneme identification on a closed-response nonsense syllable test. Paper presented at the convention of the American Speech-Language-Hearing Association, November 20–23, Houston.

Rintelmann, W. F., D. R. Schumaier, A. J. Jetty, S. A. Burchfield, D. S. Beasley, N. A. Mosher, R. A. Mosher, and E. D. Penley. 1974. Six experiments on speech discrimination utilizing CNC monosyllables. J. Aud. Res. 2(Suppl.):1–30.

Rittmanic, P. A. 1962. Pure-tone masking by narrow-noise bands in normal and impaired ears. J. Aud. Res. 2:287–304.

Robinson, M., and S. Kasden. 1970. Bone conduction speech audiometry: A calibrated method to predict post-stapedectomy discrimination scores. Ann. Otol. Rhinol. Laryngol. 79:818–824.

Roe, T. G. 1965. An evaluation of the N.U. Auditory Test No. 6. Master's thesis. Vanderbilt University, Nashville, Tenn.

Rose, D. E. 1974. A 10-word speech discrimination screening test. Paper presented at the convention of the American Speech-Language-Hearing Association, November 4–6, Las Vegas.

Ross, M., D. A. Huntington, H. A. Newby, and R. F. Nixon. 1965. Speech discrimination of hearing impaired individuals in noise: Its relationship to other audiometric parameters. J. Aud. Res. 5:44–72.

Ross, M., and J. Lerman. 1970. A picture identification test for hearing impaired children. J. Speech Hear. Res. 13:44–53.

Rupp, R. R., and D. Phillips. 1969. The effect of noise background on speech discrimination function in normal hearing individuals. J. Aud. Res. 9:60–63.

Sambataro, C., and G. Pestalozza. 1952. Masking and fatigue effect of white noise in connection with speech tests. Laryngoscope 62:1197–1204.

Sanders, J. W., A. F. Josey, and M. E. Glasscock. 1974. Audiologic evaluation in cochlear and eighth nerve disorders. Arch. Otolaryngol. 100:283–289.

Sanderson-Leepa, M. E., and W. F. Rintelmann. 1976. Articulation functions and test-retest performance of normal-hearing children on three speech discrimination tests: WIPI, PBK-50, and N.U. Auditory Test No. 6. J. Speech Hear. Disord. 41:503–519.

Schubert, E. D., and E. Owens. 1971. CVC words as test items. J. Aud. Res. 11:88–100.

Schuknecht, H. F. 1954. Further observations on the pathology of presbycusis. Arch. Otolaryngol. 80:369–382.

Schultz, M. D., and E. D. Schubert. 1969. A multiple choice discrimination test (MCDT). Laryngoscope 79:382–399.

Schwartz, D. M. 1971. The usefulness of the WIPI: A speech discrimination test for preschool children. Master's thesis. Central Michigan University, Mount Pleasant, Mich.

Schwartz, D. M., F. H. Bess, and V. D. Larson. 1977. Split half reliability of two word discrimination tests as a function of primary-to-secondary ratio. J. Speech Hear. Disord. 42:440–445.

Schwartz, D. M., and R. Surr. 1979. Three experiments on the California consonant test. J. Speech Hear. Disord. 44:61–72.

Sever, J. 1973. Speech discrimination in normal hearing individuals under adverse listening conditions. Master's thesis. Central Michigan University, Mount Pleasant, Mich.

Shapiro, M. T., W. Melnick, and V. VerMeulen. 1972. Effects of modulated noise on speech intelligibility of people with sensorineural hearing loss. Ann. Otol. Rhinol. Laryngol. 81:241–248.

Shore, I., R. C. Bilger, and I. J. Hirsh. 1960. Hearing aid evaluation: Reliability of repeated measurements. J. Speech Hear. Res. 25:152–170.

Shutts, R., K. Burke, and J. Creston. 1964. Derivation of twenty-five word PB lists. J. Speech Hear. Disord. 29:442–477.

Siegenthaler, B., and G. Haspiel. 1966. Development of two standardized measures of hearing for speech by children. U.S. Department of Health, Education, and Welfare, Project No. 2372, Contract No. OE-5-10-003.

Silverman, S. R., and I. J. Hirsh. 1955. Problems related to the use of speech in clinical audiometry. Ann. Otol. Rhinol. Laryngol. 64:1234–1244.

Silverman, S. R., W. R. Thurlow, T. E. Walsh, and H. Davis. 1948. Improvement in the social adequacy of hearing following the fenestration operation. Laryngoscope 58:607–631.

Skinner, M. W. 1980. Speech intelligibility in noise-induced hearing loss: Effects of high-frequency compensation. J. Acoust. Soc. Am. 67:306–317.

Sortini, A., and C. Flake. 1953. Speech audiometry testing for pre-school children. Laryngoscope 63:991–997.

Speaks, C., and J. Jerger. 1965. Method for measurement of speech identification. J. Speech Hear. Res. 8:185–194.

Stach, B. 1979. The paired PB-50 speech discrimination test. Master's thesis. Vanderbilt University, Nashville, Tenn.

Surr, R. K. and D. M. Schwartz. 1980. Effects of multi-talker competing speech on the variability of the California Consonant Test. Ear Hear. 1:319–323.

Suter, A. H. 1978. The ability of mildly hearing-impaired individuals to discriminate speech in noise. U.S. Environmental Protection Agency, Washington, D.C.

Thompson, G., and R. Hoel. 1962. "Flat" sensorineural hearing loss and PB scores. J. Speech Hear. Disord. 27:284–287.

Thorndike, E. L., and L. Lorge. 1944, 1952. The Teacher's Word Book of 30,000 Words. Columbia University Press, New York.

Thornton, A. R., and M. J. M. Raffin. 1978. Speech discrimination scores modified as a binomial variable. J. Speech Hear. Res. 21:507–518.

Tillman, T. W. and R. Carhart. 1966. An expanded test for speech discrimination utilizing CNC monosyllabic words. Northwestern University Auditory Test No. 6. Technical Report No. SAM-TR-66-55, USAF School of Aerospace Medicine, Brooks Air Force Base, Texas.

Tillman, T. W., R. Carhart, and L. Wilber. 1963. A test for speech discrimination composed of CNC monosyllabic words. Northwestern University Auditory Test No. 4. Technical Documentary Report No. SAM-TDR-62-135, USAF School of Aerospace Medicine, Brooks Air Force Base, Texas.

Tillman, T. W., and W. O. Olsen. 1973. Speech audiometry. In J. Jerger (ed.), Modern Developments in Audiology. 2nd Ed. Academic Press, Inc., New York. pp. 37–74.

Tobias, J. 1964. On phonemic analysis of speech discrimination tests. J. Speech Hear. Res. 7:99–100.

Tobias, J. V. 1973. Effect of practice on intelligibility of masked speech. Paper presented at the 85th meeting of the Acoustical Society of America, April 10–13, Boston.

Ullrich, K., and D. Grimm. 1976. Most comfortable listening level presentation versus maximum discrimination for word discrimination material. Audiology 15:338–347.

Veterans Administration. 1976. Veterans Administration Rating procedure relative to specific issues: 50.07 rating of hearing impairment. Dept. Med. Surg. Manual. M21-1.

Weber, S., and R. C. Redell. 1976. A sentence test for measuring speech discrimination in children. Audiol. Hear. Educ. 2:25–30, 40.

Wepman, J. and W. Hass. 1969. A Spoken Word Count (Children Ages Five, Six and Seven). Language Research Association, Chicago.

White, E. B. 1952. Charlotte's Web. Harper & Row, Pubs., Inc. New York.

Wilson, M. D. 1978. Development and analysis of a simplified synthetic sentence identification test. Doctoral dissertation. Vanderbilt University, Nashville, Tenn.

Wilson, R. H., and J. K. Antablin. 1980. A picture identification task as an estimate of the word-recognition performance of nonverbal adults. J. Speech Hear. Disord. 45:223–238.

Wilson, R. H., K. E. Caley, J. L. Haenel, and K. M. Browning. 1975. Northwestern University Auditory Test No. 6: Normative and comparative intelligibility functions. J. Am. Aud. Soc. 1:221–228.

Wilson, W. R., J. M. Moore, and G. Thompson. 1976. Sound-field auditory thresholds of infants utilizing visual reinforcement audiometry (VRA). Paper presented at the convention of the American Speech-Language-Hearing Association, November 20–23, Houston.

CHAPTER 7

MEASURES OF DISCOMFORT AND MOST COMFORTABLE LOUDNESS

Donald D. Dirks and Donald E. Morgan

CONTENTS

INTRODUCTION	203
Diagnostic Applications	203
Rehabilitative Applications	204
LOUDNESS DISCOMFORT LEVEL	205
Validity	205
Reliability	207
The LDL for Speech	210
Effects of Hearing Loss on LDL	211
Clinical Use of LDL	212
MOST COMFORTABLE LOUDNESS LEVEL	217
Validity	217
Reliability	218
Stimulus Effects on MCL	220
Effects of Hearing Loss on MCL	221
Clinical Use of MCL	223
SUMMARY	225
REFERENCES	225

INTRODUCTION

The measurements of loudness discomfort level (LDL) and most comfortable listening level (MCL) have been advocated both for the diagnostic and rehabilitative assessment of patients with hearing loss. The LDL, sometimes referred to as the threshold of discomfort, threshold of tolerance, or uncomfortable loudness level, is generally defined as the sound pressure level (SPL) above which a listener reports that an auditory stimulus is uncomfortably loud. The MCL, as the nomenclature suggests, defines the intensity-level at which the loudness of an auditory stimulus is considered to be at a comfortable listening level. Practically, the results from MCL measurements reflect a range of levels within which stimuli may be described as comfortably loud. Audiologic textbooks historically have recommended the implementation of these subjective measurements, but only recently have the validity and reliability of both the LDL and MCL been explored systematically.

Diagnostic Applications

Both the MCL and LDL measurements have been proposed as indirect measures of the anatomical site of auditory impairment. The logic suggests that a limited dynamic range (difference between the threshold of hearing and the LDL) implies the presence of loudness recruitment, thus indicating a cochlear disorder. In his development of a hearing aid selection procedure, Watson (1944) was one of the earliest investigators to suggest that a narrow range of comfortable loudness or a reduced range between threshold and uncomfortable listening levels indicated the presence of loudness recruitment. Subsequent use of the LDL as a diagnostic test was infrequent, however, until the reports of Hood and Poole (1966) and Bosatra (1969) revived interest in the diagnostic application of the measurement. The use of the MCL as a diagnostic test has been suggested by Hinchcliffe (1971) and Jerger and Jerger (1974). However, substantive documentation of the application of the MCL as a diagnostic test is absent. Neither the LDL nor the MCL has gained widespread diagnostic use because of the large intersubject variability reported for these measurements (Kamm, Dirks, and Mickey, 1978; Stephens, Blegvad, and Krogh, 1977). Because intersubject variability does not necessarily detract from use of a measurement in a rehabilitative evaluation, however, the LDL and MCL may have a greater applicability in such assessments.

Rehabilitative Applications

The measurement of LDL and MCL has been used more commonly for rehabilitative purposes. Specifically, in hearing aid evaluations, the LDL has been suggested as an estimate of the maximum saturation sound pressure level (SSPL) for an amplification system. As such, the measure defines an upper limit beyond which amplified sound is uncomfortable for the listener (Berger, Rane, and Hagberg, 1979; Dirks and Kamm, 1976; Kamm et al., 1978; McCandless and Miller, 1972; Shapiro, 1975, 1976).

The MCL also has been applied to the assessment of hearing aid characteristics. For example, it has been used to estimate the optimal acoustic gain for amplification (Erber and Alencewicz, 1976; Markle and Zaner, 1966; Shapiro, 1976; Ventry and Johnson, 1978). Additionally, several investigators have suggested that the MCL be used in the evaluation of the adequacy of a specific hearing aid (Carhart, 1946; Kopra and Blosser, 1968; Watson, 1944). The specific application in these evaluation procedures typically requires that the volume control of a hearing aid be adjusted by the patient until a "comfortable level" is obtained, given a constant input signal (Carhart, 1946).

Despite widespread recommendations for the clinical use of both comfort and discomfort loudness measures in hearing aid evaluation procedures, the reliability and validity of the LDL and MCL have been questioned repeatedly. These questions have developed from several factors, including the apparent poor reliability associated with interstudy differences in LDL and MCL, and the inherent instability of the subjective criteria required in making MCL and LDL judgments. In this chapter, the major results from experiments of the LDL and MCL will be reviewed, focusing on both the potential use and limitations of each measurement. The subsequent discussion of the LDL and MCL, however, is not restricted to the use of speech stimuli. An understanding of the potential clinical applicability as well as the limitations of these two measures necessitates consideration of tonal and noise signals in addition to speech stimuli.

LOUDNESS DISCOMFORT LEVEL

Validity

A critical problem in any measure of loudness discomfort or tolerance level is the validity of the measurement; that is, whether or not the judgment is made principally on the basis of the loudness experience. Several experiments (Morgan, Wilson and Dirks, 1974; Morgan and Dirks, 1974) were conducted at the UCLA Laboratory to investigate the validity of the LDL as a loudness measure; one of which is detailed here. The LDL was obtained for pure tone stimuli at octave frequencies between 125 and 4000 Hz, and for two bands of noise (a broadband noise and a band of noise 400 Hz wide centered at 1000 Hz). These stimuli were chosen because there is considerable evidence available concerning their relative loudness. It was anticipated that LDL measured as a function of frequency would generally reflect the patterns reported from equal loudness contour data. Subjects were nine young normal listeners, sophisticated in the LDL task. Several repetitions of the LDL judgment were obtained from each subject using the method of constants, with stimuli of 300 msec duration repeated once every 2 sec.

The results in Figure 7-1 show that the LDLs were obtained at essentially identical SPLs (~108 dB) at 1000, 2000, and 4000 Hz. Below 1000 Hz the LDL increased substantially; in fact, for some subjects, LDL could not be measured within the limits of the equipment for tones at 125 Hz. Especially in the low frequencies, the results of the LDL deviate substantially from the typical equal loudness contours obtained at such high intensities. (A similar frequency effect also has been reported by Hawkins and Smith, 1979). These deviations are related to the differences between the sound pressure measured on a NBS-9A coupler during calibration and that actually generated in the ear of a subject when the supra-aural earphone and cushion are coupled

206   Dirks and Morgan

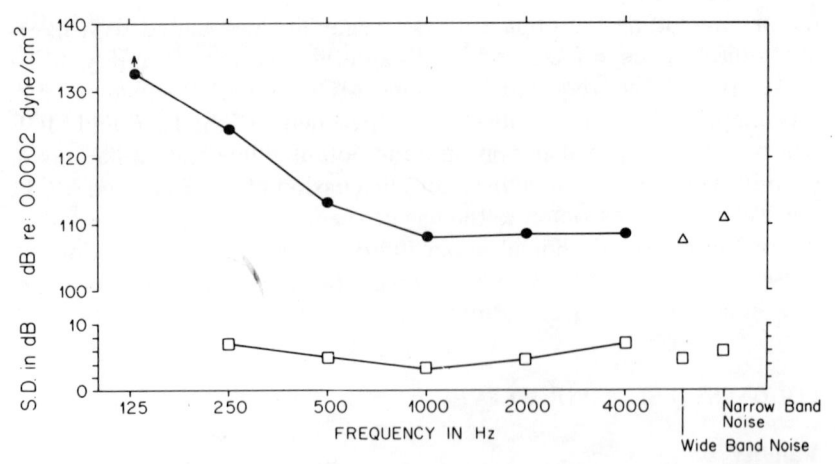

Figure 7-1. Means and standard deviations for LDL in dB SPL for six pure tones and two bands of noise. (From Morgan et al., 1974; reproduced with permission.)

to the head. As reported by Shaw (1966) there is a substantial decrease in the sound pressure actually generated in the ear canal for frequencies below 500 Hz as compared with that measured in a standard coupler. In order to account for the coupler-real ear differences, Morgan and Dirks (1974) applied a correction (derived from the real ear and coupler measurements reported by Shaw, 1966) to their mean LDL data. The corrected LDL and the equal loudness curves of Robinson and Dadson (1956) are plotted in Figure 7-2. The corrected results suggest that the LDLs closely follow the pattern established for equal loudness judgments.

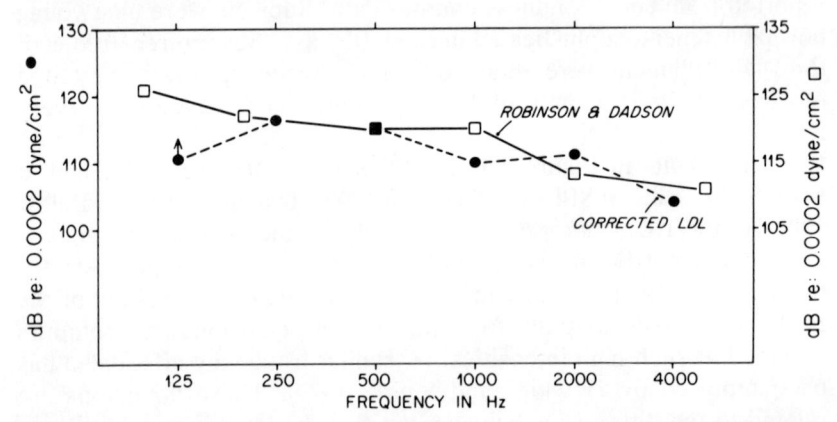

Figure 7-2. Mean "corrected" LDL in dB SPL compared with equal-loudness contour results of Robinson and Dadson (1956). (From Morgan et al., 1974; reproduced with permission.)

Now consider the LDL results for the bands of noise presented in Figure 7-1. The report of Zwicker, Flottorp, and Stevens (1957) indicates that equal loudness between a broadband noise and a narrow band noise centered at 1000 Hz occurs at an intensity discrepancy of 4 to 7 dB. In Figure 7-1, the LDL for broadband noise was 107 dB SPL, whereas for narrow band noise the LDL was measured at 111 dB SPL, a difference of 4 dB.

These results, together with those for pure tones, suggest that the relationship among the stimuli for LDL measurements approximates that observed for other measures of loudness. This observation leads to the conclusion that the LDL can be considered principally a loudness experience, at least under the conditions of the experiments noted above.

Reliability

Several factors have been identified as influencing the reliability of the LDL. Specifically, such variables as subject response criteria, psychophysical method of measurement, and parametric characteristics of the stimuli employed will be discussed in detail.

Instructions The measurement of the LDL is fundamentally dependent on the instructions used. In recognition of this fact, in most experiments, the instructions are devised purposely to dictate the desired response criterion. There is no uniform set of instructions agreed upon by investigators and clinicians, and the response instructions have ranged from defining the level at which a sound is considered initially uncomfortable (Berger, 1976; Hood and Poole, 1966; McCandless, 1973) to extremely uncomfortable (Holmes and Woodford, 1977; Silverman, 1947; Wallenfels, 1967). Several investigators (McCandless and Miller, 1972; Ritter, 1978) have demonstrated that when a group of subjects is given a series of different instructional sets, systematic changes in the LDL are observed.

The effects of instructional set on the LDL are confounded by apparent changes in the response criterion with repeated trials or exposures to loud sound. Silverman (1947) demonstrated a systematic elevation in the threshold of discomfort among subjects exposed to high intensity speech for only several minutes a day over a 3- to 4-week period. He concluded that such an exposure paradigm resulted in a systematic elevation in the threshold of discomfort. Results from a study by Morgan and Dirks (1974) also suggest that the LDL may be elevated for normal listeners with repeated high intensity exposures. Figure 7-3 shows the changes in LDL over repeated test sessions for six subjects under a variety of presentation and stimulus conditions. The method of constant stimuli was used to obtain the results, with

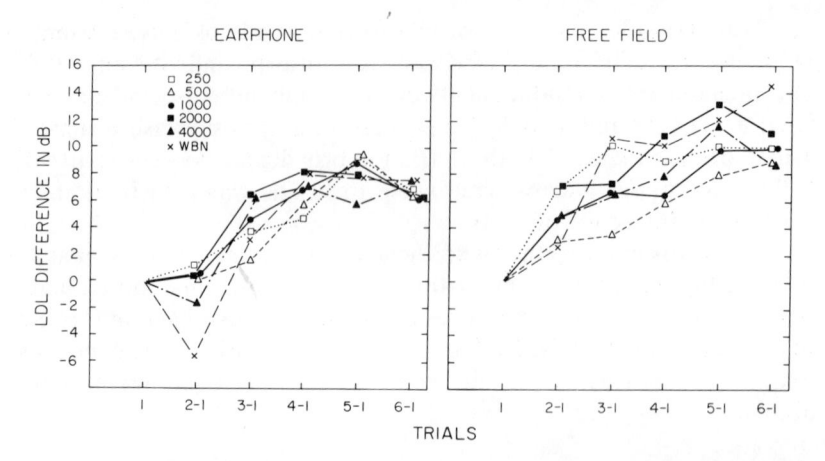

Figure 7-3. Mean LDL difference in dB between trial 1 and each successive trial over six trials for earphone and free-field LDL measurements. (From Morgan et al., 1974; reproduced with permission.)

each estimate of LDL determined from 60 stimulus presentations. Thus, each subject received numerous exposures to high intensity stimuli during the several weeks of testing. The general pattern observed for stimuli under earphones and in the free field reveals a systematic increase of 6 to 8 dB in the level at which the LDL was obtained during the initial four test runs. Thereafter, the LDL reached an asymptotic level for a majority of the stimuli. The results are in agreement with Silverman's earlier report suggesting that a subject's response criterion for LDL can be affected during the course of a lengthy experiment.

In an attempt to investigate the contention that LDL can be elevated through exposure to loud sounds, Schmitz (1969) exposed 20 subjects with sensorineural hearing loss to high intensity speech at regular intervals over 3- or 4-week periods. No change in the level of discomfort was observed for these patients. Whether or not the LDL for individuals with sensorineural hearing loss can be raised by systematic exposure to loud sounds is not yet resolved.

In view of the fact that a subject's response criteria may change over the course of experimental sessions, it is imperative that the instructions be maintained constant throughout an experiment. Any comparisons of results of LDL measures among different groups of investigators are meaningful only if similar instructions are used or changes due to the different instructions can be assessed adequately.

Psychophysical Method The psychophysical methods used for determination of the LDL vary widely among investigators and clinicians. In two studies (Morgan et al. 1974; Stephens and Anderson, 1971) the effects of several psychophysical procedures on the LDL were compared systematically. For naive listeners, Stephens and Anderson observed that LDLs were consistently measured at higher SPLs when Bekesy tracking procedures were used as compared with a manual ascending method of limits. Little or no difference in LDL was observed with these techniques when experienced listeners were subjects. Morgan et al. (1974) found that tracking and constant stimuli methods resulted in similar LDL judgments for tests repeated during six separate sessions. However, a method of adjustment initially yielded lower LDLs than the other methods, but with repeated judgments, the LDL increased. Because of the higher reliability of the method of constant stimuli, this procedure was used in several of the early laboratory studies at UCLA. However, this method is time-consuming and not conveniently adapted for use in a clinic setting.

In more recent experiments (Dirks and Kamm, 1976; Kamm et al., 1978) the simple up-down adaptive procedure for estimating the 50 percent point on the psychometric function (Levitt, 1971) was found to be especially useful in measuring the LDL. With appropriate procedural modifications (transformed up-down procedures), other points (29.3 and 70.7 percent) on the LDL response curve also can be estimated. By way of illustration, Figure 7-4 shows one data record in which the simple up-down procedure was used for obtaining LDL.

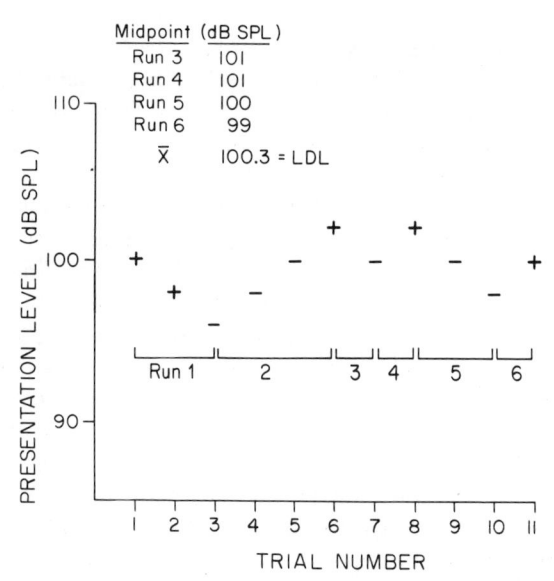

Figure 7-4. Illustration of a data record for obtaining the LDL using the simple up-down adaptive procedure.

Presentation level of the stimulus is plotted on the ordinate and the test run is on the abscissa. The starting level is determined using 10-dB steps ascending from a SPL of ≈50 or 60 dB until a positive response (stimulus is considered uncomfortable) is reported. Each such presentation (and subsequent judgment) constitutes a trial. In the example the starting level was 100 dB SPL. Because the first response was positive (+), the next stimulus was lowered 2 dB. The response was positive again but on the third presentation (96 dB SPL) the subject indicated the stimulus was comfortable (−). The direction of intensity change of the stimulus was reversed (that is, the stimulus was increased by 2 dB) to begin the second test run. A run consists of a series of trials between two consecutive reversals. To obtain stable results and precise estimates, a complete test ordinarily consists of six runs. The initial two reversals are eliminated from the derivation of the LDL estimate in order to reduce bias due to the initial stimulus level. The midpoints of the last four runs are averaged for the estimation of the 50 percent point on the psychometric function. The potential implementation of adaptive procedures in audiology has been thoroughly reviewed by Levitt (1978). The measurement of the LDL and MCL seem ideally suited for adaptive procedures and can be implemented successfully in the clinic using score sheets (as suggested in Figure 7-4) to record the sequential judgments of a subject.

The LDL for Speech

We already have indicated several sources (response criterion, psychophysical method, and stimulus frequency and bandwidth) that may affect the SPL at which the LDL is measured. Because speech is the signal of significance in most communication settings, there has been an understandable interest in the determination of the LDL for speech stimuli. Several experiments (Morgan et al., 1979) were conducted at UCLA to measure the LDL for a variety of representative speech samples. The stimuli were 24 nonsense syllables containing consonant-vowel-consonant clusters and for comparison a speech spectrum and wideband noise. The method of constant stimuli was used to obtain the LDL. Results for 11 normal listeners are shown in Figure 7-5. Despite differences in the duration and other physical characteristics of these speech samples, the LDL was consistently measured at levels of ≈100 dB SPL. These tests were not conducted over long periods of time and therefore, the changes that may be observed with repeated exposure (see Figure 7-3) were absent. This fact explains the lower LDL (re: the data of Figure 7-1) and the comparability to the levels reported by Hood and Poole (1966).

In a subsequent experiment, spondaic words and sentence materials were used as stimuli (Morgan et al., 1979). The LDL remained essentially the same as observed with the nonsense syllables (see Figure 7-5). A similar finding also was reported by Edgerton, Beattie, and Cager (1978) for normal and sensorineural hearing loss listeners. Those investigators measured LDL for a variety of speech stimuli, including running speech, spondaic words, and monosyllables. In that study, as well as the Morgan et al. (1979) experiment, the intensity of the speech stimuli was specified by measurement of the SPL of a 1000-Hz calibration tone, the intensity of which resulted in the same volume unit (VU) meter reading as the transient peak energy of the various speech stimuli. Given the limitations of this calibration procedure, the LDL was obtained at similar SPLs for various types of speech stimuli, and at levels comparable to those measured for pure tones within the speech frequency range (Dirks and Kamm, 1976; Hood and Poole, 1966).

Effects of Hearing Loss on LDL

As previously noted, Silverman (1947) was among the earliest investigators to compare discomfort levels between normal and hearing-impaired listeners. His early work and the report of Davis et al. (1946) were investigative sources for the initial clinical assumptions that: 1) LDLs were quite high for all individuals (>120 dB SPL); 2) hearing loss subjects had higher LDLs than normal-hearing subjects; and 3) "practice" resulted in significant increases in the measured tolerance level. Specifically, Silverman's (1947) results indicated that the discomfort level for normal listeners rose from 109.9 dB SPL during the initial test session to 120 dB SPL during the sixth (final) test session.

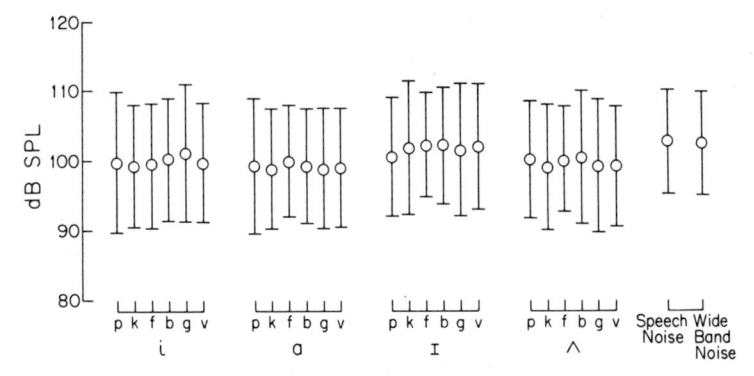

Figure 7-5. Mean LDL (o) and standard deviations (I) in dB SPL for 24 CVC clusters, speech spectrum and wide-band noise stimuli. (From Morgan et al., 1979; reproduced with permission.)

The hearing-impaired subjects revealed discomfort levels for pure tones which rose from 118.4 to 129.5 dB SPL between the first and sixth sessions. We previously have alluded to the importance of the effects of instructions and method of procedure on the measured LDL. Of even greater significance in understanding these early data is the fact that Silverman's hearing-impaired subjects included individuals with conductive lesions. Hood and Poole (1966) observed that subjects with conductive or nerve VIII impairments have substantially higher LDLs than normal listeners or those with cochlear disorders.

Between the early reports (Davis et al., 1946; Silverman, 1947) and that of Hood and Poole (1966), there were no published investigations of the LDL among normal or hearing-impaired individuals. The literature throughout this 2-decade period, therefore, reflects the conclusion drawn by Silverman and Davis et al., although clinical experience with subjects having sensorineural hearing loss surely must have implied that many individuals experienced discomfort at levels well below 120 dB SPL. In fact, after the report of Hood and Poole, 1966, subsequent LDL investigations comparing normal listeners to those with sensorineural (primarily cochlear) hearing loss have revealed that in many instances the LDLs are nearly equivalent among the two populations.

Recently, the LDL was measured for three stimulus conditions (500 Hz, 2000 Hz, and spondaic words) on 178 ears of 103 patients with well documented sensorineural hearing loss (Kamm et al., 1978). Figure 7-6 shows scatter plots of the individual LDL data. The curve of best fit drawn through the data were nonlinear least square functions. The data for 2000 Hz (middle of the figure) are, in general, representative of the results. Notice that the LDLs at 2000 Hz remain relatively constant for subjects with hearing loss less than 50 dB HL and then increase gradually as the hearing loss increases above 50 dB.

Although there is substantial variability in the LDL among individuals with the same amount of hearing loss, the results of Figure 7-6 demonstrate a nonlinear relationship between LDL and magnitude of the hearing loss. Because of the large intersubject variability, the results imply that the LDL cannot be predicted with high accuracy from the magnitude of the hearing loss and thus the LDL needs to be measured directly.

Clinical Use of LDL

LDL and Acoustic Reflex Threshold There has been interest in the prediction of LDL from measures of the acoustic reflex threshold (ART). In particular, McCandless and Miller (1972) suggested that the LDL could be predicted from ART measurements. Efforts to corro-

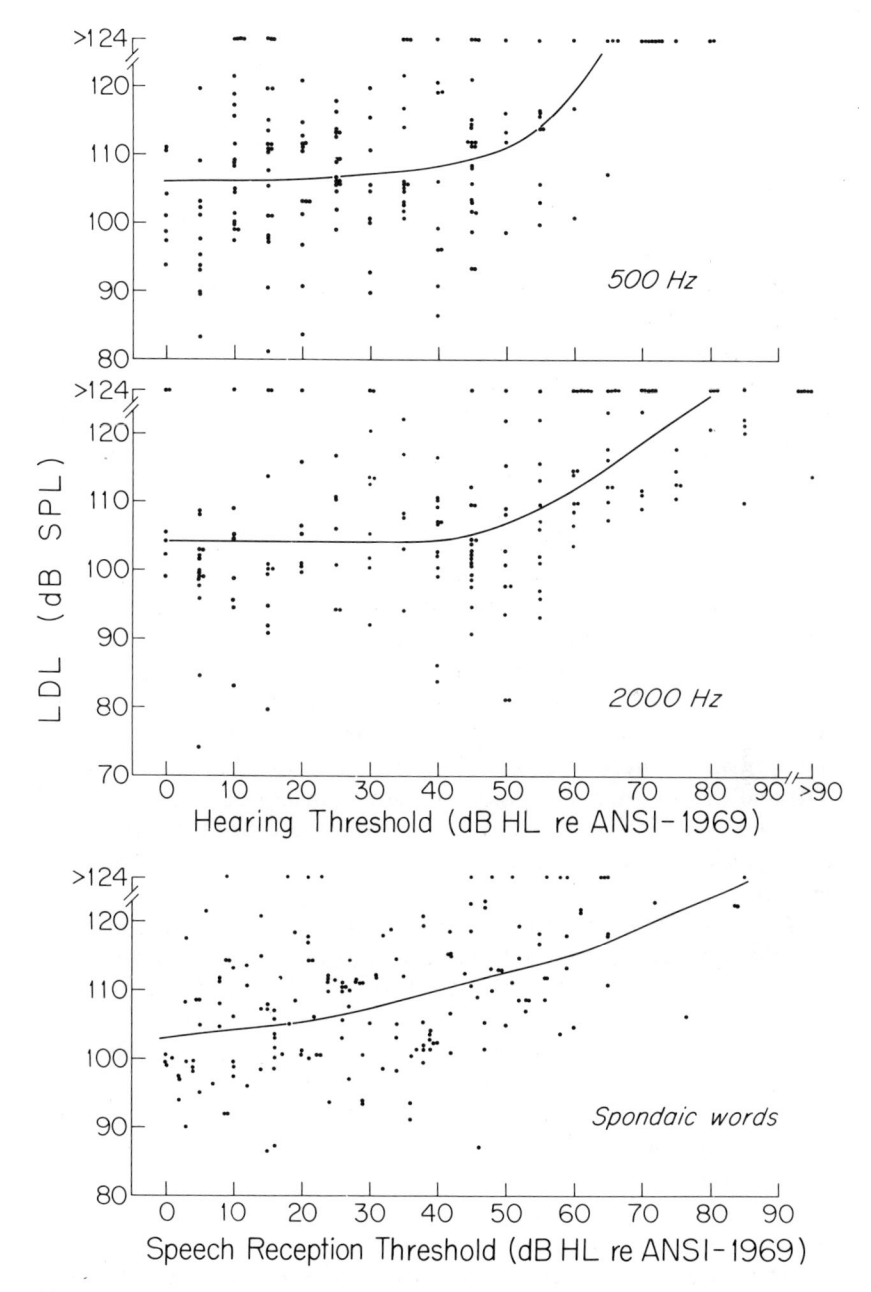

Figure 7-6. Scatter plots of individual data and computer-generated best fit curves for LDL as a function of hearing threshold for 500 Hz, 2000 Hz, and spondaic words. (From Kamm et al., 1978; reproduced with permission.)

borate their results for both normal listeners (Denenberg and Altschuler, 1976; Olson and Hipskind, 1973) and individuals with sensorineural hearing loss (Berger et al., 1979; Denenberg and Altschuler, 1976; Holmes and Woodford, 1977; Woodford and Holmes, 1977) have indicated that the difference between the two measures is characterized by wide intersubject variability. Data from Morgan et al. (1979) also demonstrated that, whereas mean differences between LDL and ART are relatively constant for several different stimuli, there is a very low correlation between the two measures. That is, the rank order of subjects on the LDL is so different from their order on ART, that one measure cannot be predicted from the other. Similar findings were also observed by Ritter (1978) in a comprehensive study of the relationship between LDL and ART on both normal and hearing-impaired listeners. These results, then, suggest that the application of a procedure to predict LDL from ART is unwarranted.

From several sets of data, recent investigators (Margolis and Popelka, 1975; Popelka, Margolis and Wiley, 1976; Scharf, 1976) have concluded that the differences between acoustic reflex and loudness characteristics preclude a simple explanation of the acoustic reflex as a direct corollary of loudness. The generally poor relationship between the LDL and ART in the previously mentioned experiments is additional evidence that loudness measures and acoustic reflex threshold measures are not direct corollaries. The objective measurement of the LDL remains a desirable goal; however, the variables affecting the LDL and the absence of a predictable relationship between LDL and ART make prediction of one measure from the other clinically inappropriate. Thus, when the LDL is of clinical interest, it should be measured directly.

LDL and SSPL It often is recommended that the LDL be used clinically for specifying the saturation sound pressure level for a hearing aid (see Alpiner, 1975; Berger, 1971; Ross, 1978; as examples). The LDL data of Morgan and Dirks (1974) taken under earphone and in free-field conditions suggest that there are several problems to be considered regarding the relationship between LDL and SSPL.

Figure 7-7 includes average LDL results as a function of stimulus frequency for conditions of earphone and free field listening. The data are from normal listeners. The LDL was observed at lower SPLs for the free field than for the earphone presentation, although the absolute difference in LDL varied as a function of frequency.

The observed difference in the LDL between earphone and free field may be explained on the basis of the known differences between conventional calibration procedures and the SPL actually occurring at the eardrum as measured by probe tube methods. Morgan and Dirks

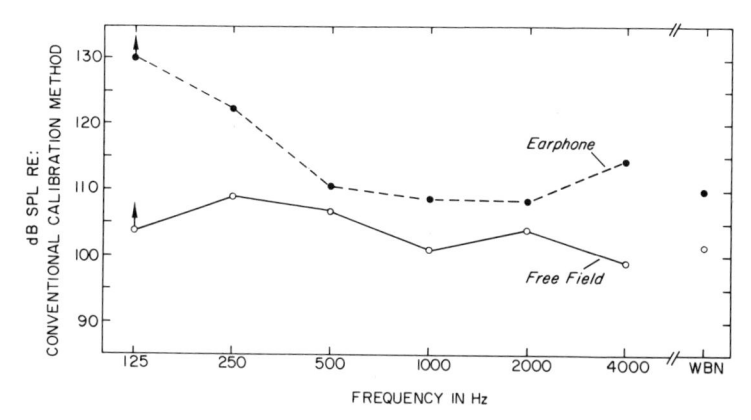

Figure 7-7. Mean LDL in dB SPL for normal listeners re the conventional calibration method for free field and earphone conditions at octave frequencies between 125 and 4000 Hz and for a wide-band white noise stimulus. (From Morgan and Dirks, 1974; reproduced with permission.)

(1974) determined the SPL in the ear canal for both the earphone and loudspeaker presentation conditions, using a probe microphone located at the entrance to the ear canal. The decibel difference between the standard calibration intensity level and the probe tube measurement intensity level was then applied to the LDL results. The corrected data are shown in Figure 7-8. Except for some inaccuracy at 4000 Hz, there is no difference between LDLs obtained under earphones or in the sound field when real ear measures are used to specify signal SPLs. However, the difference in LDL between earphone and free field, shown in Figure 7-7, will be observed when the signal level is specified by conventional calibration procedures.

Clinically, it often is desirable to determine the LDL under earphone and, from that measurement, to specify the SSPL for a hearing

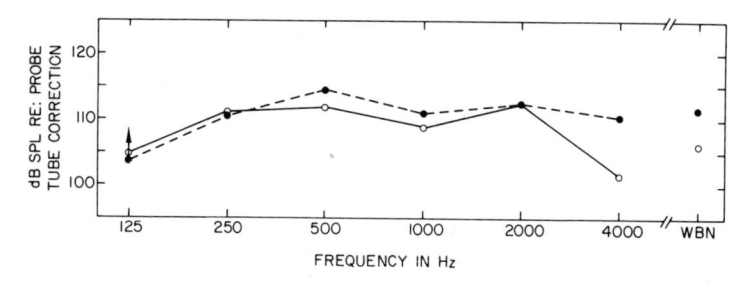

Figure 7-8. Mean LDL for free field and earphone conditions in dB SPL corrected by the relative difference in dB derived from loudness balance data on same subjects as reported in Figure 7-7. (From Morgan and Dirks, 1974; reproduced with permission.)

aid (for example, Shapiro, 1976). There would be a direct relationship between measurements of LDL and SSPL if one could specify the difference in SPL generated at the eardrum under the earphone and under the hearing aid receiver/earmold.

Typically, the earphone is calibrated in a 6 cm^3 coupler. At least between the frequencies of 400 and 2000 Hz, the coupler SPL accurately reflects that developed at the eardrum under the earphone. However, the hearing aid is calibrated, typically, in a 2 cm^3 coupler. The SPL developed in the 2 cm^3 coupler is known to deviate substantially in SPL from that measured at the eardrum of an "average" human ear (Lybarger, 1975; Sachs and Burkhard, 1972). Recently, Zwislocki (1970) has reported the development of an ear simulator, which more closely approximates the "average" human ear response. Unfortunately, no standard coupler provides a method of determining the physical changes imposed by the earmold when the hearing aid receiver is coupled to the earmold and the entire "system" is coupled to an individual's ear. In fact, recent evidence (Egolf, Tree, and Feth, 1978; Gilman, 1979) demonstrates that the effect of individual ear impedance, ear canal geometry, hearing aid receiver impedance, and earmold characteristics all interact in complex ways to determine the SPL delivered to the eardrum of a patient. As a consequence, deciding on the SSPL of a hearing aid from earphone or even loudspeaker LDL measurements is not yet straightforward.

Average corrections can be made for the apparent difference in SPL between earphone and sound field conditions, but as yet we cannot accurately estimate, for the individual case, the changes in SPL imposed by the receiver-earmold combination when coupled to the individual ear. That is, we can specify the level (dB SPL; re: a standard calibration procedure) at which the LDL occurs, as well as the SSPL of a hearing aid in a standard coupler, but we cannot specify empirically the SPL at which the LDL occurs when the hearing aid is worn by an individual. Therefore, those procedures suggesting that specification of hearing aid characteristics (measured in a standard coupler) be made on the basis of measurements either under earphone (6 cm^3 coupler calibration) or in the sound field (substitution method calibration) will not result in an accurate determination of the SPL at the eardrum when the hearing aid is worn.

Two reports (Cox, 1981; Hawkins, 1980) have been published recently suggesting clinical methods for specifying the LDL under calibration conditions comparable to those used for specifying the characteristics of a hearing aid. Specifically, each method employs a standard insert receiver coupled to a specified tubing length. The receiver-tubing combination is then calibrated in a standard HA-2 coupler, the same coupler currently in use for specifying hearing aid characteristics. Loudness discomfort levels for an individual subject are determined by delivering the test signals to the insert receiver coupled to the subject's own earmold and tubing. In this manner, the measured LDL can be converted directly into equivalent HA-2 coupler intensity levels. Because the SSPL characteristics of a hearing aid are specified from HA-2 coupler measurements, this method provides a more direct measurement of the effects of earmold tubing influences on the LDL than can be predicted from either earphone or loudspeaker LDL measurements. More importantly, this method provides a directly comparable calibration procedure for specification of the LDL of the subject and SSPL of a hearing aid.

Two notable variables are not completely accounted for in the methods of Cox (1981) and Hawkins (1980). First, as identified by Cox (1981), there are differences between the impedance of the standard insert receiver and the impedances of the various hearing aid receivers employed among available hearing aids. The effects of the impedance differences will vary depending on the load to which the individual receiver is coupled. Second, ear canal geometry and middle ear impedance will vary from subject to subject. Thus, it is not possible to account for 1) the effects of individual ear load differences on the delivered SPL under the standard receiver condition and 2) the effects on each of the various hearing aids that might be employed during a clinical evaluation session.

Until procedures are developed to account in the individual case for the interactive effects of individual ear impedance, ear canal geometry, hearing aid receiver impedance, and earmold characteristics, one must demonstrate empirically that an adequate, although unspecifiable SSPL has been chosen. This complex problem notwithstanding, the LDL measurement provides the clinician with a definitive measure of the target SSPL for the hearing aid.

MOST COMFORTABLE LOUDNESS LEVEL

Validity

Despite widespread recommendation for the use of the MCL as a clinical measure in quantifying the gain characteristics of a hearing aid, the systematic study of the MCL has been limited. Ventry and Johnson (1978) recently considered the problem of validity by noting there are "no standards, no criteria against which MCL measures can be compared" (p. 156). They, and other investigators, depend on content validity established by a "rational, logical examination of the components or contents of a test to insure that these components are suitable for the measurements . . . in question" (Ventry and Johnson, 1978, p. 156). The first comprehensive study of comfort listening levels for pure tone stimuli was described by Pollack (1952). Results of that study established the overall similarity in interfrequency relationships between comfort levels and equal loudness contours at moderate intensity levels for normal-hearing subjects. Byrne and Christen have investigated the relationship between MCLs and 60-phon equal loudness judgments for narrow band stimuli (Christen and Byrne, in press); and between MCLs (for speech) and the calculated loudness of complex signals (Byrne and Christen, 1979). The conclusion in each report is that MCL depends fundamentally on the loudness of the signal. From these observations it may be inferred that judgments of comfortable listening levels are in general agreement with other loudness measurements at comparable sound pressure levels.

Reliability

As with the LDL measurement, the MCL is affected by such variables as response criteria (i.e., instructions), psychophysical method of measurement, and parametric characteristics of the stimuli employed. The capability to quantify the individual contribution of each of these variables on the overall reliability of the measure of MCL is limited, however, by the overriding influence of a more fundamental characteristic of the MCL. Specifically, in contrast to the LDL, which (depending on the instructions employed) may be defined within a very restricted intensity range, the MCL encompasses a broad range of intensities within which a stimulus will be considered "comfortably loud." Evidence of the existence of a comfortable loudness range can be extrapolated from early reports, but only recently has enjoyed widespread recognition. Pollack (1952) was perhaps the first to report a "range of comfortable listening levels" based upon measures of the upper and lower limits an individual will accept as comfortable. The observed ranges for normal-hearing subjects varied from $\approx$20 dB at low test frequencies to $\approx$35 dB in the middle frequency region. Subsequently, Berger and Lowry (1971) concluded that the MCL should be considered a range of intensities.

A recent systematic attempt to quantify the range of intensities limiting the MCL was reported by Dirks and Kamm (1976). These investigators described the range of comfortable listening levels from the psychometric functions for most comfortable loudness using several adaptive strategies. The MCL results demonstrated two distinct functions, one with a positive slope and a second with a negative slope. Mean results from three normal listeners for 500- and 2000-Hz tones and for spondaic words are shown in Figure 7-9. For function A, the probability of a MCL judgment increased with stimulus intensity as the subject discriminated levels softer than MCL from those in the general MCL range. For function B, the probability for most comfortable loudness judgments decreased as stimulus intensity increased until LDL was approached. The appearance of the two functions may be due to a change in the internal reference criteria of subjects produced by the direction (increasing or decreasing) of the intensity increment after the subjects' initial most comfortable loudness judgment. Thus, function A may represent a lower bound, whereas function B may be considered an upper bound for MCL. The upper and lower limits for the MCL encompassed a range of ≈20 dB. Other investigators have reported similar or larger ranges of comfort listening for normal listeners (Pollack, 1952; Woods, Ventry, and Gatling, 1973) and patients with sensorineural hearing loss (Ventry and Johnson, 1978).

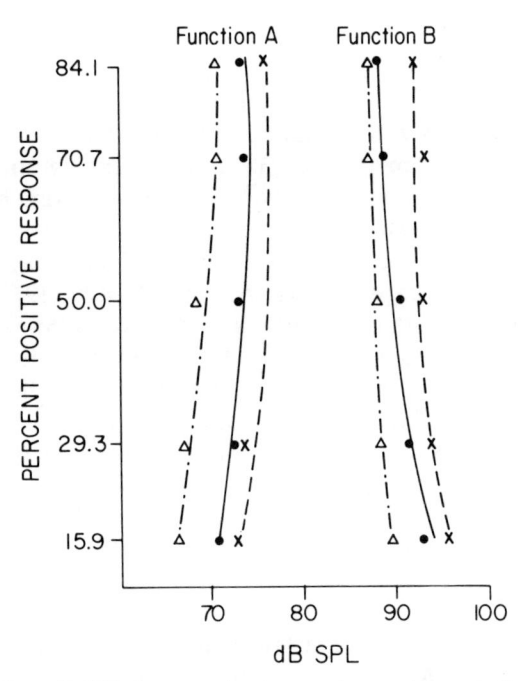

Figure 7-9. Mean dB SPL for several points on the psychometric functions for MCL. Results are from three normal listeners for 500 (×) and 2000 Hz (○) tones and for spondaic words (△). (From Dirks and Kamm, 1976; reproduced with permission.)

These observations that the MCL represents a range of intensities, as opposed to a specific intensity level, provide some insight into the historic observation that MCL judgments are characterized by wide intersubject variability. Early investigators directed subjects to choose a single level as MCL. Unquestionably, some of the variability in MCL measures must be due to the dilemma forced upon the subject who is required to choose the most comfortable level, when any one of several intensities in a range will meet the suggested criterion. This fact probably contributes to the high variability reported by investigators who have not specified the MCL as a range (Hochberg, 1975; Kopra and Blosser, 1968; Ventry et al., 1971). However, even investigators cognizant of this concept have reported high inter- and intrasubject variability for comfort level measurement (Kamm et al., 1978; Stephens et al., 1977; Ventry and Johnson, 1978).

Clearly, the recent results suggest the MCL must be viewed as a range of levels over which an individual will judge a stimulus to be comfortably loud. Reliability will be affected by the instructions to the subject, but no reports conclude that the MCL will be characterized by the same level of stability observed for other suprathreshold loudness measures.

Stimulus Effects on MCL

Because adequate speech reception is of primary concern in the rehabilitation of persons with sensorineural hearing loss, the MCL often is measured with speech stimuli (Martin and Pennington, 1971). The choice of the speech stimulus has varied among experimenters. When judgments of MCL are desired for connected discourse, the speech material recorded from a radio broadcast ("Top of the News" by Fulton Lewis, Jr.) often is used (Berger and Lowry, 1971; Ventry et al., 1971). In other instances (Dirks and Kamm, 1976; Kamm et al., 1978; Ventry and Johnson, 1978) in which a response is required for each stimulus presentation, spondaic words have been chosen because of their homogeneity and availability in tape and disc recorded form. When speech is used to obtain MCL, intersubject variability is large, but no greater than that reported using pure tones.

Ventry et al. (1971) indicated that the MCL for connected discourse is found at a SPL similar to that for a 1000-Hz tone for normal listeners, whereas Berger and Lowry (1971) and Dirks and Kamm (1976) have observed differences between MCL levels for speech and tonal stimuli. Dirks and Kamm (1976) found statistically significant differences between MCLs for speech and tones using the adaptive procedure as described previously. Recall that Figure 7-9 shows psychometric functions for MCL-A and -B for these stimuli. Although there is some disagreement about the interpretation (Ventry, 1977), these results are considered to be consistent with expected effects of loudness summation. To explain, Zwicker et al. (1957) demonstrated that loudness increases as stimulus bandwidth increases (provided the critical bandwidth has been exceeded) and that the amount of loudness summation is dependent on intensity. In the Dirks and Kamm (1976) investigation, a wide-band stimulus, such as speech, would be expected to be judged louder than a pure tone of the same intensity. Thus, judgments of comfortable loudness would be made at slightly lower SPLs for speech than for pure tone stimuli, the result observed in those data. The fact that the difference between results for speech and tonal stimuli diminished with increases in intensity is supported by the Zwicker et al. (1957) data, which demonstrates more summation for stimuli at SPLs between ≈40 dB and 80 dB than for stimuli above or below this range. At higher intensities at which LDL is found, the differences could be small, as reported earlier in this chapter. The relative SPLs at which speech and tonal MCLs are observed is controversial because the physical specification of speech is usually established in reference to a 1000-Hz calibration tone whose root mean squared (rms) level corresponds to the peaks or other characteristics of the speech; whereas, the rms level of tonal stimuli is measured directly. These issues complicate the relationship and have been discussed elsewhere (Dirks and Kamm, 1977).

Finally, large intersubject variability characterizes the MCL for both speech and tonal stimuli (Shapiro, 1975; Ventry and Johnson, 1978). As a result the MCL cannot be predicted accurately from the measured hearing threshold but requires direct measurement when used to determine gain in hearing aid evaluation procedures.

Effects of Hearing Loss on MCL

MCL measurements obtained from subjects with sensorineural hearing loss generally have been observed at higher SPLs than those obtained from normal-hearing subjects (Dirks and Kamm, 1976; Kamm et al., 1978; Martin, Stevenson, and Grover, 1978; Shapiro, 1975; Ventry and Johnson, 1978). Figure 7-10 includes data from 38 subjects with sensorineural hearing loss. The figure summarizes MCL ranges, threshold of hearing, and LDL. The MCL results are best-fit functions derived from estimates of the 50 percent points on the ascending (MCL-A) and descending (MCL-B) psychometric function. As observed by several investigators, the range of most comfortable listening levels does not divide the auditory space equally between threshold and LDL. Rather, the most comfortable listening range lies somewhat closer to the LDL than to threshold. The data indicate that the intensities defining the

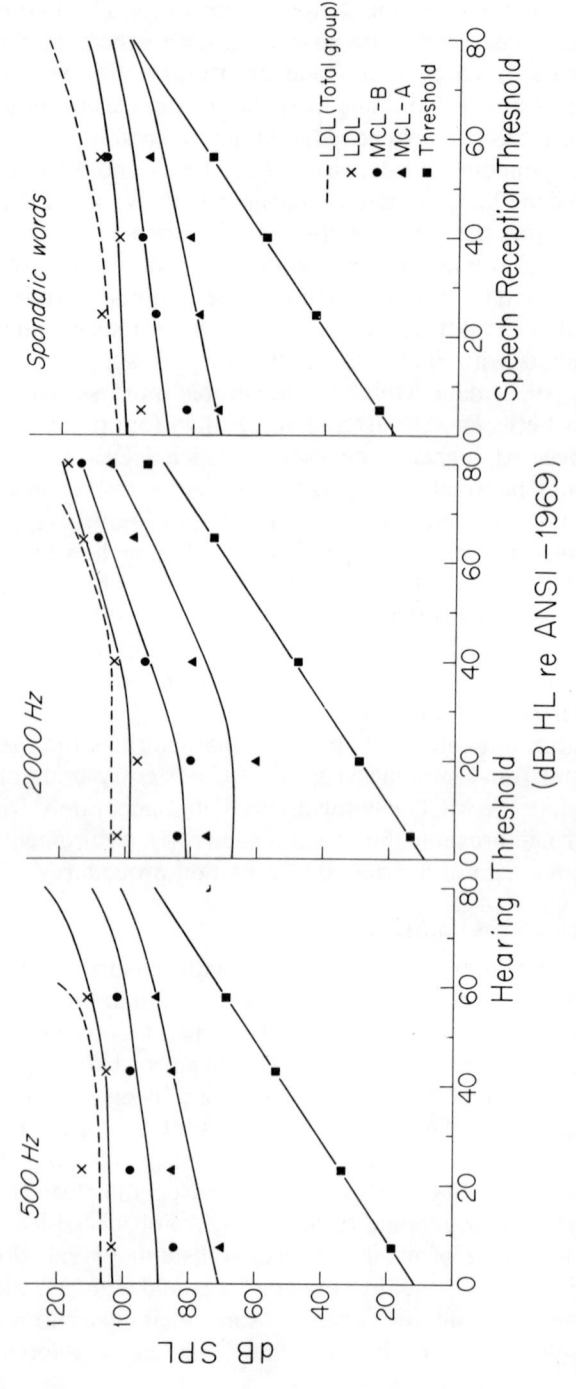

Figure 7-10. Median results and best-fit functions for MCL-A, MCL-B, and LDL for 38 subjects as a function of hearing threshold for 500 Hz, 2000 Hz, and spondaic words. Also illustrated are the median hearing threshold levels for the subjects and the LDL best-fit functions for a larger group of listeners with sensorineural hearing loss. (From Kamm et al., 1978; reproduced with permission.)

MCL range increase with hearing loss but not as rapidly as does the loss in threshold sensitivity. This characteristic is reminiscent of the LDL for persons with sensorineural hearing loss and is further evidence of the decrease in functional range available to the person with moderately severe sensorineural hearing loss.

Clinical Use of MCL

Audiology textbooks are nearly unanimous in suggesting that a most comfortable level judgment should be required of subjects during a hearing aid evaluation (Hodgson and Skinner, 1977; Pollack, 1975; Ross, 1978). This recommendation is made despite the recognized problems of validity and reliability which limit both the application and interpretation of the measurement. The majority of systematic investigations of the MCL have concentrated on parametric variables (instructional differences, methodological changes, and stimulus type) and their effects on the most comfortable level. Fundamental issues regarding the use of the MCL measurement in hearing aid evaluations remain essentially unresolved. These include the question of validity, recognition that comfortable listening levels encompass a range of intensities, and development of a defensible rationale for the application of the MCL.

Two examples of the simplistic nature of the recommendations for the application of the MCL may be illustrative. First, it has been suggested (e.g., Shapiro, 1975, 1976; Victoreen, 1960) that MCL be the basis upon which gain of the hearing aid is chosen. This suggestion is apparently made without regard for the differences in the SPL developed in the ear canal between an earphone/supra-aural cushion and a hearing aid receiver/earmold arrangement. The problems related to such coupler/real-ear measurements were developed in the LDL section of this chapter and are equally applicable to the MCL. A single report exists (Cox and Wark, 1978) in which an attempt has been made to quantify the difference in SPL between aided and unaided MCL measurements. In that study, probe tube measures were used to determine the SPL near the eardrum under aided conditions.

When such care is taken to determine the eardrum SPL, these authors concluded that the MCL judgments observed under the two conditions (aided and unaided) are made at a constant SPL at the eardrum. However, it is important to note that probe tube measurements were required to account adequately for the differences in eardrum SPL under the two conditions. The Cox and Wark report provides evidence that the judgment of MCL will be made at approximately the same SPL under unaided and aided conditions. Typically, however, gain of a hearing aid is chosen based on MCL measurements made under earphones or in the sound field and there is no recognition of coupler/real-ear differences. Until such time as a practical method of determining the SPL at the eardrum in the individual case is available, determination of appropriate hearing aid gain from unaided MCL measurements will be inherently inaccurate and of limited clinical value.

A second example may be extrapolated from recent reviews of hearing aid evaluation procedures (e.g., Elpern, 1979; Ross, 1978). None of the procedures reviewed by these authors includes recognition of the fact that comfort levels encompass a range of intensities and cannot be characterized as a single level. Typically, the procedures call for setting the functional gain of the hearing aid at a "most comfortable level" whereas the input signal is maintained constant (usually at a level equivalent to that of soft speech). A hearing aid often is judged to be adequate if the volume control, when set at mid-range, allows for "comfortable listening." Such a procedure recognizes neither the fact that a range of intensities will meet the criteria of comfort, nor that speech in real life situations encompasses a range from ≈ 55 to 85 dB SPL.

Christen and Byrne (1980) have discussed the current limitations in application of the MCL for making specific decisions regarding electroacoustic characteristics of hearing aids. Specifically, the authors identified the high intrasubject (over time) and intersubject variability as the primary limiting characteristics of the MCL as a basis for decisions regarding: 1) hearing aid candidacy; 2) hearing aid over-all gain requirements; or 3) frequency gain requirements. They concluded that there is little experimental evidence from which to justify use of the MCL for hearing aid selection purposes.

Superficial attempts have been made to determine whether or not a relationship exists between the MCL and the intensity level at which speech recognition is maximal. The data from two attempts to determine if PB-Max occurs at the same level as MCL (Clemis and Carver, 1967; Posner, 1974) led to the conclusion that a one-to-one relationship does not exist. To date, however, no one has investigated the potentially more intriguing question of the relationship between the range of intensities over which speech is comfortable and the range of intensities over which speech is maximally understood.

All of these problems notwithstanding, procedures to measure MCL in hearing aid evaluations are embraced by many. It appears that comfort level judgments have become an integral part of hearing aid evaluation procedures without regard for the inconsistencies among results of investigations and without a well documented rationale for the application of the measurement. Interestingly, the clinical literature does not suggest that use of the MCL in hearing aid evaluation leads consistently to inappropriate choices of gain. The reasons for this may be related to the following factors: 1) comfort level is a range; 2) conversational speech occurs within a range; and 3) the wearer can adjust the functional gain of a hearing aid (volume control adjustment) over a wide range. Thus, it is probable that considerable inaccuracy in the application of MCL measurements to gain characteristics of a hearing aid can be tolerated before deleterious effects on the performance of the wearer become obvious. However, insistence on the use of the MCL as the measure of choice in specifying hearing aid gain is no more justifiable than the choice of some "target" intensity level based on reasonable assumptions regarding input level range and measured tolerance levels. In fact, such a procedure has been suggested by McCandless (1976).

In summary, until such time as individuals concerned with hearing aid evaluation procedures resolve the fundamental issues regarding the application of the MCL, the insight provided by such measures will continue to be severely limited. Likewise, the problems related to specifying the level (dB SPL) at the tympanic membrane of the person wearing a hearing aid deserve concentrated investigation.

SUMMARY

In this chapter the relevant literature concerning the clinical application of LDL and MCL measurements has been reviewed. This review suggests that the LDL may be a reliable measure in defining the upper limit of usable hearing. The application of the LDL in determining SSPL for a hearing aid is limited by the absence of a practical method for accurately predicting the SPL in the ear of a patient wearing a hearing aid. Application of the MCL for determining gain likewise requires resolution of the coupler/real-ear problem. Consideration of MCL as a range of intensities rather than a single level may lead to a more insightful understanding of the ways in which the measure could be applied clinically.

REFERENCES

Alpiner, J. G. 1975. Hearing aid selection for adults. In M. Pollack (ed.), Amplification for the Hearing Impaired, pp. 145–205. Grune & Stratton, New York.

Berger, K. W. 1971. Speech audiometry. In D. E. Rose (ed.), Audiological Assessment, pp. 227–228. Prentice-Hall, Inc. Englewood Cliffs, N.J.

Berger, K. W. 1976. The use of uncomfortable loudness level in hearing aid fitting. Maico Audiological Library Series, XV:2.

Berger, K. W. and J. F. Lowry. 1971. Relationships between various stimuli for MCL. Sound 5:11–14.

Berger, K. W., R. L. Rane, and E. N. Hagberg. 1979. Comparisons of uncomfortable loudness levels and acoustic reflex thresholds. Audiol. Hear. Ed. 5:11–16.

Bosatra, A. 1969. On the seismeiological value of loudness discomfort level. Int. Audiol. 8:164–171.

Byrne, D. and R. Christen. 1979. Preferred listening levels and loudness of filtered speech: Determinants of acceptable hearing aid gain settings. Austral. J. Audiol. 1:32–40.

Carhart, R. 1946. Volume control adjustment in hearing aid selection. Laryngoscope 56:510–526.

Christen, R. and D. Byrne. 1980. Variability of MCL measurements: Significance for hearing aid selection. Austral. J. Audiol. 2:10–18.

Christen, R. and D. Byrne. Preferred listening levels for bands of speech in relation to hearing aid selection. Scand. Audiol. In press.

Clemis, J. D. and W. F. Carver. 1967. Discrimination scores for speech in Menicre's disease. Arch. Otolaryngol. 86:614–618.

Cox, R. M. 1981. Using LDLs to establish hearing aid limiting levels. Hear. Instr. 32:16–20.

Cox, R. M. and D. J. Wark. 1978. MCL at the eardrum in aided and unaided conditions. AsHA, 20:759(abstract).

Davis, H., C. W. Hudgins, R. J. Marquis, R. H. Nichols, C. E. Peterson, D. A. Ross, and S. S. Stevens. 1946. The selection of hearing aids. Laryngoscope 56:85–135.

Denenberg, L. J. and M. W. Altshuler. 1976. The clinical relationship between acoustic reflexes and loudness perception. J. Am. Aud. Soc. 2:79–82.

Dirks, D. and C. Kamm. 1976. Psychometric functions for loudness discomfort and most comfortable loudness levels. J. Speech Hear. Res. 19:613–627.

Dirks, D. and C. Kamm. 1977. Reply to Ventry's letter. J. Speech Hear. Res. 20:814–815.

Edgerton, B. J., R.C. Beattie, and D. W. Cager. 1978. LDL: Effects of speech materials on normal and sensorineural listeners. Asha 20:747(Abstract).

Egolf, D. P., D. R. Tree, and L. L. Feth. 1978. Mathematical predictions of electroacoustic frequency response of *in situ* hearing aids. J. Acoust. Soc. Am. 63:264–272.

Elpern, B. S. 1979. Hearing aids. In V. Goodhill (ed.), Ear Diseases, Deafness and Dizziness, pp. 740–754. Harper & Row, New York.

Erber, N. P. and C. M. Alencewicz. 1976. Audiologic evaluation of deaf children. J. Speech Hearing Disord. 41:256–267.

Gilman, S. 1979. The effect of hearing aid components on the acoustic properties of the external auditory system. Doctoral dissertation. University of California, Los Angeles, Calif.

Hawkins, D. B. 1980. Loudness discomfort levels: A clinical procedure for hearing aid evaluations. J. Speech Hear. Disord. 45:3–15.

Hawkins, D. B. and M. J. Smith. 1979. LDLs: Signal type, methodology, and reliability. Paper presented at the convention of the American Speech-Language-Hearing Association, November, Atlanta.

Hinchcliffe, R. 1971. Examen otoneurologique pour le diagnostic des neurinomes acoustiques. Acta Oto-rhinolaryngol. Belg. 27:770–778.

Hochberg, I. 1975. Most comfortable listening for the loudness and intelligibility of speech. Audiology 14:27–34.
Hodgson, W. R. and P. H. Skinner. 1977. Hearing Aid Assessment and Use in Audiologic Habilitation. Williams & Wilkins Company, Baltimore.
Holmes, D. W. and C. M. Woodford. 1977. Acoustic reflex threshold and loudness discomfort level: Relationships in children with profound hearing losses. J. Am. Audi. Soc., 2:193–196.
Hood, J. D. and J. P. Poole. 1966. Tolerable limit of loudness: Its clinical and physiological significance. J. Acoust. Soc. Am. 40:47–53.
Jerger, J. and S. Jerger. 1974. Diagnostic value of Bekesy comfortable loudness tracings. Arch. Otolaryngol. 99:351–360.
Kamm, C., D. Dirks, and R. Mickey. 1978. Effect of sensorineural hearing loss on loudness discomfort level. J. Speech Hear. Res. 21:668–681.
Kopra, L. L. and D. Blosser. 1968. Effects of method of measurement on most comfortable loudness level for speech. J. Speech Hearing. Res. 11:497–508.
Levitt, H. 1971. Transformed up-down methods in psychoacoustics. J. Acoust. Soc. Am. 49:467–477.
Levitt, H. 1978. Adaptive testing in audiology. Scand. Audiol. 6(Suppl.):241–292.
Lybarger, S. F. 1975. Comparison of earmold characteristics measured on the 2 cc coupler, the Zwislocki coupler and real ears. Scand. Audiol. 5(Suppl.):65–86.
McCandless, G. 1973. Hearing aids and loudness discomfort. Paper presented at Oticongress 3, Copenhagen, Denmark.
McCandless, G. 1976. Special considerations in evaluating children and the aging for hearing aids. IN M. Rubin (ed.), Hearing Aids, pp. 171–182. University Park Press, Baltimore.
McCandless, G. A. and D. L. Miller. 1972. Loudness discomfort and hearing aids. Nat. Hear. Aid J. 25:7, 28, 32.
Margolis, R. and G. Popelka. 1975. Loudness and the acoustic reflex. J. Acoust. Soc. Am. 58:1330–1332.
Markle, D. and A. Zaner. 1966. The determination of acoustic gain in fitting of hearing aids: A new method. J. Aud. Res. 6:371–379.
Martin, M. C., B. C. Stevenson, and B. C. Grover. 1978. Some aspects of auditory space, speech perception and the use of hearing aids. Scand. Audiol. 6(Suppl.):141–162.
Martin, F. M. and Pennington, C. D. 1971. Current trends in audiologic practice. Asha 13:671–679.
Morgan, D. and D. Dirks. 1974. Loudness discomfort level under earphone and in the free field: The effects of calibration methods. J. Acoust. Soc. Am. 56:172–178.
Morgan, D., D. Dirks, D. Bower, and C. Kamm. 1979. Loudness discomfort level and acoustic reflex threshold for speech stimuli. J. Speech Hear. Res. 22:849–861.
Morgan, D. E., R. H. Wilson, and D. D. Dirks. 1974. Loudness discomfort level: Selected methods and stimuli. J. Acoust. Soc. Am. 56:577–581.
Olson, A. E. and N. M. Hipskind. 1973. The relation between levels of pure tones and speech which elicit the acoustic reflex and loudness discomfort. J. Aud. Res. 13:71–76.
Pollack, I. 1952. Comfortable listening levels for pure tones in quiet and in noise. J. Acoust. Soc. Am. 24:158–162.

Pollack, M. C. 1975. Amplification for the Hearing Impaired. Grune & Stratton, New York.

Popelka, G., R. Margolis, and T. Wiley. 1976. Effect of activating-signal band width on acoustic-reflex thresholds. J. Acoust. Soc. Am. 59:153–159.

Posner, J. 1974. Relationships between comfortable loudness levels for speech and speech discrimination in sensorineural hearing loss. Doctoral dissertation. Teachers College, Columbia University, New York.

Ritter, R. 1978. The effect of instructional patterns on the relationship between loudness discomfort levels and acoustic reflex threshold levels. Doctoral dissertation. University of Denver, Denver, Colo.

Robinson, D. W. and R. S. Dadson. 1956. A re-determination of the loudness relations for pure tones. Br. J. Appl. Phys. 7:166–181.

Ross, M. 1978. Hearing aid evaluation. In J. Katz (ed.), Handbook of Clinical Audiology, pp. 524–543. Williams & Wilkins Company, Baltimore.

Sachs, R. M. and M. D. Burkhard. 1972. Zwislocki coupler evaluation with insert earphones. Indust. Res. Prod. Inc. (Knowles Elect. Inc.). Report No. 20022-1, Nov.

Scharf, B. 1976. Acoustic reflex, loudness summation and the critical band. J. Acoust. Soc. Am. 60:753–755.

Schmitz, H. 1969. Loudness discomfort level modification. J. Speech Hear. Res. 12:807–817.

Shapiro, I. 1975. Prediction of most comfortable loudness levels in hearing aid evaluation. J. Speech Hear. Disord. 40:434–438.

Shapiro, I. 1976. Hearing aid fitting by prescription. Audiology 15:163–173.

Shaw, E. A. G. 1966. Ear canal pressure generated by circumaural and supra-aural earphones. J. Acoust. Soc. Am. 39:471–479.

Silverman, S. 1947. Tolerance for pure tones and speech in normal and defective hearing. Ann. Otol. Rhinol. Laryngol. 56:658–677.

Stephens, S. D. and C. M. Anderson. 1971. Experimental studies on the uncomfortable loudness level. J. Speech Hear. Res. 14:262–270.

Stephens, S. D. G., B. Blegvad, and H. J. Krogh. 1977. The value of some suprathreshold auditory measures. Scand. Audiol. 6:213–221.

Ventry, I. M. 1977. Comment on comfortable loudness levels for pure tones and speech. J. Speech Hear. Res., 20:813.

Ventry, I. M. and J. I. Johnson. 1978. Evaluation of a clinical method for measuring comfortable loudness for speech. J. Speech Hear. Disord. 43:149–160.

Ventry, I. M., R. W. Woods, M. Rubin, and W. Hill. 1971. Most comfortable loudness for pure tones, noise and speech. J. Acoust. Soc. Am. 49:1805–1813.

Victoreen, J. A. 1960. Hearing Enhancement. Charles C Thomas Publisher, Springfield, Ill.

Wallenfels, H. G. 1967. Hearing Aids on Prescription. Charles C Thomas Publisher, Springfield, Ill.

Watson, L. A. 1944. Certain fundamental principles in prescribing and fitting hearing aids. Laryngoscope 54:531–558.

Woodford, C. M. and D. W. Holmes. 1977. Relationship between loudness discomfort level and acoustic reflex threshold in a clinical population. Audiol. Hear. Ed. 3:9–12.

Woods, R. W., I. M. Ventry, and L. W. Gatling. 1973. Effect of ascending and descending measurements methods on comfortable loudness levels for pure tones. J. Acoust. Soc. Am. 54:205–206.

Zwicker, A., G. Flottorp, and S. S. Stevens. 1957. Critical band width in loudness summation. J. Acoust. Soc. Am. 29:548–557.

Zwislocki, J. J. 1970. An acoustic coupler for earphone calibration. Special Report—Lab for Sensory Comm., Syracuse Univ., LSC-S-7, Grant No. NGR-3-022-091, NASA.

CHAPTER 8

SPEECH STIMULI FOR ASSESSMENT OF CENTRAL AUDITORY DISORDERS

William F. Rintelmann and George E. Lynn

CONTENTS

MONAURAL TESTS	234
Undistorted Speech	234
Filtered Speech	235
Time-Compressed Speech	236
Speech-in-Noise	239
Synthetic Sentence Identification-Ipsilateral Competing Message	240
BINAURAL TESTS	241
Synthetic Sentence Identification-Contralateral Competing Message	242
Northwestern University Auditory Tests Numbers 2 and 20	243
Competing Sentence Test	244
Staggered Spondaic Word Test	244
Digits	245
Syllables	247
Filtered Speech	248
Rapidly Alternating Speech Perception Test	249
Masking Level Differences for Speech	250
AUDITORY PERCEPTUAL PROBLEMS IN CHILDREN	251
NONSPEECH MEASURES	261
ILLUSTRATIVE CASES	264
CONCLUSIONS	275
REFERENCES	276

Since the middle 1950s a major focus of clinical research in audiology has been on the development and application of auditory tests for the assessment of anatomical site of lesion. These research efforts have provided clinicians with several audiologic tests for eliciting response patterns peculiarly associated with damage to a particular anatomical site within the peripheral auditory system, namely, the middle ear, cochlea, and nerve VIII. Less success, however, has been achieved in efforts to devise auditory tasks for assessing lesions in the central auditory nervous system (CANS).[1] Primarily, three reasons account

---

[1] The central auditory nervous system consists of two crossed and two uncrossed neuroanatomical pathways with multiple connections and crossover tracts coursing from the nerve VIII ganglion of the organ of Corti to the cerebral cortex. From a functional standpoint, however, the CANS is viewed as beginning at the synapse between first-

for this difficulty: 1) the lack of availability of precisely documented CANS lesions in patients seen by audiologists; 2) the redundancy of conventional auditory test signals; and 3) most importantly, the resistance of the CANS to exhibit breakdown on auditory tasks due to the structural complexity of the central auditory pathways.

To illustrate the difficulty in assessing CANS lesions, clinical studies with hemispherectomized patients have demonstrated that pure tone thresholds and word recognition (discrimination) scores obtained with high fidelity monosyllables can be essentially normal in both ears (Goldstein, Goodman, and King, 1956; Goldstein, 1961; Hodgson, 1967). As a consequence, in order to assess lesions in the central auditory pathways, the auditory task must be made sufficiently difficult to overcome the combined effect of redundancy of both the auditory system and the acoustic signal. The intrinsic CANS redundancy stems from the bilateral representation of each ear to each side of the brain via the system's multiple network of pathways and crossings, nuclear centers, intertract, and interhemispheric connections, and projections to primary and secondary cortical areas. This highly complex system results in multiple mapping or processing of auditory information within the brain. In addition, auditory signals contain varying degrees of extrinsic redundancy. Both tonal stimuli (e.g., pure tones) and high-fidelity speech signals (whether single words or connected discourse) are so redundant that the central auditory system is not taxed in persons with normal peripheral auditory systems. Bocca and his colleagues recognized this fact (Bocca, Calearo, and Cassinari, 1954; Bocca et al., 1955) and theorized that central auditory disorders could be detected by reducing the redundancy of speech stimuli by distorting (degrading) the speech. They used low-pass filtered, phonetically balanced words and found that in patients with documented auditory cortex lesions word recognition performance was reduced substantially in the ear contralateral to the lesion compared to the ipsilateral ear. Subsequently, in addition to low-pass filtering, investigators have attempted to reduce the redundancy of speech by distorting it in a variety of ways; for example, periodic interruption, acceleration, or presentation at low sensation levels (Bocca, 1958; Calearo and Lazzaroni, 1957; de Quiros, 1964; Matzker, 1959).

The acoustic features of speech that are important to perceptual processing of speech stimuli are frequency, time, and intensity. Each

---

and second-order neurons located at the ventral and dorsal cochlear nuclei of the brainstem. Hence, based on this classification system, the auditory branch of nerve VIII (first-order neuron) is considered as part of the peripheral auditory system. For further details refer to Beasley and Rintelmann (1979), Durrant and Lovrinic (1977), and Snow et al. (1977) among other sources.

of these features has been discussed in Chapter 3. Efforts to degrade (distort) speech in order to develop tasks for evaluating the integrity of the CANS have focused on manipulating either singly or in some combination the frequency, time, and intensity characteristics of speech.

An additional consideration is that speech stimuli may be presented in either monaural or binaural listening tasks. Under binaural presentation conditions, the identical stimuli can be presented simultaneously to both ears (*diotic*) or a different segment of the message, or different messages, can be delivered to each ear (*dichotic*). Normal everyday listening to a single talker in a "quiet" environment is illustrative of the diotic condition; whereas, listening to one or more talkers(s) in the presence of background noise (speech or nonspeech competition) is one form of dichotic listening. Beginning with the findings of Calearo (1957) and Matzker (1957, 1958), several investigators (Antonelli, 1970; Linden, 1964; Ohta, Hayashi, and Morimoto, 1967) found that patients with central auditory deficits have difficulty in their ability to "fuse" binaural, diotic speech messages. Subsequent investigations (Berlin and Lowe, 1972; Kimura, 1967; Studdert-Kennedy and Shankweiler, 1970) have demonstrated that patients with central auditory lesions show a "breakdown" in performance on dichotic (different signals to each ear) listening tasks. These investigations have resulted in the development and application of speech tests involving binaural integration and summation, and competing message tests.

Because the focus of this text is on the application of speech signals to the assessment of auditory function, this chapter is restricted primarily to a discussion of speech stimuli. Nevertheless, it should be pointed out that with a few notable exceptions (e.g., brainstem-evoked response measures) efforts to use signals other than speech stimuli for the assessment of central auditory disorders have been either untried or relatively unsuccessful.

In this chapter the application of both high fidelity and distorted speech signals to monaural listening tasks will be discussed first. Next, the use of various types of degraded speech stimuli under binaural diotic and dichotic listening conditions will be presented. Subsequently, a section of the chapter is devoted to a discussion of the assessment of auditory perceptual (processing) problems in children. The importance of appropriate test materials based on adequate normative data on children is stressed. Next, brief consideration is given to tests that consist of nonspeech stimuli. Thereafter, the profile from a battery of test results will be illustrated for several patients. It is beyond the scope of this chapter to present either a description of specific procedures for administering the various central auditory tests or detailed information concerning interpretation of results. Instead, the goals of this chapter are to present brief descriptions of several commonly employed tests, to show some illustrative case findings, and to provide an indication of the utility of the various tests for assessing central auditory disorders based upon our experiences with such measures along with appropriate literature citations.

MONAURAL TESTS

Word recognition tests administered under monaural conditions have been degraded (made more difficult) by modifying one or more of the important acoustic features of speech; namely, the intensity, frequency, or time domain. For each of the tests discussed in this section the reader should note which feature of speech has been manipulated.

Undistorted Speech

In addition to the employment of various types of degraded speech tasks, some use has been made also of undistorted speech tests administered in quiet.

PB Max Results from undistorted word recognition tests, usually obtained at a single high sensation level with phonetically balanced word lists (PB Max), have proven to be of limited value in the detection of CANS lesions. Such patients typically exhibit normal scores bilaterally on this type of test (Jerger, 1960a, b; 1964; Lynn and Gilroy, 1972, 1977; Noffsinger and Kurdziel, 1979).

Performance-Intensity Functions Word recognition scores can be obtained with high-fidelity phonetically balanced (PB) words or other types of monosyllables at several sensation levels (SL), ranging from low (e.g., 5 dB SL) to high (e.g., 80 dB SL). In this manner, a performance-intensity (PI) function can be plotted to demonstrate the listener's change in word recognition over a broad intensity range. Data plotted in this fashion also have been called intelligibility or articulation functions. Jerger, Speaks, and Trammell (1968) suggested that performance-intensity functions obtained with PB words (PI-PB) in quiet could prove useful in the identification of retrocochlear lesions. Although the use of PI-PB functions has been advocated both as a screening test and as a measure for assessing the extent of a central auditory disorder (Jerger and Jerger, 1971; Jerger, 1973), this measure of auditory function has proven more sensitive for detecting nerve VIII lesions than for assessing CANS disorders (Jerger and Jerger, 1975a). The PI-PB functions of such patients frequently exhibit a *rollover phenomenon*; that is, successively higher scores as sensation level is increased until a maximum score (e.g., PB Max) is reached, followed by poorer scores at still higher sensation or intensity levels (to a maximum of 110 dB sound pressure level). A rollover ratio can be calculated from the PI function (see Chapter 6 for details). The presence of "rollover" has been observed frequently on the ipsilateral ear of patients with nerve VIII lesions (Jerger and Jerger, 1971; Jerger and Jerger, 1975a), but only occasionally on either the contralateral ear or both ears of patients with brainstem lesions and even less frequently on either the ipsilateral or contralateral ear of patients with temporal lobe disorders (Jerger and Jerger, 1975a). These findings also are consistent with our experience of obtaining PI functions on patients with nerve VIII, brainstem, or cortical lesions.

Filtered Speech

Speech can be distorted by eliminating a portion of the frequency spectrum via electronic filtering. For example, a word recognition test can be recorded through a low-pass filter to remove a certain amount of high-frequency acoustic information normally present to permit good understanding of the test words. The difficulty of the test, that is, the amount of distortion, depends upon the cutoff frequency (e.g., 500 Hz) and the rejection rate (e.g., 18 dB/octave) of the filter. For this reason, plus the fact that word recognition tests vary in difficulty according to both the talker and the test material, normative data must be available before a particular filtered speech test can be applied to a pathologic population. This principle, of course, holds for all auditory tests.

Although speech can be processed through a low-pass, high-pass, or a band-pass (both low and high) filter system, most applications of monaural filtered speech tasks have used low-pass filtering. Bergman (1980) used low-pass filtered speech as one of several measures to study the effects of aging on the perception of speech. He demonstrated that filtering signal energy above 2000 Hz sharply reduced the word recognition ability of geriatric adults compared to young normal listeners. Several studies have shown that word recognition for monaurally presented low-pass filtered speech is poorer on the ear contralateral to the temporal lobe lesion compared to the ipsilateral side (Bocca, 1958; Bocca et al., 1954; Bocca et al., 1955; Hodgson, 1967; Jerger, 1960a, b; 1964; Korsan-Bengtsen, 1973; Lynn et al., 1972; Lynn and Gilroy, 1972, 1977), but is not affected substantially in cases with involvement of the transverse interhemispheric auditory pathways that cross from one hemisphere to the other via the corpus collosum (Gilroy and Lynn, 1974; Lynn et al., 1972; Lynn and Gilroy, 1971, 1972, 1975, 1977; Musiek, Wilson, and Pinheiro, 1979). Considerably less consistent findings have been obtained with low-pass filtered speech on patients with brainstem lesions (Calearo and Antonelli, 1968; Lynn and Gilroy, 1977). It has been observed that test scores for some patients were abnormal in the ear contralateral to the side of the brainstem primarily involved, and in other cases the ipsilateral or both ears showed abnormal results. Lynn and Gilroy (1977) pointed out that because brainstem lesions are often diffuse or bilateral, it is sometimes difficult to establish good correlation between test results and the locus of the brainstem pathology. Hence, the primary usefulness of this test is in identifying lesions of the central auditory system. Low-pass filtered speech, however, when used as part of a battery of tests is useful in attempting to localize the level of involvement.

Time-Compressed Speech

As stated in Chapter 3 and earlier in this chapter, temporal features of the acoustic signal play an important role in speech perception. Hence, the use of distortion in the time domain of speech has considerable potential as a measure for assessing CANS disorders. The terms accelerated speech and time-compressed speech often have been used interchangeably in the literature to describe an increase in the rate of verbal material. This is inappropriate because these two methods of temporal alteration have substantially different effects on the acoustic properties of speech. Accelerated speech most commonly is accomplished by increasing the playback speed of a tape recorder. This method not only changes rate, but also produces an upward frequency shift of the speech signal. In contrast, the technique of time compression (Fairbanks, Everitt, and Jaeger, 1954) increases rate by discarding portions of the speech signal and abutting together the remaining acoustic energy so that there are no silent intervals within the words. Thus, rate is altered (speeded) without shifting frequency; but, because some acoustic energy is removed, a proportionate amount of acoustic information is discarded also. Thus, although both acceleration and time compression have been used to alter the temporal characteristics of speech, these two methods clearly produce different types of degraded speech tasks, and hence both should not be classified as *time-compressed* speech tests.

Based on the initial findings of Bocca (1958) and his associates in Italy (Calearo and Lazzaroni, 1957), other investigators (de Quiros, 1964; Quaranta and Cervellera, 1977) also have employed accelerated speech (usually sentence material) as a means of evaluating central auditory disorders. The findings of these studies suggest that for patients with lesions in the auditory cortex accelerated speech reduces substantially speech recognition in the ear contralateral to the lesion. Patients with diffuse central lesions tend to exhibit decreased scores in both ears. For patients with brainstem involvement, Calearo and Antonelli (1968) found reduced performance in 14 of 23 cases with usually only one ear affected. Quaranta and Cervellera (1977) found, however, that of nine patients with brainstem vascular lesions all showed normal performance on the accelerated speech test.

Regarding the effect of aging on accelerated speech task performance, Calearo and Lazzaroni (1957) found that when the talking rate of Italian sentences was increased to two and a half times faster than normal speed (from 140 to 350 words per minute), persons over 70 years of age showed substantial breakdown in performance compared to young adults. However, Bergman (1980) also used an acceleration rate of two and a half times faster than normal speed and found only a slight reduction in the understanding of everyday sentences among aged subjects (70 to 89 years old) compared to young (20 to 29 years old) adults.

A collaborative series of studies has been conducted using the Fairbanks et al. (1954) method of electromechanically time compressing a monosyllabic word test, Northwestern University Auditory Test Number 6 (NU #6) (Tillman and Carhart, 1966), which was recorded by a male talker (Rintelmann et al., 1974a). The test materials used for each study in the series of investigations were taped copies of the same master tape recording. The goal of this series of investigations was two-fold: 1) to establish normative data for normal listeners and for individuals with peripheral (sensorineural) hearing disorders; and 2) to evaluate and apply this test to patients with central auditory disorders.

In the normative studies word recognition scores were obtained at several sensation levels (e.g., 8 to 40 dB in 8-dB steps) for each of several time compression ratios (e.g., 30 to 70 percent in 10 percent intervals). The findings with normal listeners (Beasley, Forman, and Rintelmann, 1972a; Beasley, Schwimmer, and Rintelmann, 1972b) demonstrated that word recognition was inversely related to time-compression ratio and directly related to sensation level. In other words, as the percentage of time compression was increased, performance decreased, and scores improved as sensation level was increased. Furthermore, the decrease in word recognition was gradual from 30 to 60 percent; however, at 70 percent time compression a dramatic breakdown in performance occurred. In the study involving noise-induced sensorineural hearing-impaired subjects (Kurdziel, Rintelmann, and Beasley, 1975) some variability in performance was found; however, in general, scores for time-compression ratios plotted as a function of sensation level were parallel to those of normal listeners but with lower word recognition scores. Konkle, Beasley, and Bess (1977) selected aged subjects so that their thresholds for pure tones and speech and their word recognition scores at 0 percent time compression essentially were equal to normal listeners. Nevertheless, these aged subjects obtained considerably reduced word recognition scores, compared to normals, at all ratios of time compression. This reduced performance in the perception of time-compressed speech has been attributed to degenerative changes in the central auditory nervous system of the aged listeners.

Patients with cortical lesions were tested in two investigations (Kurdziel, Noffsinger, and Olsen, 1976; Rintelmann, Beasley, and Lynn, 1974b) with the above described version of time compressed monosyllables (NU#6) using 0, 40, and 60 percent time compression. In both studies patients with diffuse temporal lobe lesions (e.g., cerebral vascular accident cases) showed substantially poorer scores at 60 percent time compression or less in the contralateral ear irrespective of whether the lesion was in the right or left hemisphere (see Figures 8-3 and 8-7 for illustrative cases). Kurdziel et al. (1976) found, however, that for patients with unilateral discrete lesions, who had undergone anterior temporal lobe surgery, word recognition scores at 60 percent time compression generally were equal in both ears and only slightly poorer (about 10 percent) than scores at 0 percent time compression. Hence, based on limited data to date, it appears that time-compressed monosyllables may be more sensitive for assessing cerebral lesions that are diffuse or massive than for localized discrete lesions. This, however, is a tentative conclusion and awaits confirmation after considerably more data have been reported. For example, no data have been reported yet on this technique for patients with brainstem insults.

The interest in time-altered (compressed or expanded) speech has led to the development of improved instrumentation (Lee, 1972) and the use of test materials other than NU #6. The performance of adult normal-hearing listeners has been established for the modified rhyme test (Schwartz and Mikus, 1977); for first-order sentential approximations (Freeman and Church, 1977); for the Central Institute for the Deaf (CID) and revised CID sentence lists, and for third-order sentential approximations (Beasley, Bratt, and Rintelmann, 1980). Also, Swedish sentences have been time compressed for identifying patients with central auditory disorders (Korsan-Bengtsen, 1973; Lundborg et al., 1975). Furthermore, Bergman (1980) confirmed the findings of Konkle et al. (1977) by showing a dramatic breakdown of elderly versus young adults on a time-compressed version of a "token" test in which the subjects responded manually to simple commands (e.g., marking different colored squares and circles). Finally, the performance of young normal-hearing children has been examined on time-compressed versions of the phonetically balanced kindergarten (PBK) lists and the word intelligibility by picture identification (WIPI) test (Beasley, Maki, and Orchik, 1976). A further discussion of time-compressed speech tests applied to children with auditory perceptual problems is presented later in this chapter.

In summary, considerable research effort has been devoted to attempting to establish normative data for both children and adults on time-compressed versions of several different speech recognition tests. The task that remains, however, is to evaluate the various time-compressed test materials mentioned above when used in a patient population that has central auditory disorders.

Each test described thus far in this chapter has been based upon manipulating one or more of the crucial acoustic features of speech (e.g., intensity, frequency, or time). In contrast, a difficult listening task is achieved for the measures discussed below by mixing into a single ear some type of high fidelity speech (*primary message*) with broadband noise or some other masker/distractor (*competing message*).

Speech in Noise

A measure that has been employed by several investigators for the assessment of retrocochlear lesions is a speech-in-noise task (Dayal, Tarantino, and Swisher, 1966; Heilman, Hammer, and Wilder, 1973; Katinsky, Lovrinic, and Buchheit, 1972; Morales-Garcia and Poole, 1972; Noffsinger et al., 1972; Olsen, Noffsinger, and Kurdziel, 1975). The primary message for this test is usually monosyllables presented at a high SL (e.g., 40 dB). White noise or speech spectrum noise is presented to the same ear typically at an overall sound pressure level (SPL) equal to that of the primary message, that is, at approximately a 0-dB signal-to-noise (S/N) ratio. Normal listeners as well as hearing-impaired patients show wide variability in speech recognition scores obtained in the presence of noise, depending upon the specific primary message, type of noise, and the S/N ratio used. Under conditions such as those mentioned above, however, normal listeners typically show 20 to 40 percent poorer scores in noise than in quiet. In evaluating the scores from this task for patients suspected of CANS lesions, the primary comparison is between ipsilateral and contralateral ears in terms of the relative "breakdown" in scores from quiet to noise and the extent to which such breakdown exceeds that of normal listeners.

Abnormal findings have been reported for the speech-in-noise task in ears ipsilateral to nerve VIII lesions (Dayal et al., 1966; Katinsky et al., 1972) and peripheral brainstem disorders (Dayal et al., 1966), in one or both ears of patients with intra-axial brainstem lesions (Morales-Garcia and Poole, 1972; Noffsinger et al., 1972), in both ears of commissurotomized ("split brain") patients but with poorer scores on the left compared to the right ear (Musiek et al., 1979), and in ears contralateral to temporal lobe disorders (Heilman et al., 1973; Morales-

Garcia and Poole, 1972). Recognizing that no previous investigation had compared the performance of a broad-spectrum patient population (e.g., patients with cochlear, nerve VIII, brainstem, or cortical lesions) on a single speech-in-noise test, Olsen et al. (1975) conducted a definitive investigation designed to examine this interaction. They employed the NU #6 test at 40 dB SL both in quiet and in white noise (0 dB S/N ratio). They established normative data on a large group of normal listeners and also tested several groups of patients with cochlear, nerve VIII, and CANS disorders. Based on their findings, Olsen et al. (1975) stated that lesions anywhere in the auditory system from the cochlea through the temporal lobe can exhibit marked reduction in speech recognition scores when measured in the presence of "same ear" white noise. Thus, they concluded that this test " . . . may have some clinical usefulness in revealing abnormalities in auditory function but not in suggesting a particular site of involvement as being responsible for the dysfunction" (p. 382). This appears to be an appropriate caution regarding the limitation of the speech-in-noise test.

Synthetic Sentence Identification-Ipsilateral Competing Message

Speaks and Jerger (1965) developed the synthetic sentence identification (SSI) test, which consists of artificial sentences constructed as approximations to real English sentences based on the rules governing the probabilities of word sequence. Jerger and his associates have found the synthetic sentence identification task presented with an ipsilateral competing message (SSI-ICM) to be useful in assessing CANS dysfunction, especially brainstem lesions (Jerger, 1970a, b; Jerger and Hayes, 1977; Jerger and Jerger, 1974, 1975a, b). The particular test advocated by Jerger (1973) for evaluating patients with CANS disorders consists of ten third-order approximation sentences. Each sentence has seven words and contains nine syllables (± one syllable). The 10 sentences are presented as a closed-message set with a competing message (continuous discourse) presented to the ipsilateral ear. In general, two methods have been used for presenting this test. In one method, a constant message to competition ratio of 0 dB is used and the stimulus materials (SSI-ICM) are presented at several SLs ranging from low to high SL. In the other, more commonly used method, the primary message (synthetic sentences) is given at a constant high SL (e.g., 40 dB) and the intensity level of the competing message (continuous discourse) is varied to achieve message to competition ratios (MCRs) from about +10 dB to −20 dB in 10-dB steps. Note that in a minus MCR condition the competing message is more intense than the primary message. Both methods described above for administering the SSI-ICM task permit plotting PI functions.

According to Jerger (1973), most normal listeners perform at 100 percent when the message and the competition are at the same level, that is at a MCR of 0 dB. Normal performance drops to about 80 percent at a MCR of −10 dB, to about 55 percent at a MCR of −20 dB, and to about 20 percent at a MCR of −30 dB. It should be recognized that these expected normal responses only apply to Jerger's recorded version of this test. If another version is used (e.g., different talker or different stimulus items) norms for that version should be established before the test is applied to patients.

Responses on the SSI-ICM task are considered abnormal when the PI functions exhibit marked deficits from expected normal results in one or both ears. Abnormal performance on this task may be exhibited by patients with either brainstem or temporal lobe lesions, but occurs more commonly in the former. Brainstem lesions are displayed by depressed performance either in the contralateral ear or in both ears. Temporal lobe lesions that produce deficits on the SSI-ICM test also do so in both ears or, less often, in the contralateral ear only (Jerger and Jerger, 1975a). The most useful application of the SSI test for differentiating brainstem from temporal lobe lesions presents the competing message in both the ipsilateral and contralateral modes. This latter task is a dichotic test and is discussed below.

BINAURAL TESTS

As stated previously in this chapter, a diotic listening condition involves simultaneous presentation of the same message(s) to both ears, whereas a dichotic listening task involves the presentation of different acoustic signals to each ear. Although both types of listening tasks are employed in the assessment of CANS lesions, as revealed in the discussion below there are many more binaural tests consisting of dichotic as opposed to diotic messages.

Dichotic speech recognition tests fall into three general categories according to the listener's task. In one, the listener is required to attend only to a primary signal in one ear while attempting to ignore a competing signal in the opposite ear. Examples of this type of dichotic test are the synthetic sentence identification with contralateral competing message (SSI-CCM) (Jerger and Jerger, 1975a), Northwestern University auditory test No. 20 (Olsen and Carhart, 1967) and the competing sentence test (Willeford, 1976). In the second type of dichotic task, the listener attempts to respond to different stimuli presented to each ear. Tests in this category include the staggered spondaic word test (SSW) (Brunt, 1978; Katz, 1962) and the consonant-vowel syllable test (Berlin et al., 1968). In both abovementioned forms of dichotic listening tests, the presentation levels and signal to competing message ratios may vary over a wide range. A third type of dichotic test, typically called the *binaural fusion* or *resynthesis* task, requires the listener to respond to the presentation of different portions of the speech signal to each ear. Examples of this type of dichotic test include the rapidly alternating speech perception (RASP) test (Bocca and Calearo, 1963; Lynn and Gilroy, 1970, 1972) in which speech signals alternate rapidly between ears, and the binaural filtered speech test (Matzker, 1959) in which different filtered portions (low- and high-pass bands) of the speech material are delivered to each ear simultaneously. This filtered speech binaural fusion task may be presented also in the diotic mode, that is, with both low- and high-pass bands delivered simultaneously to both ears. Each of the above mentioned tests are discussed below.

Various types of speech and competing message dichotic tests have been developed in which the primary message consists of meaningful words or sentences or artificial sentences (e.g., SSI) and the competing message is either meaningful speech (e.g., sentences or connected discourse) or nonmeaningful speech (e.g., simultaneous multitalkers). Such tasks are relatively easy for normal listeners even when administered at a message to competition ratio of -10 dB, that is, when the primary message is 10 dB weaker than the competing message. This type of task tends to be most sensitive for showing breakdown in performance in patients with diffuse temporal lobe lesions when the primary message is presented to the contralateral ear. Three different competing message speech tests are described briefly below.

Synthetic Sentence Identification-Contralateral Competing Message

The stimulus materials for this task are identical to those of the SSI-ICM discussed above. Recall, the primary message is third-order approximations of English sentences and the competing message, presented to the contralateral ear in this task (SSI-CCM), is meaningful connected discourse (Jerger, 1970a,b; Speaks and Jerger, 1965). The procedure for administering this test is similar to that used for the SSI-ICM. Usually, the primary message (SSI) is presented at a single high SL (e.g., 40 dB) and the intensity level of the contralateral competing message (CCM) is varied to produce message to competition ratios from about 0 dB to -40 dB. Because the primary and competing messages are presented to different ears, the speech recognition scores of normal listeners on the SSI-CCM task usually are unaffected even under the most adverse (e.g., -40 dB) message to competition ratios. Patients with cortical lesions, however, exhibit breakdown in performance on this task when the primary message is delivered to the ear contralateral to the lesion. In most instances patients with brainstem disorders obtain normal scores on this task. Hence, when both the ICM and CCM modes of the SSI test are administered to the same patient, brainstem versus cortical lesion sites often can be distinguished (Jerger and Jerger, 1974; Jerger and Jerger, 1975a; Spitzer and Ventry, 1980). This illustrates that efforts to assess auditory site of lesion, whether peripheral or central, should involve the administration of a battery of tests.

Northwestern University Auditory Tests Numbers 2 and 20

Both the Northwestern University (NU #2) (Jerger, Carhart and Dirks, 1961) and the NU #20 (Olsen and Carhart, 1967) were developed as dichotic listening tasks and were used initially in studies concerned with the evaluation of binaural hearing aids. The primary message of the NU #2 contains PB monosyllables and the competing message consists of meaningful sentences from the Bell Telephone intelligibility lists. The competing sentences are aligned so that they begin before the start of the primary message carrier phrase and end after the occurrence of the PB test word. The original NU #20 test was developed with two versions (Olsen and Carhart, 1967). In both versions the primary message is the NU #6 monosyllabic words introduced by a carrier phrase. The competing message of one version, termed NU #20S, contains sentences from the Bell Telephone intelligibility lists, and hence is similar to the NU #2 except for the type of monosyllable used for the primary message. The competing signal of the other version, called NU #20N, consists of speech spectrum noise. Both the NU #2 and the NU #20S (now simply termed NU #20) have received limited use as a dichotic competing message task for assessing central auditory lesions with generally similar findings. Using the NU #2 Jerger (1964) found poorer discrimination scores when the primary message was presented to the ear contralateral to a temporal lobe lesion compared to the scores obtained when the PB words were delivered to the ear homolateral to the side of the lesion. Based on Jerger's (1964) preliminary findings, it has been recommended that the NU #2 and #20 tests be administered at a primary to competing message ratio of −10 dB with the primary message presented at a high SL (e.g., 50 dB). As with other tests of this type, normal listeners experience little or no difficulty with this task, whereas patients with temporal lobe lesions show reduced performance when the primary message is delivered to the ear contralateral to the lesion (Jerger, 1964; Noffsinger et al., 1972; Noffsinger and Kurdziel, 1979). Data from clinical reports suggest that the NU #20 test also may be useful in helping to identify disruption of the interhemispheric auditory pathways when used in a battery with other dichotic procedures (Musiek and Sachs, 1980; Musiek et al., 1979).

Competing Sentence Test

This test developed by Willeford (1976) consists of a series of 25 pairs of meaningful sentences six or seven syllables in length. The sentences in each pair are presented simultaneously, one sentence to each ear. The onset times of the sentences are not timed precisely. The listener attends to a primary sentence in one ear while attempting to ignore the competing sentence in the opposite ear. Willeford recommended the primary message be presented at 35 dB SL and the competing sentences at 50 dB SL (MCR = −15 dB). Intelligibility in percentage correct is determined for 10 primary messages for each ear.

Gilroy and Lynn (1974) and Lynn and Gilroy (1972, 1975, 1977) reported abnormal performance scores in the ear contralateral to the affected hemisphere in some adult patients with temporal lobe lesions, and in the ear ipsilateral to the dominant hemisphere for speech and language (left ear in most cases) in some patients with right or left hemisphere lesions involving the interhemispheric auditory pathways. Also, in some cases with progressive or curable lesions, serial testing demonstrated declining or improved test scores (Gilroy and Lynn, 1974). Musiek, Wilson, and Reeves (1981) reported normal scores bilaterally preoperatively and postoperatively after two-stage partial and complete sectioning of the corpus collosum in two adult patients. The application of this test to children with suspected central auditory lesions is described later in this chapter.

Staggered Spondaic Word Test

Developed by Katz in 1962, this test is a dichotic procedure in which the listener attends to messages presented to both ears. Details on administering, scoring, and interpreting the SSW have been published elsewhere (Brunt, 1978; Katz, 1968; Katz and Pack, 1975) and thus will only be reviewed briefly here. Each test item consists of a pair of spondaic words in which different spondees are presented to each ear. The onset of one of the spondees is delayed to one ear so that its first syllable coincides approximately with the start of the second syllable of the leading stimulus word in the other ear. Thus, there are two noncompeting stimulus syllables, one for each ear, and two competing stimuli.

Scoring the test involves obtaining the number of response errors for: 1) each ear under the noncompeting and competing conditions; 2) each ear for both conditions combined; and 3) both ears and conditions combined. These raw scores then are corrected by subtracting the monosyllabic word discrimination error in percent, which, according to Katz (1977), neutralizes "the effect of peripheral distortion" (p. 110). The various corrected scores are applied to normative values for interpretation. Some audiologists, including the present authors, question the validity of applying such a word recognition correction based on monosyllabic words presented in quiet to spondee words given in a totally different type of task.

Gilroy and Lynn (1974), Lynn and Gilroy (1972, 1975, 1977), Musiek and Sachs (1980), and Musiek et al. (1981) have used the SSW test as part of a battery for patients with central lesions. Their method of scoring differs from Katz's recommendation in that raw scores are not corrected for phonemic discrimination error. Instead, word recognition scores in percent correct are obtained for each ear under the noncompeting and competing conditions and the degree of asymmetry is compared to normative data which serve as the basis for determining abnormal performance.

Various reports of SSW findings in patients with central auditory nervous system lesions reveal that the test is especially sensitive to abnormalities involving auditory areas of the temporal lobes and interhemispheric auditory tracts deep in the parietal lobes (Brunt, 1978; Gilroy and Lynn, 1974; Jerger and Jerger, 1975a; Katz and Pack, 1975; Katz, 1977; Lynn and Gilroy, 1972, 1975, 1977; Musiek and Sachs, 1980; Musiek and Wilson, 1979). In temporal lobe lesions, abnormal performance typically occurs in the ear contralateral to the affected hemisphere. Patients with deep parietal or frontal lobe lesions involving the transverse interhemispheric auditory pathways of the corpus collosum or its lateral extensions often demonstrate abnormal scores in the left ear (ear ipsilateral to the dominant hemisphere for speech) regardless of the hemisphere primarily involved (Gilroy and Lynn, 1974; Lynn and Gilroy, 1977; Musiek and Sachs, 1980). In patients with lesions of the brainstem, SSW test results have been shown to vary considerably ranging from no test deficits in some cases to poor performance in others (Jerger and Jerger, 1975a; Spitzer and Ventry, 1980).

Digits

In 1961, Kimura published two papers that described an auditory test employing digits along with results obtained from a large series of patients with seizure disorders. The test consisted of groups of six digits per group in which half were presented to the left ear and half to the right ear. After each group of six numbers, the listener repeated all the numbers heard in any order. For the purpose of these studies, Kimura presented the test under three different conditions. The first was a dichotic condition based on a procedure first used by Broadbent (1956). The six digits of a group were presented in pairs *simultaneously* to the two ears, one number of a pair to the left ear and a different number to the right ear with an interval of about one-half second between each pair. There were 16 groups for a total possible score of 48 for each ear. In the second condition, the six numbers of a group were presented *alternately* to the two ears (each ear received three numbers) with about a half-second interval between each number. There were 16 groups: half of the groups started in the left ear and half in the right. The total possible score was 48 for each ear. In the third condition, the six numbers in each group were presented successively to one ear with a half-second interval between numbers. Eight groups were presented to the left ear and eight to the right for a total possible score for each ear of 48. This was the *digit span* condition and was used as a control measure.

In the first study, Kimura (1961a) administered the digits test to 71 patients with epileptic seizures including 55 with temporal or frontal lobectomy, 10 with unoperated seizure disorder of subcortical origin, five unoperated with unilateral temporal lobe seizure focus and one with an unoperated unilateral frontal lobe seizure focus. Among other things, Kimura found that recognition was impaired for digits arriving in the ear contralateral to the temporal lobectomy. Also, overall efficiency of recognition from both ears was reduced by left temporal lobectomy, but not by right temporal lobectomy. Both pre- and postoperative scores obtained from patients with left temporal lobe lesions were inferior to the scores of patients with lesions of the right temporal lobe. In the second study (Kimura, 1961b) involving 120 patients with epileptogenic lesions in various regions of the brain (107 with left cerebral dominance and 13 with right cerebral dominance) and 13 right-handed normal control subjects, Kimura found that recognition of dichotic digits was more efficient in the ear contralateral to the dominant hemisphere than in the ear ipsilateral to the dominant hemisphere. This was found in both the left and right hemisphere dominant groups and was independent of handedness and site of the epileptic activity. The results of the two studies suggested that the decussating auditory pathways are stronger than the uncrossed and that the dominant temporal lobe (left in most people) is more important than the nondominant as far as recognition of verbal material is concerned.

Since the work of Kimura in 1961, others have reported similar results with dichotic digits in patients with other type lesions (Goodglass, 1967; Musiek and Sachs, 1980; Roeser and Daly, 1974; Schulhoff and Goodglass, 1969; Sparks, Goodglass and Nickel, 1970). Also Milner, Taylor and Sperry (1968) and Sparks and Geschwind (1968) reported nearly complete suppression of dichotic digits in the left ear of patients with midline section of the cerebral commissures. Under monaural test conditions, however, scores were normal for each ear. Similar findings were reported also by Musiek and Wilson (1979) and Musiek et al. (1979) in four cases with complete section of the corpus collosum and hippocampal commissure. In contrast, Musiek et al. (1981) obtained normal dichotic digit scores bilaterally pre- and postoperatively in two patients who had undergone a two-stage sectioning of the corpus collosum.

Thus, although two decades have elapsed since Kimura (1961a,b) first demonstrated the value of using digits as stimuli for measuring central auditory dysfunction, the findings of recent studies have resulted in a renewed interest in the employment of dichotic digits for identifying disruption of the central auditory system.

Syllables

Competing message tests using simultaneous pairs of nonsense consonant-vowel syllable (CVs) were developed by Berlin et al. (1968). The syllables consisted of the English stop plosives with the vowel /a/, that is, /pa/, /ba/, /ta/, /da/, /ga/, /ka/, which were recorded on tape with onset times rigorously controlled within ± 2.5 msec.

Each of the initial consonants was paired in all possible combinations. In a series of experiments, Berlin and his associates (1972) found that under dichotic listening conditions, right ear scores were better than left ear scores. Further, voiceless stop consonants were identified more correctly than voiced when presented dichotically. Under monotic listening conditions, no right ear effect was found and there was no clear superiority favoring voiceless consonants.

Porter, Shankweiler, and Liberman (1969) used CVs to show that when the onset of signals was delayed in time to one ear, perception of the lagging stimuli was better than for leading syllables in the dichotic listening mode. Lowe et al. (1970) confirmed this observation and found that when the CV pairs were separated by 15, 30, 60, and 90 msec, the right ear scores for the lagging stimulus were consistently superior to left ear scores for the leading signals, and as the lag increased in the right ear, there was a consistent improvement in right ear scores. When the 30-msec lagging stimulus was heard in the left ear, however, left ear scores were about the same as the right ear leading score. With 60- and 90-msec lag times in the left ear, lag scores became somewhat better than lead scores in the right ear; however, the difference was not statistically significant. Right ear lag scores were superior to left ear lag scores at 15, 30, and 60 msec. At 90 msec, scores of the two ears were virtually the same.

Berlin et al. (1972) reported results of dichotic testing with CVs from four patients with documented temporal lobe lesions. One had a gunshot wound and the other three had temporal lobectomies. Perception of the CVs was impaired significantly in the ear contralateral to the lesion in all four patients. Lynn and Gilroy (1977) reported dichotic CV test results in a patient with a large cystic astrocytoma of the left temporal lobe. Other test results including pure tone thresholds, undistorted and low-pass filtered monosyllabic PB word recognition, rapidly alternating speech perception (RASP), SSW, and competing sentences, were normal bilaterally. There was no evidence from these auditory tests of temporal lobe dysfunction; however, with CVs, right ear performance was consistently and significantly inferior to that of the left ear on all test conditions. Clearly, in this case, the CV material was more sensitive to the effects of the lesion than any of the other tests. Lynn and Gilroy (1977) reported that for clinical use, the dichotic CV test often is very difficult for many patients with brain lesions. In the experience of these authors, it is most appropriate in selected cases who have excellent hearing levels, normal phonemic discrimination and minimal neurologic deficit.

Filtered Speech

The use of filtered speech signals under monaural listening conditions was presented earlier in this chapter. This method of distorting speech by electronically filtering (eliminating) segments of the frequency spectrum can be employed also for dichotic and diotic listening tasks. Matzker (1959) is credited as the first clinical investigator to use both low-pass (500 to 800 Hz) and high-pass (1815 to 2500 Hz) bands of filtered speech (German two-syllable PB words) in a binaural resynthesis (fusion) task as a measure of brainstem integrity or pathology. Matzker presented the binaural filtered speech test in two different modes: 1) dichotic, low-pass band to one ear and simultaneously high-pass band to the other ear; and 2) diotic, both low- and high-pass bands presented simultaneously to both ears. The procedure used was to first present the dichotic task, next the diotic task, and then to repeat the first (dichotic) task. Matzker reported that for the first dichotic presentation, normal listeners obtained higher scores than patients with brainstem lesions. In the second task, scores improved compared to the first test for both normal hearers and patients with brainstem lesions. In the third task, normals demonstrated improved scores over the first dichotic presentation, whereas patients with brainstem pathology did not obtain such improvement. Based on these findings, Matzker (1959) concluded that this filtered speech test was useful for assessing brainstem lesions involving the auditory pathways. He further postulated that patients with unilateral lesions involving the auditory cortex should not exhibit abnormal results. Because synthesis of this dichotic task is presumed to take place at the level of the brainstem, Matzker reasoned that the intact hemisphere should receive sufficient information for relatively normal performance on this test.

Several other investigators have used binaural filtered speech tasks with low- and high-band pass filter characteristics that differed somewhat from study to study and with various types of speech stimuli (Hayashi, Ohta, and Morimoto, 1966; Linden, 1964; Lynn and Gilroy, 1972; Musiek et al., 1981; Ohta, Hayashi, and Morimoto, 1967; Palva and Jokinen, 1975; Smith and Resnick, 1972; Tillman, Bucy, and Carhart, 1966). Although Matzker's (1959) findings were not corroborated by all of the above-cited studies, most of these investigations presented evidence to support the notion that fusion or resynthesis of dichotic (low- and high-band pass) filtered speech signals takes place at the level of the brainstem. Hence, patients with brainstem lesions tend to exhibit breakdown in performance on the dichotic task compared to scores obtained in the diotic mode of presentation. By the same token, patients with cortical lesions usually do not show such a performance deficit. It appears, therefore, that dichotic and diotic filtered speech tests can be employed to help distinguish brainstem from more central lesions.

Rapidly Alternating Speech Perception Test

The use of speech material alternating rapidly between the two ears to assess central auditory deficit (Bocca and Calearo, 1963) was based on methodology proposed initially by Cherry and Taylor (1954) and Hennebert (1955). Bocca and Calearo referred to their test as *swinging speech* in which spoken sentences oscillated back and forth between ears for equal periods of time. Bocca and Calearo (1963) reported that normal listeners and patients with isolated pathology of the temporal auditory cortex demonstrated no reduced performance for any period of oscillation ranging from 2 to 40 alternations per second. However, in some cases with diffuse cerebral pathology and in patients with brainstem lesions, poor scores occurred with low rates of alternation of about three or four oscillations per second up to about eight or 10. Calearo and Antonelli (1968) reported that nine cases out of 22 (45 percent) with brainstem lesions at various levels of the neuro-axis had decreased swinging speech scores compared to normal listeners.

In 1970, Lynn and Gilroy developed a modified version of Bocca and Calearo's swinging speech test called the rapidly alternating speech perception test. In this procedure, speech (sentences) alternated rapidly between ears in bursts of 300 msec with 10-msec rise time and 50 percent duty cycle. Normal data (Adams, 1973; Lynn and Gilroy, 1975) obtained with this test under three different rates of alternation (200-, 300-, and 400-msec bursts) showed that when performance scores were calculated only for the portion of the alternating message heard in one ear, average monaural scores did not exceed 11.7 percent correct. Under binaural listening conditions with the message alternating rapidly between ears, mean scores ranged 95 to 100 percent correct for the three alternating rates. Lynn and Gilroy (1977) found that in patients with lesions of the central auditory system, RASP scores averaged 38 percent correct for six patients with pontine lesions (cerebello-pontine angle in one and intra-axial in five). This score was significantly lower than the mean scores of 82 and 94 percent correct for nine patients with upper brainstem lesions and 32 patients with unilateral cerebral hemisphere lesions, respectively. In a study cited earlier, Musiek et al. (1981) found normal RASP scores before and after corpus collosum section in two patients. These findings suggested that poor RASP scores may be a sign of abnormal binaural fusion indicating the presence of an abnormality of the pons in patients with normal phonemic discrimination and no evidence of bilateral cerebral lesions.

Masking Level Differences for Speech

Ever since the early reports of Licklider (1948) and Hirsh (1948) it has been known and confirmed in a variety of experiments that binaurally masked thresholds for pure tones or speech improve substantially in normal-hearing persons when the phase relationship of either the signal (S), tones, or speech, or noise (N) at the two ears is reversed 180 degrees ($S_\pi N_o$ or $S_o N_\pi$) compared to the condition in which the interaural phase relationship is the same ($S_o N_o$). The decibel difference in thresholds is called the masking level difference (MLD) or release from masking, which in normal listeners ranges from about 8 to 12 dB, depending on the type of signals and whether the signal or noise is out of phase interaurally. Wilson and Margolis discuss details of this phenomenon in Chapter 5.

Recent clinical studies have shown that the normal MLD may be reduced significantly in patients with certain types of peripheral auditory lesions causing either conductive or sensorineural hearing loss (Olsen, Noffsinger, and Carhart, 1976; Olsen and Noffsinger, 1976; Schoeny and Carhart, 1971). In contrast to these peripheral effects on the MLD, the studies of Cullen and Thompson (1974) and Olsen and Noffsinger (1976) have shown that the MLDs in patients with cerebral level lesions are not significantly different from the normal MLD. Other studies (Noffsinger et al. 1972; Olsen, Noffsinger, and Carhart, 1976; Noffsinger, Kurdziel, and Applebaum, 1975) have shown, however, that MLDs in patients with multiple sclerosis and other types of lesions involving subcortical structures are reduced significantly in size compared to the normal MLD. Thus, Olsen et al. (1976) suggested "that MLDs are mediated at levels below the auditory cortex," and "that small MLDs in multiple sclerosis patients implicate lesions in the brainstem or midbrain, or both" (p. 299).

More recently, Lynn et al. (1981) reported binaural speech detection MLD data from 26 normal-hearing patients with confirmed lesions at various levels of the central nervous system. Mean MLDs for 12 patients with cerebral level lesions (group 1) and five patients with lesions involving the upper pons, midbrain, or thalamic regions (group 2) ranged from 10.4 to 12.2 dB for the $S_\pi N_o$ antiphasic condition and 8.4 to 10.2 dB for the $S_o N_\pi$ antiphasic condition. Average MLDs for these two groups were not significantly different from a normal control group. However, mean MLDs for nine patients with ponto-medullary level lesions (Group 3) (2.4 and 2.3 dB for the $S_\pi N_o$ and $S_o N_\pi$ antiphasic conditions, respectively) were significantly different statistically from the other two patient groups and the normal control group at the 0.001 level. The findings from this study support the hypothesis that MLD phenomena involve some form of binaural auditory processing that correlates information from each ear and that the region of the cochlear nucleus and the superior olivary complex in the caudal pons is the anatomical area that probably mediates this process. Moreover, the data further suggest that tests of the binaural speech MLD may be used effectively to differentiate level of involvement of auditory centers and pathways of the brainstem.

AUDITORY PERCEPTUAL PROBLEMS IN CHILDREN

Although the number of published reports providing auditory test results on adult patients with well-documented lesions of the central auditory nervous system is limited, similar data on children are essentially nonexistent. As a consequence, the literature devoted to this topic in children is focused on efforts to assess central auditory processing dysfunction in children typically labeled as *learning disabled*. The rationale for this approach is based on the assumption that such children have auditory perceptual processing disorders resulting from *minimal brain dysfunction*. Children so classified have normal intelligence, do not have visual deficits or other measurable physical disabilities or emotional disturbances, yet they exhibit one or more specific learning disabilities that may involve disorders of speech and language, writing, spelling, reading, or arithmetic. It should be recognized that anatomical or direct physiologic verification of central auditory pathway pathology simply cannot be obtained with this method of clinical investigation. Nevertheless, keeping this limitation in mind, carefully designed and executed clinical studies showing the relationship between performance on a battery of central auditory tests (properly normalized on children) and specific types of learning disabilities should contribute to our understanding of central auditory dysfunction in children.

Willeford and Billger (1978) have pointed out that whereas interest in central auditory processing disorders in children has increased substantially in recent years, especially among speech pathologists and educators, serious clinical research efforts by audiologists and other hearing scientists have been lacking regarding this problem.

In order for audiologists to achieve success in assessing auditory perceptual processing disorders, it is important to know something about normal auditory perceptual processing, what the common types of auditory processing dysfunctions are and which tests are sensitive to identifying specific problems. Unfortunately, these are concepts and issues that presently are only vaguely understood (Rees, 1981). Also, it is beyond the scope of this chapter to discuss such information in detail. Hence, only brief consideration of this topic will be given here. For further discussion refer to Beasley and Rintelmann (1979), Dempsey (1977), Katz and Illmer (1972), Rees (1981), and Willeford and Billger (1978), among other sources. To date much remains unknown about the underlying mechanisms and the neurophysiologic complexity related to auditory perceptual dysfunction. Hence, efforts to describe and classify common types of processing abilities and problems leaves one vulnerable both to oversimplification and omission. Recognizing this danger, Musiek and Guerkink (1980) nevertheless briefly described the following common types of processing problems: 1) selective listening; 2) binaural separation; 3) binaural integration; 4) temporal sequencing; and 5) interhemispheric interaction. They also suggested which type of auditory test(s) should be sensitive to identifying specific processing problems and they presented a few illustrative cases. Keith (1981) also has categorized specific tests of "auditory neuromaturational level" that he feels assess fundamental auditory abilities.

In general, most of the central auditory tests described earlier in this chapter that are employed to assess lesions of the central auditory nervous system in adults are used also to identify or assess auditory perceptual disorders in children. In some instances the linguistic stimuli used in these tests have been adapted to the speech and language level of young children. Unfortunately, in some cases, however, tests that have proven useful in assessing central auditory lesions in adults simply have been applied without modification to children in an effort to measure auditory perceptual disturbances. Also, a serious criticism of much of the literature on this topic is that frequently the findings on central auditory tests applied to children are reported as abnormal without documenting what constitutes the range of normal behavior for children on such auditory measures. An equally serious criticism of such clinical investigations is that sometimes normative values are simply stated without giving the reader any information about how the norms were obtained. Moreover, some reports do not even provide a reference(s) to permit the interested reader to learn how these norms were established, and hence to what age levels and how such tests should be properly administered and interpreted. When reading the literature on the application of central auditory tests to children, the above criticisms and cautions should be kept in mind.

A brief review follows concerning the application of central auditory tests using speech stimuli to identify or assess auditory perceptual problems in children. The Flowers-Costello test of central auditory abilities was developed to identify children with auditory problems that cannot be attributed to an intellectual or psychologic deficit, or a peripheral hearing loss. As Costello (1977) clearly stated, this test "was not designed to locate or specify lesions in the auditory system" (p. 259). After a series of pilot studies that began in the early 1960s the Flowers-Costello test of central auditory abilities was produced and made available commercially with normative data based on 249 kindergarten-age children (see Flowers, Costello, and Small, 1970). This tape-recorded test consists of two auditory tasks: low-pass filtered speech (24 sentences); and a monaural competing message test with 24 sentences as the primary message and a story recorded by the same talker as the competing signal at a message to competition ratio of 0 dB. A closed-message set method of responding is used for both tasks, in that the child points to one of the three pictures (in a set) that completes the sentence. The findings from several studies using the Flowers-Costello test on various samples of children with speech, language, and/or learning problems have been summarized by Costello (1977) who reported that this test has proven useful in identifying many children with central auditory dysfunction.

Willeford (1976) developed a competing sentence test described briefly earlier in this chapter in terms of its application as a site of lesion test for adult patients having lesions involving the central auditory pathways. Normative data on children between 5 and 9 years of age (40 subjects at each age level) have been reported by Willeford (1977) based on a message to competition ratio of -15 dB with the primary message (sentences) presented at 35 dB SL and the competing sentences given at 50 dB SL. Results from this normative study demonstrated a substantial ear difference with higher percentage scores for the right ear at all age levels. Interestingly, a systematic reduction in the performance difference between ears was found as a function of age. To illustrate, Willeford (1977) reported that in the 5-year-old group, average correct scores were 28.0 percent for left ears and 91.6 percent for right ears. By age 9 this dramatic ear difference was nearly eliminated, in that mean left ear scores were 93.0 percent compared to average scores of 98.8 percent via the right ear. This right ear advantage was so consistent that among the 200 children in the normative study there were only 11 children who showed higher scores on the left ear compared to the right. Based on such large right ear superiority scores obtained in the normative study by Willeford (1977), one might question the advisability of applying and attempting to interpret the findings of this competing sentence test on children below the age of 8 or 9 who are suspected of having auditory perceptual disorders. This test, however, has been applied by Willeford (1976, 1977) and others (e.g., Pinheiro, 1977; White, 1977) to learning-disabled children under age 8. According to Willeford (1977) some children, even in the lower age groups, may achieve scores of 100 percent in each ear. He stated that one should be concerned if a child fails to give a high score in one ear or if the poorer ear score (usually left) does not improve as a function of maturation.

In addition to the competing sentence test, Willeford (1977) has reported *preliminary* (small sample) normative data for adults and for children between 5 and 9 years of age on three other central auditory tests that have been discussed earlier in this chapter. These are: 1) monaural low-pass filtered speech (with a band width from 300 to 500 Hz at a rejection rate of 18 dB per octave) using consonant-nucleus-consonant (CNC) words presented at 50 dB SL relative to the speech reception threshold (SRT) or pure tone average; 2) binaural fusion (dichotic) test consisting of simultaneous presentation of low-pass (500 to 700 Hz) and high-pass (1900 to 2100 Hz) filtered spondees at 30 dB SL re pure tone threshold at 500 Hz and 2000 Hz for the low-pass and high-pass bands, respectively; and 3) the alternating speech test in which simple sentences presented at a 30 dB SL alternate every 300 msec between the left and right ears. This test is similar to the RASP test developed by Lynn and Gilroy (1970), except that different stimulus items are used.

Based on Willeford's (1977) preliminary norms for the monaural low-pass filtered speech test and the binaural fusion test, the normal range of performance scores is wide at all age levels (5 through 9 years) and, as expected, scores improve as age increases. For the alternating speech test, however, at all age levels (including 5 year olds) scores were high and in a fairly restricted range (90 to 100 percent). See

Willeford (1977) for his suggested preliminary norms. It should be noted that the binaural fusion and RASP tests were developed as measures of "binaural synthesis," yet for both of these tests Willeford (1977, 1980) has advocated reporting scores for each ear independently. On the binaural fusion task he considers the test ear to be the one that receives the low-pass band. On the alternating speech test the ear in which the stimulus is initiated (lead ear) is regarded as the test ear. Although some audiologists have adopted these arbitrary methods of reporting both right and left ear scores for these two tests, considering the nature of both tasks, the most appropriate score is a *single binaural measure*.

Findings obtained from administering the above described battery of four tests to 150 learning-disabled children have been summarized by Willeford and Billger (1978). Although specific failure criteria for each test were not reported, they stated that more than 90 percent of the children failed one or more of the tests in the battery. The distribution of reported abnormal findings in percent by test was: binaural fusion, 64 percent; low-pass filtered speech, 57 percent; competing sentences, 48 percent; and alternating speech, 18 percent. Hence, the task most often failed was binaural fusion, whereas the test least often failed was alternating speech.

Several other investigators have employed the four above described auditory tests, sometimes referred to as the Willeford test battery, for assessing auditory perceptual abilities in children. Pinheiro (1977) investigated the central auditory processing difficulties in 14 learning-disabled children using a battery of seven tests. She administered the four tests discussed above plus a simultaneous sentences test. In this dichotic task the child is asked to repeat two simultaneous but different sentences delivered to the two ears at 50 dB SL relative to the SRT for each ear. The other two tasks used were the staggered spondee word (SSW) test (Katz, 1962) and a pitch pattern test developed by Pinheiro (1977). This latter test consists of six different combinations of three tone bursts, but only two different frequencies are used, for example, high-low-high. Refer to Pinheiro (1977) and the section on nonspeech measures of this chapter for further details regarding the pitch pattern test. Concerning her findings, Pinheiro (1977) reported that all of the learning-disabled children showed similar test result profiles, in that all showed reduced performance on the same tasks with scores varying only in amount of difficulty. She reported that the simultaneous sentences and pitch pattern tests were of the greatest value in assessing auditory processing problems.

Katz (1962) reported that children as young as 8 years of age can demonstrate normal adult responses to the SSW test. Subsequently, Katz and Illmer (1972) reported tentative normative data on the SSW test for children between the ages of 5 and 12 years and they suggested that this test might be useful in the evaluation of children with learning disabilities. Within the past few years some clinicians have shown interest in applying this test to children with auditory perceptual disorders, yet definitive data regarding the sensitivity of this measure to such problems remains sparse. White (1977) administered both the SSW test and the four tests of the Willeford battery to 31 learning-disabled children and found that 11 children responded within normal ranges on all tests. In testing the remaining 20, the SSW and the Willeford tests appeared to be about equally effective in demonstrating auditory processing deficits. Brunt (1978) concluded that due to the variability in performance of children under 11 years (compared to the norms), and because young children show a significant ear laterality effect favoring the right ear, the results from the SSW test should be interpreted with caution on children younger than 11 years. Recently, Johnson, Enfield, and Sherman (1981) administered the SSW test to 91 normal and 76 learning-disabled children between 6 and 12 years of age. Based on group data (means and standard deviations), they found that for the 7- to 10-year-old children, the learning-disabled groups could be distinguished from the normal groups; however, the SSW test did not adequately separate the learning-disabled from the normal children in either the youngest (6 year) or the oldest (11 and 12 year) age groups. Furthermore, the authors stressed that even though group differences were found at some age levels, their findings do not permit using the SSW test for identifying auditory disorders in individual children. Hence, caution should be observed in interpreting the results of the SSW test when it is administered to children suspected of having auditory perceptual problems.

The word intelligibility by picture identification (WIPI) test (Ross and Lerman, 1970) has received some application as a measure of central auditory function in children. The WIPI test items have been distorted by filtering (Martin and Clark, 1977; Plakke, Orchik, and Beasley, 1981) and by time compression (Beasley, Maki, and Orchik, 1976). A group of 11 young, normal children was compared to a group of equal numbered language learning-disabled children by Martin and Clark (1977) on filtered versions of the WIPI test: monaural low-pass, and binaural low- and high-band pass presented in both diotic and dichotic modes. They reported that the two groups performed essentially the same on the monaural task, but that the language learning-disabled group exhibited significantly greater improvement in diotic over dichotic scores compared to the normal group. Plakke and associates (1981) studied binaural fusion ability on the WIPI test by presenting low- and high-band pass filtered words to 108 normal-hearing children (4, 6, and 8 years old) in three presentation modes: dichotic$_1$, diotic, and dichotic$_2$. They investigated the effect of three varying bandwidth conditions (100, 300, and 600 Hz) and two sensation levels (30 and 40 dB). They found that word recognition scores improved with increasing age, filter bandwidth, and sensation level. Diotic scores were higher than dichotic scores for the two narrower bandwidth conditions, but this diotic enhancement effect was substantially reduced in the widest bandwidth (600 Hz) condition. Plakke et al. (1981) concluded that whereas the binaural fusion task appears to hold promise as a method for assessing central auditory processing ability, they cautioned that the variability in scores obtained by normal children is too great to warrant using such data as "norms" against which to compare the scores of individual clinical patients.

Sanderson-Leepa and Rintelmann (1976) compared the performance of 60 normal-hearing children, divided equally between the ages 3½, 5½, 7½, 9½, and 11½ years, on high fidelity (undistorted) tape recoreded versions of the WIPI, phonetically balanced kindergarden (PBK-50) and the Northwestern University No. 6 (NU #6) word recognition tests. They found that the WIPI test resulted in the highest scores, the PBK-50 was intermediate and the NU #6 was most difficult. Time-compressed versions of the Sanderson-Leepa and Rintelmann (1976) recordings of both the WIPI and the PBK-50s were constructed by Beasley et al. (1976) and administered to young, normal-hearing children (4, 6, and 8 years of age). They found that scores improved as a function of increasing age and sensation level, and became poorer as a function of greater amounts of time compression. Furthermore, the findings of Beasley et al. (1976) supported those of Sanderson-Leepa and Rintelmann (1976), who suggested that the closed-message set task of the WIPI was markedly easier for young children than the open-message set task of the PBK-50. Hence, the WIPI test appears to be more appropriate for use with young children, whereas the PBK-50 test can be used effectively with older children. The same version of the time-compressed WIPI test was presented by Orchik and Oelschlaeger (1977) to 48 young normal-hearing children (5 and 6 years of age) who were divided into three groups according to their speech articulation ability. They found significant differences in word recognition scores among the three groups and as a function of the amount of time compression. The authors concluded that children with multiple articulation errors appear to be developmentally delayed in their ability to process time-compressed speech. Ormson and Williams (1975) presented the Beasley et al. time-compressed version of the WIPI test to 40 normal-hearing children (6 to 8 years of age). Thirty of these children exhibited either speech articulatory disorders, reading problems or both articulatory and reading impairments. Ten children without such learning problems comprised the normal control group. When the findings of this study are viewed in terms of difference scores between 0 and 60 percent time compression, the time-compressed WIPI test clearly distinguishes normal children from those with specific learning (articulation and reading) problems.

The Beasley et al. (1976) time-compressed version of the PBK-50 test was given by Manning, Johnston, and Beasley (1977) to 20 children reported to have auditory perceptual problems. The authors stated that the children with auditory perceptual disorders performed more poorly at both 0 percent (control condition) and at 60 percent time compression compared to the normative data of Beasley et al. (1976).

The use of sentential approximations (synthetic sentences) was discussed earlier in this chapter as a means of assessing central auditory pathway lesions. Normal-hearing children's perception of sentential approximations and temporally distorted meaningful sentences was investigated by Beasley and Flaherty-Rintelmann (1976). They found that as order of sentential approximations was increased to full grammatical sentences, recall accuracy improved; but recall accuracy became poorer as sentence length was increased from three to five words. Also, as the silent interstimulus interval was made longer (from 200 to 400 msec), recall accuracy decreased. In general, as grade level increased (from second to fourth grade) performance improved on all measures. Freeman and Beasley (1978) compared the performance of normal-reading to reading-impaired children on a time-compressed version of the Beasley and Flaherty-Rintelmann (1976) stimuli and on the time-compressed WIPI test presented both with and without pictures. They reported that children with reading problems could be differentiated from normal readers based on scores obtained with these auditory tasks.

As discussed above, a limited amount of data for "normal" children is available on time-compressed versions of the WIPI test, the PBK-50 test, and on speech tasks involving sentential approximations. Furthermore, these measures appear to be sensitive to differentiating children with certain specific learning disabilities, for example, speech articulatory disorders or reading problems. Based on the studies reported to date, the most fruitful application of the various time-compressed speech tasks is to administer these tests at 0 and 60 percent time compression at a 24-dB sensation level or higher and to compare difference scores (between 0 and 60 percent) with the comparable values obtained from "normal" children. For example, a normal-hearing child who obtains a difference score (0 to 60 percent time compression) of greater than 10 percent on the WIPI test given in the usual closed-set format at 24 dB SL, according to Beasley and Freeman (1977), "should be followed closely for possible auditory processing difficulties" (p. 160).

The dichotic consonant-vowel syllable task (Berlin et al., 1968), described earlier in this chapter as a measure for assessing cortical lesions in adults, also has received some application to children. Berlin et al. (1973) administered this test to 150 right-handed children (15 males and 15 females in each age group of 5, 7, 9, 11, and 13 years). All children had normal hearing and adequate speech and language for their age. The test consisted of six English stop syllables (pa, ba, ta, da, ka, and ga) which were precisely aligned on two channels of magnetic tape. These CVs were presented simultaneously in pairs, one to each ear. Each child received sixty CV pairs so that each CV was presented an equal number of times in each ear. Based on the findings of this investigation, Berlin et al. (1973) concluded: ". . . dichotically presented nonsense syllables with strict acoustic and phonetic control of the stimuli, generate a right ear advantage that is essentially fixed by 5 years of age. What seems to change with age in our sample is total accuracy, phonetic content and nature of the errors, and . . . 'capacity' of the hypothesized left hemisphere speech processor" (p. 401). A few years later Mirabile et al. (1978) extended the Berlin et al. (1973) findings on the CV syllable task. They administered this dichotic test to 150 right-handed children (15 males and 15 females in each age group of 7, 9, 11, 13, and 15 years) in both a simultaneous and time-staggered (15, 30, 60, and 90 msec) mode. Their results for the simultaneous-onset condition agreed with previous findings of a "right ear advantage" (higher right compared to left ear scores) and improvement in performance as a function of age. Also, in the time-staggered mode of stimulus presentation they found a "lag effect" similar to earlier reported findings for adults, that is, more accurate identification of the lagging compared to the leading item of a dichotic pair. These investigators further found: ". . . age- and sex-related differences in the rate of performance increase as asynchronies (time-staggered differences) were increased, suggesting that consonant-vowel processing may take longer for younger children, especially males, than for adults" (p. 277). At the time of this writing only a few investigators have reported using the dichotic CV syllable task with children classified as having auditory processing problems. Dermody et al. (1975) presented the Berlin et al. (1973) tape-recorded dichotic CV stimuli to 24 learning-disabled children between 8 and 14 years of age. They found that the learning-disabled children performed as well as normal children when scores were viewed in terms of single correct responses for either right or left ear; however, the learning-disabled children scored poorer than normals on double correct responses, that is, when CVs were identified correctly in both ears. In a subsequent study, Dermody and Noffsinger (1976) presented the dichotic CV task to four different groups, including 15 children with learning disabilities between 8 and 14 years of age. Three dichotic conditions were used: both ears simultaneously; left ear lead by 90 msec; and right ear lead by 90 msec. In each of the three conditions, the learning-disabled children demonstrated poorer performance than, in this case, an adult normal control group. Tobey et al. (1979) conducted two experiments with the dichotic CV syllable task in which they compared the performance of two small groups of learning-disabled children with auditory processing disorders (age range from 7 to 12 years) to two groups of matched control subjects. In the simultaneous-onset condition, the findings of Tobey et al. (1979) were similar to those of Dermody et al. (1975) mentioned above; that is, learning-disabled children performed equally well as matched normal controls on single correct responses and showed a right ear advantage, but they scored poorer than normals on double correct responses. Furthermore, in conditions in which stimulus onsets were separated by 30, 90, and 150 msec, analysis of single correct responses demonstrated that all subjects (learning disabled and normal) achieved higher performance on lagging compared to leading stimuli. As the temporal onset between CV syllables increased, however, the ability of normal children to identify correctly both leading and lagging stimuli approached equality, whereas the learning-disabled children showed little improvement in the identification of leading CVs even when stimuli were separated by 150 msec. Hence, whereas Tobey et al. (1979) found that children with auditory processing disorders exhibited an overall performance deficit on the dichotic CV task compared to matched controls, this reduced performance was attributable to dichotic trials resulting in either both-correct or neither-correct responses. Thus, based on these above-reported studies, it appears that the dichotic CV task may be a sensitive measure for assessing auditory processing problems in children. At any rate, further investigation is warranted.

In concluding this section on assessing auditory perceptual disorders in children, two cautions should be kept in mind. First, the studies reported herein concern children with normal peripheral auditory systems. If a central auditory problem is suspected in a patient with a concomitant peripheral disorder, interpretation of the central auditory test results is a difficult, if not impossible task (Miltenberger, Dawson, and Raica, 1978). A second caution that should be contemplated concerns the use of "normative data" against which to compare the test results of any child suspected of exhibiting an auditory perceptual disorder. The results of any auditory test can be influenced by a multitude of variables related to the specific stimuli used, test procedures, and the acoustic environment. The importance of this fact is discussed and illustrated in other chapters of this text and elsewhere (e.g., White, 1977) and hence is not amplified here. It is sufficient to stress that one should not use the norms developed in someone else's laboratory unless the same recorded stimuli are employed with identical test procedures. Even under these circumstances it is appropriate to gather sufficient normative data to permit one to compare one's "local norms" to previously reported norms. If a difference is found, and the local norms were properly collected, in most instances it would be appropriate to use the local norms.

Finally, one may question what can be done after a child has been identified as having an auditory perceptual processing disorder. Unlike an adult with a central auditory nervous system lesion whereby a diagnosis often is followed by medical treatment and/or surgery, remedial procedures for children with central auditory problems involve auditory training or other forms of therapy (Musiek and Guerkink, 1980). Hence, it is not sufficient simply to identify such children. The primary goal must be to attempt to evaluate and analyze the specific auditory processing problems exhibited by such children in order to devise appropriate remedial programs to meet each child's individual needs. Based on the present-day state of the art, considerable knowledge remains to be gained prior to fully reaching this goal—and it can be accomplished only by an intensive interdisciplinary effort involving audiologists, speech and language pathologists, learning disability specialists, and pediatric neurologists among others.

NONSPEECH MEASURES

Although the focus of this chapter is on the various types of speech measures that are used for the assessment of central auditory disorders, brief mention is made of certain tests in which auditory stimuli other than speech are used for assessment. As noted earlier (Snow et al., 1977), most past efforts concerned with the application of signals other than speech for the assessment of central auditory lesions have been largely unsuccessful with a few exceptions. The recent application, however, of certain techniques appears promising. Four such tests are discussed briefly in this section. These are: 1) the frequency (pitch) pattern perception test; 2) the pure tone masking level difference task; 3) the acoustic reflex threshold measurement; and 4) the auditory brainstem response measurement.

A monaural tonal task developed by Pinheiro (1976, 1977), called the *pitch pattern test*, appears to be sensitive for identifying disruption of the interhemispheric auditory pathways. This task typically consists of 30 monaural presentations of a series of three successive tone bursts with one differing in frequency from the other two by being lower or higher. Hence, only two frequencies (880 and 1122 Hz) are presented in six different patterns (e.g., high-low-high, low-high-low, etc.) at a high SL (e.g., 40 or 50 dB). The recommended stimulus parameters are a tonal duration of 150 msec with a 200-msec interval between tones. The listener's task is to verbally label the pattern (e.g., high-high-low) or to imitate the three-tone sequency by "humming." The findings on this task have been reported recently in a series of small sample case studies cited earlier in this chapter in connection with various speech tasks. Musiek and Sachs (1980) reported that in a patient with right frontal lobe abscess and presumed secondary interhemispheric auditory tract involvement, before treatment the patient could not perform the pitch pattern task for either ear. After treatment, however, the patient could do the task, but the scores for both ears were somewhat below normal. Musiek, Pinheiro, and Wilson (1980) found that sectioning the corpus collosum in three patients dramatically affected their ability to report pitch patterns verbally, but they could "hum" correctly the pitch patterns presented. In contrast to the above findings, Musiek et al. (1981) reported that when two patients received commissurotomy in two stages (with about 2 months between operations) their ability to perform the pitch pattern task was not changed post surgically compared to preoperative scores. One patient's scores were normal bilaterally whereas the other patient's scores were slightly below the normal range. Hence, the case findings reported by Musiek and his associates demonstrate that the frequency (pitch) pattern perception task appears to serve a useful role in the CANS test battery by helping to identify dysfunction of the interhemispheric auditory pathways.

Based on evidence reported within the past few years, a binaural tonal task that holds promise for identifying brainstem and nerve VIII lesions and for distinguishing brainstem from higher central auditory pathway disorders is the pure tone MLD task (Clemis, Noffsinger, and Derlacki, 1977; Olsen and Noffsinger, 1976; Olsen, Noffsinger, and Carhart, 1976; Noffsinger et al., 1972, 1975). A description of the pure tone MLD task may be found in Chapter 5 of this text; recall that the application of the MLD test using speech signals for the assessment of CANS disorders was presented earlier in this chapter. Among normal listeners the absolute MLD size varies somewhat according to specific measurement procedures used and reduced MLDs have been found in some patients with peripheral auditory disorders (Quaranta and Cervellera, 1974; Schoeny and Carhart, 1971). Nevertheless, the MLD task with low frequency (e.g., 500 Hz) pure tones is useful also in assessing CANS disorders. Patients with brainstem lesions who have normal pure tone thresholds frequently exhibit reduced (7 dB or less for the $S_\pi N_o$ antiphasic condition) or absent MLDs, compared to normals (mean MLD of 11 dB for the $S_\pi N_o$ condition), whereas patients with cortical lesions typically obtain normal-size MLDs (Olsen et al., 1976). Hence, the findings with pure tone MLDs are in agreement with, but somewhat less sensitive than the reported results from studies using speech MLDs.

The measurement of middle ear muscle reflexes using tonal or noise stimuli and brainstem evoked responses using clicks are especially valuable because voluntary responses from the patient are not required. Both of these measures, and especially the latter, are quite sensitive techniques for assessing nerve VIII lesions. Furthermore, both methods also hold promise for evaluating CANS disorders (Jerger, 1981).

The neural pathways of the acoustic reflex arc consist of a three- or four-neuron tract situated in the lower brainstem. Further, because the neuronal organization of the crossed reflex pathways is more complex than that of the uncrossed pathways, a comparison of crossed versus uncrossed reflex thresholds may aid in localizing the site of lesion. Specifically, patients with nerve VIII lesions frequently exhibit abnormal (elevated or absent) acoustic reflex thresholds for both crossed and uncrossed test conditions. Patients with intra-axial brainstem disorders often show abnormal reflex thresholds on both ears to contralateral (crossed) stimulation, but normal ipsilateral (uncrossed) reflex thresholds. Also, some evidence shows that patients with temporal lobe disorders usually have normal contralateral and ipsilateral acoustic reflex thresholds. For a detailed discussion of this topic including appropriate literature citations refer to Jerger (1980).

The final nonspeech procedure to be mentioned is measurement of brainstem-evoked response (BSER) recently termed auditory brainstem response (ABR) audiometry. This technique involves recording brainstem-evoked potentials with surface electrodes commonly placed on the vertex and mastoid. Evoked responses from a large number of stimuli (usually clicks) are recorded and the corresponding electrical activity is averaged with a computer. The normal waveform pattern contains five positive peaks that appear within 10 msec after click stimulation and are labeled I through V in their order of occurrence. According to Buchwald and Huang (1975), these waves are thought to be generated from nerve VIII (wave I) and successive brainstem auditory nuclei and tracts to the level of the inferior colliculus (wave V). Although this may be a generally useful overview, it is undoubtedly an oversimplified description of a highly complex auditory neural pathway (Starr and Achor, 1975; Achor and Starr, 1980a,b). Clinical interpretation is based on the waveform shape and expected latency, or time interval from presentation of the signal to the occurrence of the peak response. Evidence shows that patients with brainstem lesions exhibit distorted waveforms with delayed peak latencies or an absence of one or more of the expected peaks (waves). Patients with temporal lobe disorders, however, usually display normal results (Rowe, 1981). For further discussion of auditory evoked potentials (responses) refer to Berlin and Dobie (1979), Rowe (1981), or Skinner (1978), among other sources.

In summary, although the emphasis of this chapter is on the use of speech stimuli for the assessment of CANS disorders, various types of nonspeech measures have been employed for this purpose. Measurement of acoustic reflex thresholds and brainstem-evoked responses should prove especially valuable because both of these techniques can be used with patients (e.g., infants and young children) who cannot be tested with those procedures that require behavioral responses.

ILLUSTRATIVE CASES

In this section of the chapter auditory test findings are presented for seven patients (five adults and two children) seen because of neurologic abnormalities suggesting a brain lesion which subsequently was confirmed. The cases were selected to illustrate test findings that can occur in patients with lesions at various locations and levels of the brain, including the lower and upper brainstem, the temporal lobes of both the right and left cerebral hemispheres, and the interhemispheric auditory pathways deep in the parietal lobes of both hemispheres. These cases also illustrate test results from many (but not all) of the central auditory tests discussed in the preceding sections of this chapter. The reader should recognize, moreover, that the cases illustrated are neither exhaustive of the varieties of CANS lesions one may encounter nor of the auditory tests used for assessing dysfunction of the central auditory pathways. Furthermore, these illustrative cases do not represent all possible patterns of test findings.

The primary criterion applied to the test findings to determine abnormality on the monaural low redundancy and dichotic tests is the significance of the degree of asymmetry in the scores of the two ears. Absolute scores may vary over a wide range among patients depending on variables having little to do with the effects of CANS lesions. This makes the level of the absolute scores of the two ears for a given patient less useful for identification and localization of CANS lesions than the difference in test scores between the two ears. Abnormality on the binaural fusion tests (RASP and Matzker's low-band and high-band pass test) is determined on the basis of whether or not binaural performance is substantially improved compared to monaural performance for the portion of the total message received in just one ear.

Case 1 Forty-five-year-old-female. When seen initially, this patient's test findings (Figure 8-1) revealed normal sensitivity for pure tones and normal speech recognition for undistorted PB material, bilaterally. Monaural understanding of low-pass filtered words was considerably poorer in the right ear (56 percent) compared to the left (76 percent). Also, on the simultaneous binaural condition of the dichotic SSW test, the right ear score (78 percent) was clearly inferior to that of the left (98 percent). There was no abnormality in either ear (100 percent) on the dichotic competing sentence test. Moreover, the binaural score (100 percent) on the RASP test was substantially improved over the monaural scores (0 percent), thus revealing no abnormality in binaural fusion of alternating messages.

Neurologic and radiologic findings revealed the presence of an expanding mass in the left hemisphere, subsequently confirmed as an astrocytoma. The patient expired 8 months after audiologic studies were completed. Postmortem findings, as revealed in the coronal section of the brain (Figure 8-2), showed the presence of a large left hemisphere tumor extending anteriorly into the caudate nucleus and internal capsule, posteriorly into the occipital lobe and laterally into the temporal lobe compressing the lateral ventricle, third ventricle, and temporal lobe.

Patients with involvement of the temporal lobe, as in this case, usually demonstrate abnormal monaural low redundancy and dichotic test

ASTROCYTOMA, LEFT TEMPORAL LOBE

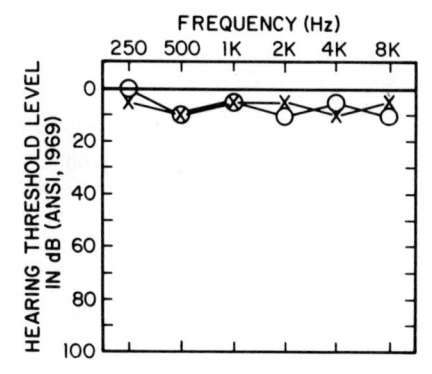

	UD PB	LPF PB	ALT BIN	SIM BIN	COMP SENT
RE	100	56	83	78	100
LE	100	76	100	98	100

	RASP
RE	0
LE	0
BIN	100

Figure 8-1. Case 1. Auditory test findings in a 45-year-old female with an astrocytoma involving the left temporal lobe. Results are shown for: pure tone thresholds; monaural speech recognition scores for undistorted PB (UD PB) words and low-pass filtered PB (LPF PB) words; dichotic speech recognition scores for the alternate binaural (ALT BIN) and simultaneous binaural (SIM BIN) conditions of the SSW test; competing sentence (COMP SENT) test; and the rapidly alternating speech perception (RASP) test in both monaural and binaural modes.

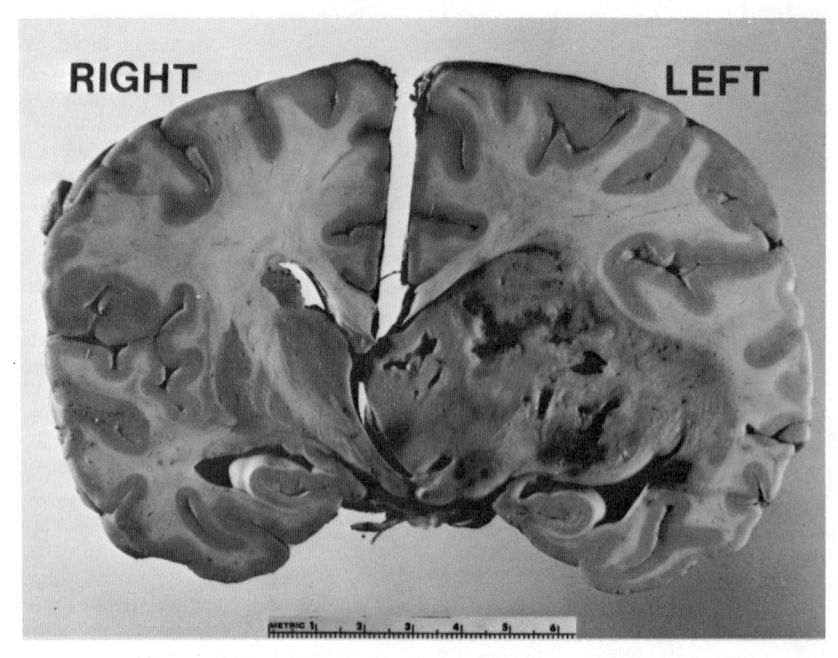

Figure 8-2. Case 1. Coronal section (anterior surface) of the brain of a 45-year-old female with an astrocytoma involving the left temporal lobe. The left cerebral hemisphere was enlarged. The tumor involved the caudate nucleus, internal and extreme capsules, occipital and temporal lobes with compression of the lateral ventricle, third ventricle, and temporal lobe.

scores in the ear contralateral to the involved hemisphere. This has been called the contralateral ear effect. However, in some cases with left temporal lobe abnormality, ipsilateral ear scores also may be depressed, but to a lesser extent than in the contralateral ear. Understanding of speech alternating rapidly between the two ears usually is normal, as this case showed, unless there is associated secondary involvement of the pons or bilateral involvement of the cerebral hemispheres. In this case there was no neurologic or radiologic evidence of brainstem or bilateral cerebral involvement at the time of testing.

Case 2 Forty-five-year-old male. Two years before testing, this patient had a cerebral infarction involving the right hemisphere. Subsequently, right-sided atrophy of the brain developed in the region of the right lateral ventricle. This was accompanied by focal seizure activity, right temporo-parietal region. Test findings (Figure 8-3) showed the presence of a high-frequency sensorineural hearing loss above 2000 Hz, greater in the left ear than in the right. It could not be determined whether this hearing loss was associated with the known brain abnormality. Speech recognition for undistorted PB material was normal bilaterally. There was, however, substantial left ear dysfunction compared to right ear performance (contralateral ear effect) on monaural low-pass filtered tests

(48 percent) and with 40 and 60 percent time compression (74 and 42 percent), the dichotic simultaneous binaural condition of the SSW test (65 percent) and on the competing sentence test (0 percent). Binaural recognition of rapidly alternating speech between the two ears was mildly impaired (70 percent), which could have been due, in part, to the high-frequency sensorineural hearing loss. However, the binaural score was substantially improved over the monaural scores (20 and 10 percent for right and left ears, respectively). Scores of 10 and 20 percent are normal for the RASP monaural test conditions. There were no neurologic or radiologic signs of brainstem abnormality in this case. Even though the undistorted speech recognition scores (UD PB) were normal bilaterally, the marked high-frequency sensorineural loss above 2000 Hz in the left ear could have contributed somewhat to the reduced left ear scores on the monaural low redundancy and dichotic test procedures (Miltenberger et al., 1978; Speaks, 1980). It is unlikely, however, that the entire left ear deficit was due solely to the high frequency sensorineural hearing loss in that ear.

Case 3 Twenty-three-year-old female. When this patient was seen for audiometric tests there was neurologic and radiologic evidence of a mass lesion located in the left parietal lobe involving interhemispheric pathways of the brain. Auditory test findings (Figure 8-4) revealed a mild high frequency sensorineural hearing loss at 4000 Hz, not exceeding 30 dB hearing level (HL). Word recognition scores for undistorted PB material

CEREBRAL INFARCTION, RIGHT HEMISPHERE
POST STROKE HEMIATROPHY, RIGHT LATERAL VENTRICAL
SEIZURE DISORDER, RIGHT TEMPORO-PARIETAL REGION

SPEECH RECOGNITION IN % CORRECT

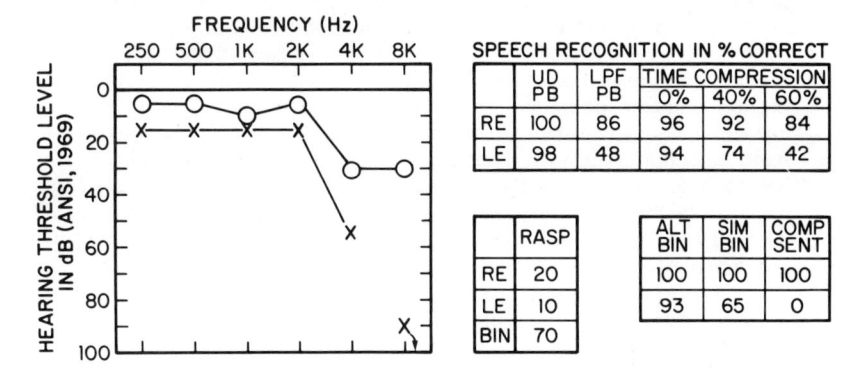

	UD PB	LPF PB	TIME COMPRESSION		
			0%	40%	60%
RE	100	86	96	92	84
LE	98	48	94	74	42

	RASP
RE	20
LE	10
BIN	70

	ALT BIN	SIM BIN	COMP SENT
	100	100	100
	93	65	0

Figure 8-3. Case 2. Auditory test findings in a 45-year-old male with an infarction involving the right cerebral hemisphere, post stroke hemiatrophy of the right lateral ventricle, and seizure disorder from the right temporo-parietal region of the brain. Results are shown for: pure tone thresholds; monaural speech recognition scores for undistorted PB (UD PB) words, low-pass filtered PB (LPF PB) words, and CNC monosyllables at 0, 40, and 60 percent time compression; dichotic speech recognition scores for the alternate binaural (ALT BIN) and simultaneous binaural (SIM BIN) portions of the SSW test, competing sentence (COMP SENT) test; and the rapidly alternating speech perception (RASP) test in both monaural and binaural modes.

ASTROCYTOMA, LEFT PARIETAL LOBE

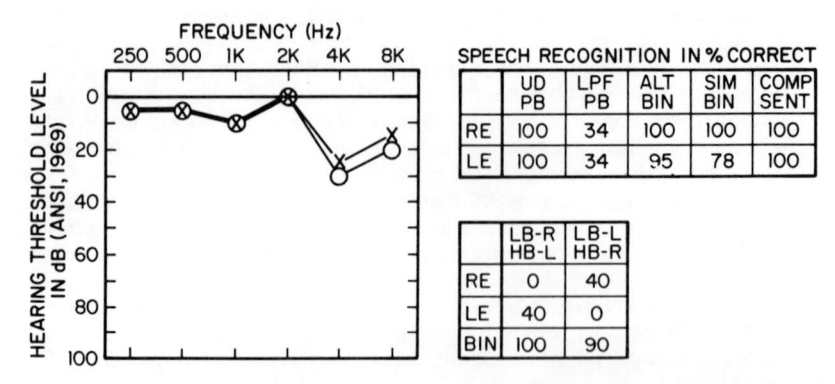

	UD PB	LPF PB	ALT BIN	SIM BIN	COMP SENT
RE	100	34	100	100	100
LE	100	34	95	78	100

	LB-R HB-L	LB-L HB-R
RE	0	40
LE	40	0
BIN	100	90

Figure 8-4. Case 3. Auditory test findings in a right-handed 23-year-old female with an astrocytoma deep in the left parietal lobe of the brain. Results are shown for: pure tone thresholds; monaural speech recognition scores for undistorted PB (UD PB) words and low-pass filtered PB (LPF PB) words; dichotic speech recognition scores for the alternate binaural (ALT BIN) and simultaneous binaural (SIM BIN) conditions of the SSW test and competing sentence (COMP SENT) test; the filtered speech test with low-band (LB) and high-band (HB) pass filtered spondees administered both monaurally with only one band of filtered speech to right or left ear and also binaurally with one band to each ear.

and low-pass filtered word lists presented monaurally were normal bilaterally, and identical for each ear. However, performance on the simultaneous binaural condition of the SSW test was definitely poorer in the left ear (78 percent) compared to the right (100 percent). There was no difference between ears on the dichotic competing sentence test. Perception of low-band and high-band pass filtered speech was tested under three conditions. Monaural scores did not exceed 40 percent correct with the low-band or high-band pass material heard in either the right or the left ear. Under the binaural condition, however, when the low- and high-band pass materials were heard in the two ears simultaneously, scores improved greatly (90 and 100 percent correct). These results demonstrated integrity of binaural fusion processes thought to occur at the brainstem level. There was no neurologic or radiologic evidence of brainstem involvement in this case at the time of testing.

At autopsy, 4 months after testing, the left parietal lobe was found to be enlarged compared to the right as shown in the coronal brain section (Figure 8-5). The tumor was hemorrhagic and extended deeply in the parietal lobe above the Sylvian fissure to involve the lateral extension of the corpus callosum in the left hemisphere. This lesion undoubtedly involved the interhemispheric auditory pathways that course between the two hemispheres via the corpus callosum. The coronal section of the brain also showed evidence of downward pressure on the left temporal lobe; however, there was no evidence of this on the arteriogram or audiologic studies at the time of testing.

The auditory findings in this case demonstrated 1) a deficit in recognition of dichotic material in the left ear, which is the ear ipsilateral to the dominant hemisphere for speech and language, and 2) no asymmetry in monaural speech recognition of frequency distorted material which usually occurs in patients with temporal lobe abnormality. This pattern of abnormality with monaural low redundancy and dichotic tests is seen frequently in patients with involvement of the interhemispheric auditory pathways due to lesions in either the right or left hemispheres. Recognition of this pattern often is helpful in differentiating interhemispheric pathway involvement from temporal lobe dysfunction in cases with no known brainstem disturbance.

Case 4 Fifty-nine-year-old male. Test findings (Figure 8-6) showed the patient had a mild bilateral high frequency sensorineural hearing loss not exceeding 45 dB in the left ear. His ability to understand high-fidelity monosyllabic PB material (UD PB) was normal bilaterally as was his ability to understand the same type of material when low-pass filtered (LPF). This was shown by the close agreement in test scores (within 4 percent) for the two ears. Under dichotic test conditions, however, left ear performance was substantially poorer than that for the right ear with both the alternate (85 percent) and simultaneous (50 percent) binaural conditions of the SSW test and the competing sentence test (70 percent). Left ear scores ranged from 15 to 48 percent poorer than right ear scores on these dichotic measures. The RASP test score of 100 percent correct

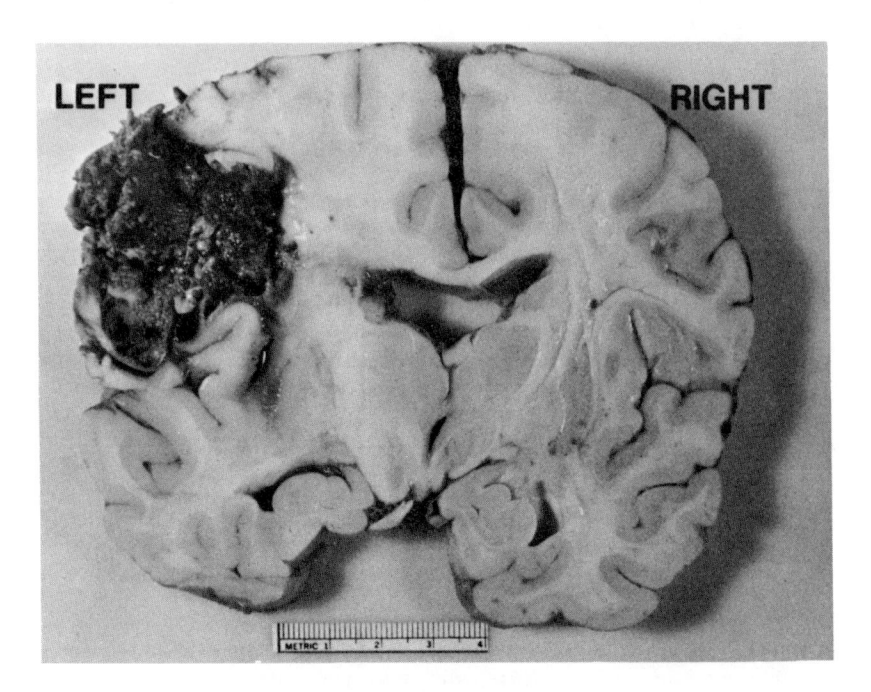

Figure 8-5. Case 3. Coronal section (posterior surface) of the brain of a 23-year-old female with an astrocytoma, left parietal lobe. The left parietal lobe was enlarged. The tumor was hemorrhagic and involved the lateral extension of the corpus callosum above the Sylvian fissure in the left hemisphere.

ASTROCYTOMA, RIGHT PARIETAL LOBE

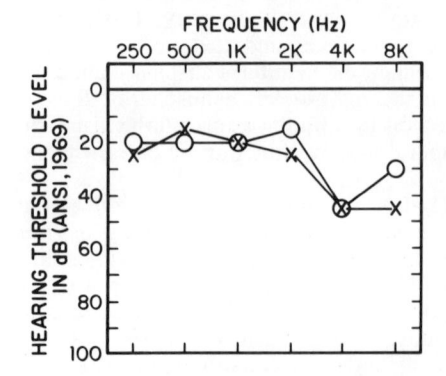

SPEECH RECOGNITION IN % CORRECT

	UD PB	LPF PB	ALT BIN	SIM BIN	COMP SENT
RE	96	56	100	98	100
LE	94	60	85	50	70

	RASP
RE	0
LE	0
BIN	100

Figure 8-6. Case 4. Auditory test findings in a right-handed 59-year-old male with an astrocytoma of the right parietal lobe. Results are shown for: pure tone thresholds; monaural speech recognition scores for undistorted PB (UD PB) words and low-pass filtered PB (LPF PB) words; dichotic speech recognition scores for the alternate binaural (ALT BIN) and simultaneous binaural (SIM BIN) portions of the SSW test and the competing sentence (COMP SENT) test; and the rapidly alternating speech perception (RASP) test in both monaural and binaural modes.

under the binaural alternating condition was normal. When compared to the monaural scores of 0 percent correctly understood, the normal binaural score indicted the absence of disturbance in binaural fusion processes.

This patient had neurologic and radiologic signs of mass lesion deep in the right parietal lobe of the brain which was confirmed as an astrocytoma. Its location would have interfered with the interhemisphere transfer of information from one side of the brain to the other. As in Case 3, audiologic findings showed a deficit in the left ear performance with dichotic material (ear ipsilateral to the dominant hemisphere) but no apparent deficit in understanding of monaural frequency distorted test material. Findings are consistent with the effects of a lesion involving the interhemispheric auditory pathways.

Case 5 Fifty-five-year-old female. This patient had a hemorrhage involving the parietooccipital region of the left cerebral hemisphere. Test findings (Figure 8-7) revealed the patient's audiogram was essentially normal bilaterally although high-frequency sensitivity was slightly elevated in the right ear. Understanding of undistorted and 0 percent time-compressed monosyllables was normal bilaterally. When these words were time compressed 40 and 60 percent, however, right ear performance (70 and 56 percent) was considerably reduced compared to the left ear (92 and 96 percent). Similarly, monaural performance for the right ear on the synthetic sentence identification task with competing messages in the same ear at a message-to-competition ratio of 0 dB was reduced to 0 percent correct in comparison to the perfect performance for the left ear (100 percent). Thus, the two monaural tests (time compression and synthetic sentence identification with ipsilateral competing messages) revealed a right ear performance deficit. A similar right ear abnormality for synthetic sentences was seen under dichotic conditions in which the competing message was heard in the non-test ear (SSI-CCM). Right ear scores were 50 and 60 percent poorer than left ear scores with 0 and −30 dB competing message ratios, respectively.

This case demonstrates a substantial deficit in the understanding of degraded material in the right ear when presented monaurally and dichotically. Assuming the absence of brainstem involvement for which there was no neurologic evidence, these audiologic signs suggest left temporal lobe involvement as well as the parieto-occipital abnormality which was demonstrated neurologically and radiographically.

Case 6 Ten-year-old female. Test results (Figure 8-8) showed the patient's hearing sensitivity for pure tones and word recognition scores for undistorted PB material were normal bilaterally. Understanding of monaural low-pass filtered PB material and performance on the alternate and simultaneous binaural conditions of the SSW test was 12 to 15 percent poorer in the left ear than in the right. The dichotic competing sentence test results were normal bilaterally. Rapidly alternating speech perception findings were normal on the binaural alternating condition (80 percent) showing substantial improvement over the monaural scores (0 percent).

Audiometric findings in this case demonstrated left ear abnormality with monaural frequency distorted (LPF) and dichotic (SSW) tests. The patient had an intra-axial tumor involving both sides of the brainstem at the ponto-mesencephalic level. The auditory findings in this case are indistinguishable from the expected findings in patients with right temporal lobe abnormality. In other words, it was not possible with these tests to

HEMORRHAGE, LEFT HEMISPHERE
PARIETO-OCCIPITAL REGION

	UD PB
RE	96
LE	96

TIME COMPRESSION		
0%	40%	60%
96	70	56
96	92	96

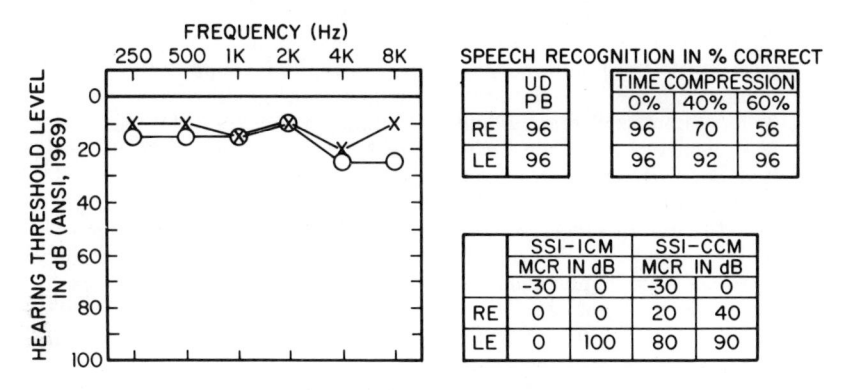

	SSI-ICM		SSI-CCM	
	MCR IN dB		MCR IN dB	
	−30	0	−30	0
RE	0	0	20	40
LE	0	100	80	90

Figure 8-7. Case 5. Auditory test findings in a 55-year-old female with a hemorrhage involving the parieto-occipital region of the left cerebral hemisphere. Results are shown for: pure tone thresholds; monaural speech recognition scores for undistorted PB (UD PB) words and CNC monosyllables at 0, 40, and 60 percent time compression; synthetic sentence identification (SSI) with ipsilateral competing message (ICM) and contralateral competing message (CCM) scores were obtained at message to competition ratios (MCR) of 0 and −30 dB.

INTRA-AXIAL BRAINSTEM ASTROCYTOMA, PONTO-MESENCEPHALIC REGION, BILATERAL

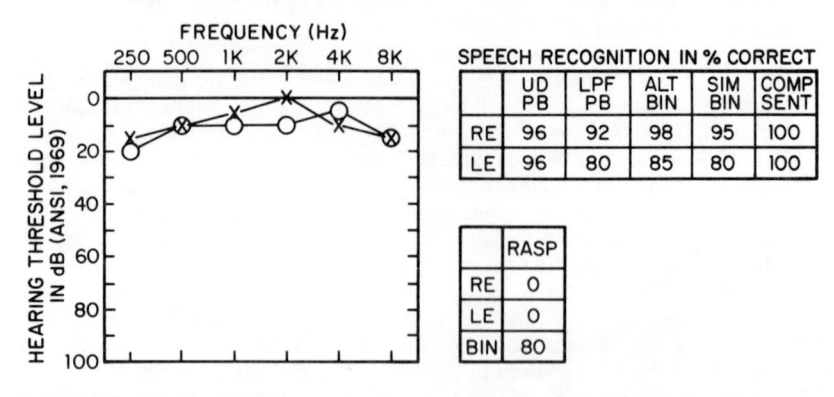

	UD PB	LPF PB	ALT BIN	SIM BIN	COMP SENT
RE	96	92	98	95	100
LE	96	80	85	80	100

	RASP
RE	0
LE	0
BIN	80

Figure 8-8. Case 6. Auditory test findings in a 10-year-old female with an intra-axial brainstem astrocytoma, bilateral, ponto-mesencephalic region. Results are shown for: pure tone thresholds; monaural speech recognition scores for undistorted PB (UD PB) words and low-pass filtered PB (LPF PB) words; dichotic speech recognition scores for the alternate binaural (ALT BIN) and simultaneous binaural (SIM BIN) conditions of the SSW test, competing sentence (COMP SENT) test; and the rapidly alternating speech perception (RASP) test in both monaural and binaural modes.

identify correctly the level of involvement of the auditory system in this case. Furthermore, this patient had diffuse bilateral involvement of the upper part of the brainstem, yet the auditory abnormality occurred only in the left ear. This points out the difficulty that may be encountered in attempting to differentiate brainstem from cerebral level lesions with the test battery used in this case.

Case 7 Ten-year-old male. This patient had an intra-axial astrocytoma localized to the ponto-medullary level of the brainstem on the left side. Figure 8-9 shows the audiometric findings. The patient's audiogram was within the normal range bilaterally, although sensitivity for the left ear was slightly poorer than for the right but not in excess of 10 dB at any frequency. Recognition of undistorted PB words was severely impaired (12 percent correct) in the left ear. Thus, recognition of monaural low-pass filtered PBs was not tested The dichotic tests (SSW, competing sentence, and RASP) were administered because the speech stimuli of these tasks are linguistically different from the distorted monosyllabic PB words. Hence, potentially higher scores might have been obtained on these tasks than for monosyllables. Under dichotic conditions (alternate and simultaneous binaural modes of the SSW and competing sentence test), left ear performance was markedly abnormal. Rapidly alternating speech perception also was abnormal binaurally, thus showing no binaural improvement over monaural scores.

This patient demonstrated essentially normal hearing for pure tones bilaterally and a severe deficit in the left ear for speech under monaural undistorted, rapidly alternating, and dichotic conditions. All of these findings could be explained on the basis of either 1) an intrinsic ponto-

INTRA-AXIAL BRAINSTEM ASTROCYTOMA, PONTO-MEDULLARY REGION, LEFT

SPEECH RECOGNITION IN % CORRECT

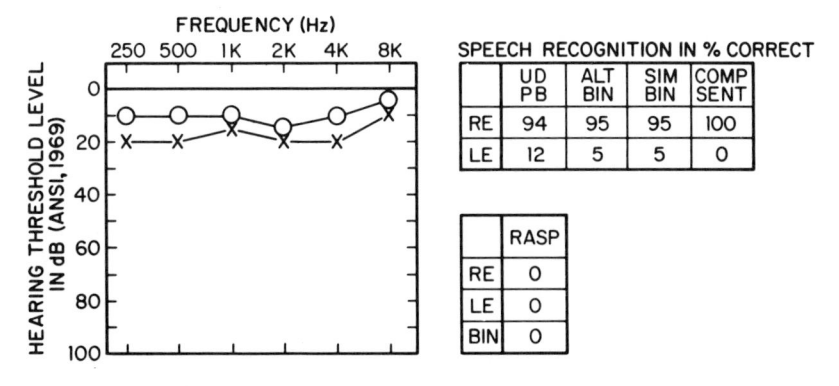

	UD PB	ALT BIN	SIM BIN	COMP SENT
RE	94	95	95	100
LE	12	5	5	0

	RASP
RE	0
LE	0
BIN	0

Figure 8-9. Case 7. Auditory test findings in a 10-year-old male with an intra-axial brainstem astrocytoma, ponto-medullary region, left side. Results are shown for: pure tone thresholds; monaural speech recognition scores for undistorted PB (UD PB) words; dichotic speech recognition scores for the alternate binaural (ALT BIN) and simultaneous binaural (SIM BIN) conditions of the SSW test, competing sentence (COMP SENT) test; and the rapidly alternating speech perception (RASP) test in both monaural and binaural modes.

medullary level lesion on the left side, or 2) possible cranial nerve VIII or extrinsic brainstem lesion in the region of the left cerebello-pontine cistern. In our experience and that of others (see Chapter 6) the latter would be less likely because pure tone hearing sensitivity was so well preserved. As in Case 6, it is difficult to be certain about the level of involvement in this case of intra-axial brainstem tumor.

In summary; the following points may be made:

1. The expected findings in patients with either right or left temporal lobe lesions are abnormal test scores in the ear contralateral to the affected hemisphere with monaural low redundancy *and* dichotic speech recognition tests. In some cases with left temporal lobe abnormality test scores may be reduced in both ears, but more so in the contralateral ear. Areas of involvement may include the auditory thalamo-cortical projects as well as the auditory cortex. Involvement may be primary to the temporal lobe or may represent associated secondary effects, such as from pressure or edema resulting from lesions located elsewhere in the brain. The ear showing the abnormal auditory function is not dependent on cerebral dominance.

2. Patients with lesions involving the transverse interhemispheric auditory tracts may be expected to yield abnormal performance with dichotic tests in the ear ipsilateral to the dominant language hemisphere, which in most patients is the left ear. In some left-handed

patients who may be right cerebral dominant, the abnormal dichotic performance may be in the right ear. Speech recognition scores for monaural low redundancy tests remain normal (bilaterally symmetrical) unless auditory areas of the temporal lobe on one side or the other are also involved to a substantial extent. Thus, the distinction between temporal lobe (including the thalamo-cortical projections and cortex) and interhemisphere auditory pathway involvement may be made in some cases on the basis of whether or not understanding of monaural low redundancy tests is abnormal, meaning asymmetrical, along with abnormal dichotic test performance in the left ear (or in the right ear in the rare patient with right cerebral dominance). Involvement of the transverse interhemispheric auditory tracts frequently is found in patients with deep right or left parietal lobe lesions involving the lateral extensions of the corpus callosum. Also, the secondary effects of expanding lesions (pressure, edema, or infiltration) located in the frontal, occipital, or temporal lobes of the brain, right or left side, may affect function of the interhemispheric pathways. In some cases it may not be possible to differentiate between temporal lobe and interhemispheric auditory pathway involvement. For example, a left ear deficit on dichotic and monaural low redundancy tests may occur from a right temporal lobe lesion or a right parietal lobe lesion with secondary effects on the right temporal lobe.

3. Lesions of the temporal lobe may be localized to either of the cerebral hemispheres in cases with unilateral lesions; however, the hemispheres primarily involved in cases with lesions of the interhemispheric pathways cannot be identified on the basis of the dichotic abnormality alone. For example, a left ear deficit with dichotic tests could be associated with a lesion involving either the right temporal lobe, the right parietal lobe, or the left parietal lobe. The abnormal ear on dichotic tests in cases with interhemispheric pathway lesions may be either ipsilateral or contralateral to the affected hemisphere, depending on which side of the brain the lesion is located.

4. Patients with brainstem lesions involving the decussating and ascending tracts on one or both sides of the brainstem often demonstrate inconsistent laterality findings with respect to anatomical localization of the lesion. Some cases may demonstrate deficits on monaural low redundancy and dichotic tests in the ear ipsilateral or contralateral to the lesion, whereas other cases may demonstrate bilateral ear dysfunction (but often asymmetrical) in apparent unilateral brainstem lesions or even unilateral ear deficits in bilateral lesions. The nature, region, and extent of the brainstem involvement are important factors contributing to apparent "inconsistent" test scores with regard to lo-

calization of brainstem abnormalities. Abnormal scores with binaural fusion tests, such as RASP, MLDs, and the SSI-ICM and CCM tests may be helpful in identifying involvement of the brainstem in cases in which either peripheral or diffuse bilateral cerebral level abnormalities can be ruled out.

CONCLUSIONS

Several tests described in this chapter have been found to be useful in assisting to identify lesions within the central auditory nervous system. Further, by utilization of an appropriate battery of tests the site of the lesion often can be isolated to the brainstem, the interhemispheric auditory pathways, or to the auditory cortex and related structures. The degree to which lesions can be localized to more specific structures must await further research in which there is evidence of precisely documented lesions in conjunction with the results of a complete battery of auditory tests. Obviously, this requires a cooperative interdisciplinary clinical research effort. Whereas some data, although limited, have been published on adult patients with well-described, confirmed lesions of the central auditory nervous system, as mentioned earlier, such data on children are essentially nonexistent. Hence, the assessment of auditory perceptual processing dysfunction in children has been focused on studying children labeled as *learning disabled* based on the rationale that such children are presumed to have *minimal brain dysfunction*. The difficulty with such an important assumption is that there is yet no clear evidence to support a cause-and-effect relationship between specific learning disabilities and *brain dysfunction*. Moreover, the categorization of specific types of auditory processing problems (e.g., selective listening, temporal sequencing, etc.) is primarily speculative, in that there is little direct support for such classification based on any well-established models of auditory perceptual processing. A detailed discussion and critique of these issues has been provided by Rees (1981).

Another vital issue that was expressed in the text of this chapter, which is of sufficient importance to be re-emphasized, concerns the use of "normative data." The results obtained from any auditory test can be substantially affected by a multitude of variables including the specific stimuli used, the talker, test procedures, and the acoustic environment; therefore, one should not use the norms developed in someone else's laboratory unless the same recorded stimuli are employed with identical test procedures. In any event, it is appropriate to collect sufficient normative data in order to compare one's "local norms" to those previously reported. If a difference is found and the local norms were properly collected, in most instances the local norms should be used.

Furthermore, because the aging process may have a substantial impact on virtually any degraded speech task (Bergman, 1980), the interpretation of central auditory test results in elderly patients can be a challenging experience. This problem is even more complex when attempting to identify central auditory dysfunction in patients of any age who have peripheral auditory disorders.

Thus, there are many potential obstacles for clinicians who attempt to assess central auditory deficits. Nevertheless, based on today's state of the art, if central auditory tests are used with proper caution and judicious skepticism along with dedicated efforts to relate auditory test data to precise anatomical lesion findings, the future can hold a rewarding and productive alliance among audiologists, neurologists, otologists, speech and language pathologists, and others interested in normal and impaired function of the central auditory nervous system.

REFERENCES

Achor, L. J., and A. Starr. 1980a. Auditory brain stem responses in the cat. I. Intracranial and extracranial recording. Electroencephalogr. Clin. Neurophysiol. 48:154–173.

Achor, L. J., and A. Starr. 1980b. Auditory brainstem responses in the cat. II. Effects of lesions. Electroencephalogr. Clin. Neurophysiol. 48:174–190.

Adams, K. M. 1973. A test to assess the integrity of subcortical auditory pathways in the human central nervous system. Master's thesis. Wayne State University, Detroit.

Antonelli, A. 1970. Sensitized speech tests in aged people. In C. Rojskjaer (ed.), Speech Audiometry (Second Danavox Symposium), pp. 66–77. Danavox Foundation, Odense, Denmark.

Beasley, D., G. Bratt, and W. Rintelmann. 1980. Intelligibility of time-compressed sentential stimuli. J. Speech Hear. Res. 23:722–731.

Beasley, D. S., and A. K. Flaherty-Rintelmann. 1976. Children's perception of temporally distorted sentential approximations of varying length. Audiology 15:315–325.

Beasley, D. S., B. Forman, and W. F. Rintelmann. 1972a. Intelligibility of time-compressed CNC monosyllables by normal listeners. J. Aud. Res. 12:71–75.

Beasley, D. S., and B. A. Freeman. 1977. Time-altered speech as a measure of central auditory processing. In R. W. Keith (ed.), Central Auditory Dysfunction, pp. 129–176. Grune & Stratton, New York.

Beasley, D. S., J. E. Maki, and D. J. Orchik. 1976. Children's perception of time-compressed speech on two measures of speech discrimination. J. Speech Hear. Disord. 41:216–225.

Beasley, D. S., and A. K. Rintelmann. 1979. Central auditory processing. In W. F. Rintelmann (ed.), Hearing Assessment, pp. 321–349. University Park Press, Baltimore.

Beasley, D. S., S. Schwimmer, and W. F. Rintelmann. 1972b. Intelligibility of time-compressed CNC monosyllables. J. Speech Hear. Res. 15:340–350.

Bergman, M. 1980. Aging and the Perception of Speech. University Park Press, Baltimore.

Berlin, C. I., and R. A. Dobie. 1979. Electrophysiologic measures of auditory function via electrocochleography and brainstem-evoked responses. In W. F. Rintelmann (ed.), Hearing Assessment, pp. 425–458. University Park Press, Baltimore.

Berlin, C. I., L. F. Hughes, S. S. Lowe-Bell, and H. L. Berlin. 1973. Dichotic right ear advantage in children 5 to 13. Cortex 9:394–402.

Berlin, C. I., and S. S. Lowe. 1972. Temporal and dichotic factors in central auditory testing. In J. Katz (ed.), Handbook of Clinical Audiology, pp. 280–312. Williams & Wilkins Company, Baltimore.

Berlin, C. I., S. S. Lowe, C. L. Thompson, and J. K. Cullen, Jr. 1968. The construction and perception of simultaneous messages. Asha 10:397.

Berlin, C. I., S. S. Lowe-Bell, P. J. Jannetta, and D. G. Kline. 1972. Central auditory deficits after temporal lobectomy. Arch. Otolaryngol. 96:4–10.

Bocca, E. 1955. Binaural hearing: Another approach. Laryngoscope 65:1164–1171.

Bocca, E. 1958. Clinical aspects of cortical deafness. Laryngoscope 68:301–309.

Bocca, E., and C. Calearo. 1963. Central hearing processes. In J. Jerger (ed.), Modern Developments in Audiology, pp. 337–370, Academic Press, Inc., New York.

Bocca, E., C. Calearo, and V. Cassinari. 1954. A new method for testing hearing in temporal lobe tumors. Acta Otolaryngol. 44:219–221.

Bocca, E., C. Calearo, V. Cassinari, and F. Migliavacca. 1955. Testing "cortical" hearing in temporal lobe tumors. Acta Otolaryngol. 45:289–304.

Broadbent, D. E. 1956. Successive responses to simultaneous stimuli. Quart. J. Exp. Psychol. 8:145–162.

Brunt, M. 1978. The staggered spondaic word test. In J. Katz (ed.), Handbook of Clinical Audiology, pp. 262–275. 2nd Ed. Williams & Wilkins Company, Baltimore.

Buchwald, J. S., and C.-M. Huang. 1975. Far field acoustic response: Origins in the cat. Science 189:382–384.

Calearo, C. 1957. Binaural summation in lesions of the temporal lobe. Acta Otolaryngol. 47:392–397.

Calearo, C., and A. R. Antonelli. 1968. Audiometric findings in brainstem lesions. Acta Otolaryngol. 66:305–319.

Calearo, C., and A. Lazzaroni. 1957. Speech intelligibility in relation to the speed of the message. Laryngoscope 67:410–419.

Cherry, E. C., and W. Taylor. 1954. Some further experiments upon the recognition of speech, with one and with two ears. J. Acoust. Soc. Am. 26:554–559.

Clemis, J. D., D. Noffsinger, and E. L. Derlacki. 1977. A jugular foramen schwannoma simulating an acoustic tumor recovery of retrolabyrinthine cochleovestibular function. Trans. AAOO 84:ORL 687–696.

Costello, M.R. 1977. Evaluation of auditory behavior of children using the Flowers-Costello test of central auditory abilities. In R. W. Keith (ed.), Central Auditory Dysfunction, pp. 257–276. Grune & Stratton, New York.

Cullen, J. K., and C. L. Thompson. 1974. Masking release for speech in subjects with temporal lobe resections. Arch. Otolaryngol. 100:113–116.

Dayal, V. S., L. Tarantino, and L. P. Swisher. 1966. Neuro-otologic studies in multiple sclerosis. Laryngoscope 76:1798–1809.

de Quiros, J. 1964. Accelerated speech audiometry, an examination of test results. Translated by J. Tonndorf. Transl. Beltone Inst. Hear. Res. 17, 48 pgs. Chicago.

Dempsey, C. 1977. Some thoughts concerning alternate explanations of central auditory test results. In R. W. Keith (ed.), Central Auditory Dysfunction, pp. 293–317. Grune & Stratton, New York.

Dermody, P., and D. Noffsinger. 1976. Auditory processing factors in dichotic listening. Paper presented at the 91st Meeting of the Acoustical Society of America, April, Washington, D.C.

Dermody, P., P. D. Noffsinger, C. P. Hawkins, and P. L. Jones. 1975. Auditory processing difficulties in children with learning disabilities. Paper presented at the convention of the American Speech and Hearing Association, November, Washington, D.C.

Durrant, J. D., and J. H. Lovrinic. 1977. Neurophysiology of the central auditory system. In Bases of Hearing Sciences, pp. 110–137. Williams & Wilkins Co., Baltimore.

Fairbanks, G., W. Everitt, and R. Jaeger. 1954. Methods for time or frequency compression-expansion of speech. Transactions of speech. Transactions of IRE-PGA. AU-2, pp. 7–12.

Flowers, A., M. R. Costello, and V. Small. 1970. Manual for Flowers-Costello Test of Central Auditory Abilities. Perceptual Learning Systems, Dearborn, Michigan.

Freeman, B. A., and D. S. Beasley. 1978. Discrimination of time-altered sentential approximations and monosyllables by children with reading problems. J. Speech Hear. Res. 21:497–506.

Freeman, B., and G. Church. 1977. Recall and repetition of time-compressed sentential approximations by normal-hearing young adults. J. Am. Audiol. Soc. 3:47–50.

Gilroy, J., and G. E. Lynn. 1974. Reversibility of abnormal auditory findings in cerebral hemisphere lesions. J. Neuro. Sci. 21:117–131.

Goldstein, R. 1961. Hearing and speech in follow-up of left hemispherectomy. J. Speech Hear. Disord. 26:126–219.

Goldstein, R., A. Goodman, and R. King. 1956. Hearing and speech in infantile hemiplegia before and after hemiplegia. Neurology 6:869–875.

Goodglass, H. 1967. Binaural digit presentation and early lateralized brain damage. Cortex 3:295–306.

Hayashi, R., R. Ohta, and M. Morimoto. 1966. Binaural fusion test: A diagnostic approach to central auditory disorders. J. Int. Audiol. 5:133–135.

Heilman, K. M., L. C. Hammer, and B. J. Wilder. 1973. An audiometric defect in temporal lobe dysfunction. Neurology 23:384–386.

Hennebert, D. 1955. A speech test. Acta Oto-Rhino-Laryngol. 9:344.

Hirsh, I. J. 1948. The influence of interaural phase on interaural summation and inhibition. J. Acoust. Soc. Am. 20:536–544.

Hodgson, W. 1967. Audiological report of a patient with left hemispherectomy. J. Speech Hear. Disord. 32:39–45.

Jerger, J. 1960a. Audiological manifestations of lesions in the auditory nervous system. Laryngoscope 70:417–425.

Jerger, J. 1960b. Observations on auditory behavior in lesions of the central auditory pathways. Arch. Otolaryngol. 71:797–806.

Jerger, J. 1964. Auditory tests for disorders of the central auditory mechanism. In B. R. Alford and W. S. Fields (eds.), Neurological Aspects of Auditory and Vestibular Disorders, pp. 77–86. Charles C Thomas Publisher, Springfield, Ill.

Jerger, J. 1970a. Development of synthetic sentence identification (SSI) as a tool for speech audiometry. In C. Rojskjaer (ed.), Speech Audiometry (2nd Danavox Symposium), pp. 44–65. Danavox, Odense, Denmark.

Jerger, J. 1970b. Diagnostic significance of SSI test procedures: retrocochlear site. In C. Rojskjaer (ed.), Speech Audiometry (2nd Danvox Symposium), pp. 163–175. Danavox, Odense, Denmark.

Jerger, J. 1973. Audiological findings in aging. Adv. Oto-Rhinol-Laryngol. 20:115–124.

Jerger, J., R. Carhart, and D. Dirks. 1961. Binaural hearing aids and speech intelligibility. J. Speech Hear. Res. 4:137–148.

Jerger, J., and D. Hayes. 1977. Diagnostic speech audiometry. Arch. Otolaryngol. 103:216–222.

Jerger, J., and S. Jerger. 1971. Diagnostic significance of PB word functions. Arch. Otolaryngol. 93:573–580.

Jerger, J., and S. Jerger. 1974. Auditory findings in brainstem disorders. Arch. Otolaryngol. 99:324–350.

Jerger, J., and S. Jerger. 1975a. Clinical validity of central auditory tests. Scand. Audiol. 4:147–163.

Jerger, J., C. Speaks, and J. Trammell. 1968. A new approach to speech audiometry. J. Speech Hear. Disord. 33:318–328.

Jerger, S. 1980. Diagnostic applications of impedance audiometry: Central auditory disorders. In J. Jerger and J. L. Northern (eds.), Clinical Impedance Audiometry, pp. 128–140. 2nd Ed. American Electromedics Corp., Acton, Mass.

Jerger, S. 1981. Evaluation of central auditory function in children. In R. W. Keith (ed.), Central Auditory and Language Disorders in Children, pp. 30–60. College-Hill Press, Houston.

Jerger, S., and J. Jerger. 1975b. Extra- and intra-axial brainstem auditory disorders. Audiology 14:93–117.

Johnson, D. W., M. L. Enfield, and R. E. Sherman. 1981. The use of the staggered spondaic word and the competing environmental sounds tests in the evaluation of central auditory function of learning disabled children. Ear Hear. 2:70–77.

Katinsky, S., J. Lovrinic, and W. Buchheit. 1972. Cochlear findings in VIIIth nerve tumors. Audiology 11:213–217.

Katz, J. 1962. The use of staggered spondaic words for assessing the integrity of the central auditory nervous system. J. Aud. Res. 2:327–337.

Katz, J. 1968. The SSW test: An interim report. J. Speech Hear. Disord. 33:132–146.

Katz, J. 1977. The staggered spondee word test. In R. W. Keith (ed.), Central Auditory Dysfunction, pp. 103–128. Grune & Stratton, New York.

Katz, J., and R. Illmer. 1972. Auditory perception in children with learning disabilities. In J. Katz (ed.), Handbook of Clinical Audiology, pp. 540–563. Williams & Wilkins Company, Baltimore.

Katz, J., and G. Pack. 1975. New developments in differential diagnosis using the SSW test. In M. D. Sullivan (ed.), Central Auditory Processing Disorders, pp. 85–107. University of Nebraska, Omaha.

Keith, R. W. 1981. Audiological and auditory-language tests of central auditory function. In R. W. Keith (ed.), Central Auditory and Language Disorder in Children, pp. 61–76. College-Hill Press, Houston.

Kimura, D. 1961a. Cerebral dominance and the perception of verbal stimuli. Canad. J. Psychol. 15:166–171.

Kimura, D. 1961b. Some effects of temporal-lobe damage on auditory perception. Canad. J. Psychol. 15:156–165.

Kimura, D. 1967. Functional asymmetry of the brain in dichotic listening. Cortex 3:163–178.

Konkle, D. F., D. S. Beasley, and F. Bess. 1977. Intelligibility of time-altered speech in relation to chronological aging. J. Speech Hear. Res. 20:108–115.

Korsan-Bengtsen, M. 1973. Distorted speech audiometry: a methodological and clinical study. Acta Otolaryngol. 310(Suppl.):7–75.

Kurdziel, S., D. Noffsinger, and W. Olsen. 1976. Performance by cortical lesion patients on 40% and 60% time-compressed materials. J. Am. Audiol. Soc. 2:3–7.

Kurdziel, S., W. F. Rintelmann, and D. Beasley. 1975. Performance of noise-induced hearing impaired listeners on time-compressed CNC monosyllables. J. Am. Audiol. Soc. 1:54–60.

Lee, F. 1972. Time compression and expansion of speech by the sampling method. J. Audio Engineer. Soc. 20:738–742.

Licklider, J. C. R. 1948. The influence of interaural phase relation upon the masking of speech by white noise. J. Acoust. Soc. Am. 20:150–159.

Linden, A. 1964. Distorted speech and binaural speech resynthesis tests. Acta Otolaryngol. 58:32–48.

Lowe, S. S., J. K. Cullen, Jr., C. L. Thompson, C. I. Berlin, L. L. Kirkpatrick, and J. T. Ryan. 1970. Dichotic and monotic simultaneous and time-staggered speech. J. Acoust. Soc. Am. 47:47–76.

Lundborg, T., H. Rosenhamer, T. Murray, and N. Zwetnow. 1975. Information abundance of speech and distorted speech testing in topical diagnosis within the C.N.S. Scand. Audiol. 4:9–19.

Lynn, G. E., J. T. Benitez, A. B. Eisenbrey, J. Gilroy, and H. I. Wilner. 1972. Neuro-audiological correlates in cerebral hemisphere lesions: Temporal and parietal lobe tumors. Audiol. J. Aud. Commun. 11:115–134.

Lynn, G. E., and J. Gilroy. 1970. Rapidly Alternating Speech Perception (RASP): A Test of Brainstem Dysfunction. Unpublished report. Wayne State University, Detroit.

Lynn, G. E., and J. Gilroy. 1971. Auditory manifestations of lesions of the corpus collosum. Asha 13:566.

Lynn, G. E., and J. Gilroy. 1972. Neuro-audiological abnormalities in patients with temporal lobe tumors. J. Neurol. Sci. 17:167–184.

Lynn, G. E., and J. Gilroy. 1975. Effects of brain lesions on the perception of monotic and dichotic speech stimuli. In M. D. Sullivan (ed.), Central Auditory Processing Disorders, pp. 47–83. University of Nebraska, Omaha.

Lynn, G. E., and J. Gilroy. 1977. Evaluation of central auditory dysfunction in patients with neurological disorders. In R. W. Keith (ed.), Central Auditory Dysfunction, pp. 177–221. Grune & Stratton, New York.

Lynn, G. E., J. Gilroy, P. C. Taylor, and R. P. Leiser. 1981. Binaural masking-level differences in neurological disorders. Arch. Otolaryngol. 107:357–362.

Manning, W. H., K. L. Johnston, and D. S. Beasley. 1977. The performance of children with auditory perceptual disorders on a time-compressed speech discrimination measure. J. Speech Hear. Disord. 42:77–84.

Martin, F. N., and J. G. Clark. 1977. Audiologic detection of auditory processing disorders in children. J. Am. Audiol. Soc. 3:140–146.

Matzker, J. 1957. The binaural test in space-occupying endocranial processes: A new method of otological diagnosis of brain disease. Z. Laryngol. 36:177–189.

Matzker, J. 1958. A Test of Binaural Fusion in Central Hearing Impairment. G. Thieme, Stuttgart.

Matzker, J. 1959. Two new methods for the assessment of central auditory functions in cases of brain disease. Ann. Otol. 68:1185–1197.

Milner, B., L. Taylor, and R. Sperry. 1968. Lateralized suppression of dichotically presented digits after commissural section in man. Science 161:184–185.

Miltenberger, G. E., G. J. Dawson, and A. N. Raica. 1978. Central auditory testing with peripheral hearing loss. Arch. Otolaryngol. 104:11–15.

Mirabile, P. J., R. J. Porter, Jr., L. F. Hughes, and C. I. Berlin. 1978. Dichotic lag effect in children 7 to 15. Devel. Psychol. 14:277–285.

Morales-Garcia, C., and J. O. Poole. 1972. Masked speech audiometry in central deafness. Acta Otolaryngol. 74:307–316.

Musiek, F. E., and N. A. Geurkink. 1980. Auditory perceptual problems in children: Considerations for the otolaryngologist and audiologist. Laryngoscope 90:962–971.

Musiek, F. E., M. L. Pinheiro, and D. H. Wilson. 1980. Auditory pattern perception in "split brain" patients. Arch. Otolaryngol. 106:610–612.

Musiek, F. E., and E. Sachs, Jr. 1980. Reversible neuroaudiologic findings in a case of right frontal lobe abscess with recovery. Arch. Otolaryngol. 106:280–283.

Musiek, F. E., and D. H. Wilson. 1979. SSW and dichotic digit results pre- and post-commissurotomy: A case report. J. Speech Hear. Disord. 44:528–533.

Musiek, F.E., D. H. Wilson, and M. L. Pinheiro. 1979. Audiological manifestations in "split brain" patients. J. Am. Aud. Soc. 5:25–29.

Musiek, F. E., D. H. Wilson, and A. G. Reeves. 1981. Staged commissurotomy and central auditory function. Arch. Otolaryngol. 107:233–236.

Noffsinger, P. D., and S. A. Kurdziel. 1979. Assessment of central auditory lesions. In W. F. Rintelmann (ed.), Hearing Assessment, pp. 351–377. University Park Press, Baltimore.

Noffsinger, D., S. Kurdziel, and E. L. Applebaum. 1975. Value of special auditory tests in the latero-medial inferior pontine syndrome. Ann. Otol. Rhinol. Laryngol. 84:384–390.

Noffsinger, D., W. O. Olsen, R. Carhart, C. W. Hart, and V. Sahgal. 1972. Auditory and vestibular aberrations in multiple sclerosis. Acta Otolaryngol. 303(Suppl.):1–63.

Ohta, R., R. Hayashi, and M. Morimoto. 1967. Differential diagnosis of retrocochlear deafness: Binaural fusion test and binaural separation test. J. Int. Aud. 6:58–62.

Olsen, W. O., and R. Carhart. 1967. Development of test procedures for evaluation of binaural hearing aids. In Bulletin of Prosthetics Research: Prosthetic and Sensory Aids Service, pp. 22–49. Department of Medicine and Surgery, Veterans Administration, Washington, D.C.

Olsen, W. O., and D. Noffsinger. 1976. Masking level differences for cochlear and brainstem lesions. Ann. Otol. Rhinol. Laryngol. 85:820–825.

Olsen, W. O., D. Noffsinger, and R. Carhart. 1976. Masking level differences encountered in clinical populations. Audiology 15:287–301.

Olsen, W. O., D. Noffsinger, and S. Kurdziel. 1975. Speech discrimination in quiet and in white noise by patients with peripheral and central lesions. Acta Otolaryngol. 80:375–382.

Orchik, D. J., and M. L. Oelschlaeger. 1977. Time-compressed speech discrimination in children and its relationship to articulation. J. Am. Audiol. Soc. 3:37–41.

Ormson, K., and D. Williams. 1975. Central auditory function as assessed by time-compressed speech with elementary school children having articulatory and reading problems. Paper presented at the convention of the American Speech and Hearing Association, November, Washington, D.C.

Palva, A., and K. Jokinen. 1975. The role of the binaural test in filtered speech audiometry. Acta Otolaryngol. 79:310–314.

Pinheiro, M. 1976. Auditory pattern perception in patients with right and left hemisphere lesions. Ohio J. Speech Hear. 12:9–20.

Pinheiro, M. L. 1977. Tests of central auditory function in children with learning disabilities. In R. W. Keith (ed.), Central Auditory Dysfunction, pp. 223–256. Grune & Stratton, New York.

Plakke, B., D. J. Orchik, and D. S. Beasley. 1981. Children's performance on a binaural fusion task. J. Speech Hear. Res. 24:520–525.

Porter, R., D. Shankweiler and A. Liberman. 1969. Differential effects of binaural time differences on perception of stop consonants and vowels. Proceedings of the 77th Meeting of the American Psychology Association, pp. 15–16.

Quaranta, A., and G. Cervellera. 1974. Masking level difference in normal and pathological ears. Audiology 13:428–431.

Quaranta, A., and G. Cervellera. 1977. Masking level differences in central nervous system diseases. Arch. Otolaryngol. 103:482–484.

Rees, N. S. 1981. Saying more than we know: Is auditory processing disorder a meaningful concept? In R. W. Keith (ed.), Central Auditory and Language Disorders in Children, pp. 94–120. College-Hill Press, Houston.

Rintelmann, W. F., and Associates. 1974a. Six experiments on speech discrimination utilizing CNC monosyllables J. Aud. Res. 2(Suppl.):1–30.

Rintelmann, W., D. Beasley, and G. Lynn. 1974b. Time-compressed CNC monosyllables: Case findings in central auditory disorders. Paper presented to the Michigan Speech and Hearing Association, Detroit.

Roeser, R. J., and D. D. Daly. 1974. Auditory cortex disconnection associated with thalamic tumor: A case report. Neurology 24:555–559.

Ross, M. and J. Lerman. 1970. A picture identification test for hearing-impaired children. J. Speech Hear. Res. 13:44–53.

Rowe, III., M. J. 1981. The brainstem auditory evoked response in neurological disease: A review. Ear Hear. 2:41–51.

Sanderson-Leepa, M. E., and W. F. Rintelmann. 1976. Articulation functions and test-retest performance of normal-hearing children on three speech discrimination tests: WIPI, PBK-50, and N.U. Auditory Test No. 6. J. Speech Hear. Disord. 41:503–519.

Schoeny, Z. G., and R. Carhart. 1971. Effects of unilateral Meniere's disease on masking-level differences. J. Acoust. Soc. Am. 50:1143–1150.

Schulhoff, C., and H. Goodglass. 1969. Dichotic listening, side of brain injury and cerebral dominance. Neuropsychologia 7:149–160.

Schwartz, D. M., and B. Mikus. 1977. Performance of normal hearing listeners on the time-compressed modified rhyme test. J. Am. Audiol. Soc. 3:14–19.

Skinner, P. H. 1978. Electroencephalic response audiometry. In J. Katz (ed.), Handbook of Clinical Audiology, pp. 311–328. Williams & Wilkins Company, Baltimore.
Smith, B., and D. Resnick. 1972. An auditory test for assessing brain-stem integrity: Preliminary report. Laryngoscope 82:414–424.
Snow, J., W. Rintelmann, J. Miller, and D. Konkle. 1977. Central auditory imperception. Laryngoscope 87:1450–1471.
Sparks, R., and N. Geschwind. 1968. Dichotic listening in a man after section of neocortical commissures. Cortex 4:3–16.
Sparks, R., H. Goodglass and B. Nickel. 1970. Ipsilateral versus contralateral extinction in dichotic listening resulting from hemisphere lesions. Cortex 6:249–260.
Speaks, C. 1980. Evaluation of disorders of the central auditory system. In M. M. Paparella and D. A. Shumrick (eds.), Otolaryngology, Vol. II, The Ear, pp. 1846–1860. W. B. Saunders Company, Philadelphia.
Speaks, C., and J. Jerger. 1965. Method for measurement of speech identification. J. Speech Hear. Res. 8:185–194.
Spitzer, J. B., and I. M. Ventry. 1980. Central auditory dysfunction among chronic alcoholics. Arch. Otolaryngol. 106:224–229.
Starr, A., and L. J. Achor. 1975. Auditory brain stem responses in neurological disease. Arch. Neurol. 32:761–768.
Studdert-Kennedy, M. and D. Shankweiler. 1970. Hemispheric specialization for speech perception. J. Acoust. Soc. Am. 48:579–594.
Tillman, T. W., P. C. Bucy, and R. Carhart. 1966. Monaural versus binaural discrimination for filtered CNC materials: The impaired auditory mechanism. SAM-TR-66-64, USAF School of Aerospace Medicine, Aerospace Medical Division (AFSC), Brooks Air Force Base, Tex.
Tillman, T., and R. Carhart. 1966. An expanded test for speech discrimination utilizing CNC monosyllabic words: N.U. auditory test No. 6. Technical Report SAM-TR-66-65, USAF School of Aerospace Medicine, Aerospace Medical Division (AFSC), Brooks Air Force Base, Tex.
Tobey, E. A., J. K. Cullen, Jr., D. R. Rampp, and A. M. Fleischer-Gallagher. 1979. Effects of stimulus-onset asynchrony on the dichotic performance of children with auditory-processing disorders. J. Speech Hear. Res. 22:197–211.
White, E. J. 1977. Children's performance on the SSW test and Willeford battery: Interim clinical data. In R. W. Keith (ed.), Central Auditory Dysfunction, pp. 319–340. Grune & Stratton, New York.
Willeford, J. 1976. Central auditory function in children with learning disabilities. Audiol. Hear. Educ. 2:12–20.
Willeford, J. A. 1977. Assessing central auditory behavior in children: A test battery approach. In R. W. Keith (ed.), Central Auditory Dysfunction, pp. 43–72. Grune & Stratton, New York.
Willeford, J. 1980. Central auditory behaviors in learning-disabled children. Semin. Speech Lang. Hear. 1:127–140.
Willeford, J. A., and J. M. Billger. 1978. Auditory perception in children with learning disabilities. In J. Katz (ed.), Handbook of Clincial Audiology, pp. 410–425. 2nd Ed. Williams & Wilkins Company, Baltimore.

CHAPTER 9

MASKING IN SPEECH AUDIOMETRY

Dan F. Konkle and Grant A. Berry

CONTENTS

RATIONALE FOR CONTRALATERAL MASKING 287
    Terminology 287
    Interaural Attenuation 291
    Masking Functions 295
CLINICAL APPLICATIONS OF CONTRALATERAL MASKING 302
    Selection of an Appropriate Masker 303
    When to Mask 307
    Selection of Appropriate Masking Levels 312
    Central Masking 316
CONCLUSION 317
REFERENCES 318

Assessment of auditory function with speech, as well as other forms of acoustic stimuli, frequently requires that test signals be presented monaurally. Monaural testing, which typically is accomplished by transducing the test signal via a single earphone, is especially useful in speech audiometry because it allows test findings to be interpreted independently for each ear. Indeed, discussions throughout this book stress the importance of monaural testing in virtually every phase of speech audiometry for the identification, assessment, and management of auditory disorders. The reader must recognize, however, that simply presenting a test signal to one ear does not necessarily insure monaural hearing. In certain situations it is possible for a monaurally presented signal, even when transduced via a head-worn earphone, to be perceived by the opposite ear. This phenomenon, whereby stimuli presented to one ear are heard in the contralateral (opposite) ear, commonly is termed *cross hearing*.

    Cross hearing occurs most frequently during audiologic assessment when there is either a substantial difference in threshold sensitivity between ears, or when test stimuli are presented to one ear at a relatively intense suprathreshold level. Because cross hearing allows the contralateral ear to participate in the auditory task, the listener's responses may be influenced by such participation, and hence such test results do not represent the "true" status of the ear being tested. Such invalid or erroneous test findings, of course, can result in serious misinterpretations that can culminate in misdiagnosis and subsequent mismanagement of aural disorders. It is important, therefore, that audiologists not only recognize those situations where cross hearing can compromise monaural test findings, but also employ appropriate procedures to minimize the unwanted influences of cross hearing.

When it appears that cross hearing is contributing to the listener's responses, a masking noise must be presented to the nontest ear to "block out" its perception of the test signal. This practice is termed "contralateral masking" because the masker noise is presented to the opposite (contralateral) ear with respect to the ear that receives the test stimuli. The specific goal of contralateral masking is to elevate the threshold sensitivity of the nontest ear so that it does not perceive stimuli presented to the test ear. Equally important, however, is that the contralateral masker should not be so intense that it "crosses over" and influences the sensitivity or acuity of the test ear. Otherwise stated, contralateral maskers should be of sufficient intensity to minimize the influence of cross hearing, but not so intense that they adversely influence perception in the ear being tested.

The importance of contralateral masking to the practice of audiometry has been recognized for many years. It is somewhat disconcerting, therefore, that as recently as 1978 Sanders observed, "Of all the clinical procedures used in auditory assessment, masking is probably the most often misused and least understood" (p.124). Indeed, published survey data on audiometric practices (Martin and Pennington, 1971; Martin and Forbis, 1978), in addition to the author's experiences, lend support to this observation. Moreover, the confusion associated with contralateral masking appears to be most critical for the practice of speech audiometry. Although most recent textbooks on audiology contain specific treatments of contralateral masking, these usually are focused on pure tone testing. Applications of masking in speech audiometry are either ignored completely, or are given consideration only in terms of speech threshold assessment. Consequently, many audiologists extrapolate from procedures designed to mask pure tone stimuli presented at threshold intensity levels in order to devise masking procedures for speech signals presented at suprathreshold intensities. Such extrapolations probably account, in part, for the confusion that has existed concerning the use of contralateral masking in speech audiometry.

With the exception of an excellent chapter by Studebaker (1979), the literature on masking in speech audiometry is located in numerous different sources, many of which are not commonly available. This makes it difficult for many audiologists to have access to information necessary to develop efficient and appropriate masking procedures. It is the purpose of this chapter, therefore, to present both the rationale and clinical applications of contralateral masking in speech audiometric practice. The reader should realize, however, that many of the decisions required in the practice of contralateral masking during speech audiometry depend upon available pure tone data. Fortunately, pure tone testing is conducted before speech assessment in most clinical settings. This practice is convenient for the purpose of contralateral masking in speech audiometry because it provides important information upon which to base masking procedures. This also means that the pure tone test results must be valid. Consequently, it is as important to mask appropriately during pure tone testing as when conducting speech audiometry. Because this chapter is restricted to speech audiometry, readers interested in similar information on the use of contralateral masking in pure tone assessment are directed to Martin (1981), Sanders (1978), or Studebaker (1979).

RATIONALE FOR CONTRALATERAL MASKING

The appropriate and effective use of contralateral masking during speech audiologic assessments depends upon the clinician's ability to decide when to mask, the type of masking noise to use, and the intensity level at which to present the masking noise. Answers to these questions depend upon several factors including interaural attenuation, the occlusion effect, differences in the acoustic spectra of the masker and test signal, central masking phenomena, the status of the listener's auditory system, and the nature of specific test procedures. Moreover, interactions among these variables often vary as functions of individual differences among patients, test procedures, and stimuli. Failure to understand the rationale that serves as the basis for contralateral masking can result in examiner confusion when such interactions occur. It is this confusion that can cause misapplication of masking procedures. It is imperative, therefore, that the reader have a basic understanding of the rationale for contralateral masking. Thus, before pursuing the clinical procedures advocated for contralateral masking during speech audiometry, it is necessary to devote attention to several concepts that provide the basis for masking procedures.

Terminology

The literature on contralateral masking contains a variety of different terms. Unfortunately, many of the terms useful in describing masking procedures have been defined differently by various authors. This not only is confusing, but also makes it necessary to define the terms used in this chapter. The following section, therefore, provides a description of several terms that will clarify subsequent discussions on clinical applications. The reader should realize that these terms are defined in an exact manner in order to avoid confusion and to facilitate an understanding of concepts related to contralateral masking. The reader is encouraged to understand the following terminology before attempting to read and interpret subsequent sections of this chapter.

Ears and Stimuli The process of contralateral masking involves a dichotic listening task in which different stimuli are presented simultaneously to each ear. It is convenient, therefore, to assign terms that distinguish between ears and define stimuli. The terms *test ear* and *nontest ear* are basic descriptors that are used to denote the ears to which stimuli are directed. The test ear, by convention, refers to the ear to which the test signal is directed; the opposite ear is termed the nontest ear. The reader should note that the classification of test or nontest ear is based on where the test signal is presented (i.e., the ear under test). This distinction in no way depends upon the masking noise because this stimulus may be directed to either the test or nontest ear. Moreover, the designation of test and nontest ear does not depend upon the ear that actually perceives the test or masking stimuli. Simply, the test ear is the ear to which test signals are directed.

The terms *maskee* and *masker* refer to the test signal and masking noise, respectively. Whereas by definition the maskee (i.e., the test signal) always is directed to the test ear, recall that the masker may be directed to either the test or nontest ear. The ear to which the masker is directed creates either an ipsilateral or contralateral paradigm. These paradigms are illustrated in Figure 9-1. When both the maskee and masker are directed to the same ear, an *ipsilateral paradigm* exists. Conversely, a *contralateral paradigm* is created when the maskee and masker are directed individually to opposite ears. In clinical audiologic assessment a contralateral paradigm is used to mask the nontest ear. If, however, one wanted to determine how much masking is produced by a given maskee/masker combination, it is convenient to use the ipsilateral masking paradigm. Both the contralateral and ipsilateral masking paradigms will be used frequently in the following discussions.

Masking Any definition of masking depends upon the nature of the auditory behavior under study. The definition of masking most commonly applied to clinical audiology is based on threshold concepts. Within this context, masking is defined as the amount of threshold shift, expressed in decibels, for a test signal (maskee) that is caused by the introduction of a masking noise (masker). If, for example, a listener's speech recognition threshold for spondaic words is measured as 20 dB sound pressure level (SPL) without masking, but shifts to 28 dB SPL when a masking noise is presented, the amount of masking is 8 dB (e.g., 28 dB $-$ 20 dB = 8 dB). It is important to note that this

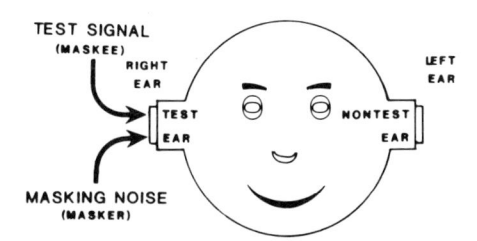

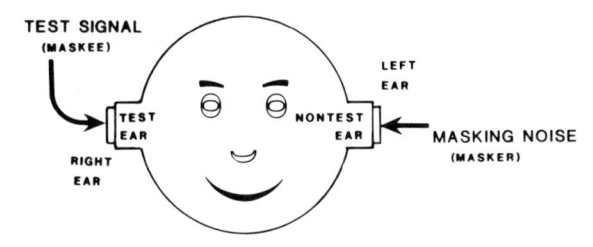

Figure 9-1. The ipsilateral and contralateral masking paradigms whereby the maskee and masker are either directed to the same ear (ipsilateral) or to different ears (contralateral).

definition of masking requires a shift in the threshold of the maskee. Given this definition, it is entirely possible to present a masker of sufficient intensity to be audible (i.e., perceived by the listener) without causing masking so long as the maskee threshold remains unchanged. Another important concept related to this definition is that the amount of masking caused by a given masker depends upon the acoustic spectra of both the masker and maskee. Whereas the intensity of the masker must be sufficient to produce a maskee threshold shift, different combinations of maskee/masker stimuli may result in varied amounts of threshold shift for the maskee, even though the maskers are presented at the same overall intensity level. Regardless of the maskee/masker combination, however, once the intensity of a specific masker causes a maskee threshold shift, additional increases in the intensity of the masker generally result in equal decibel shifts of the maskee threshold.

These relationships are illustrated in Figure 9-2 where typical maskee/masker functions are plotted for speech recognition thresholds masked by two types of noise stimuli. The data presented in Figure 9-2 were obtained with an ipsilateral masking paradigm by transducing both the maskee (spondaic words) and masker stimuli via the same TDH-39 earphone. One of the maskers was comprised of broadband

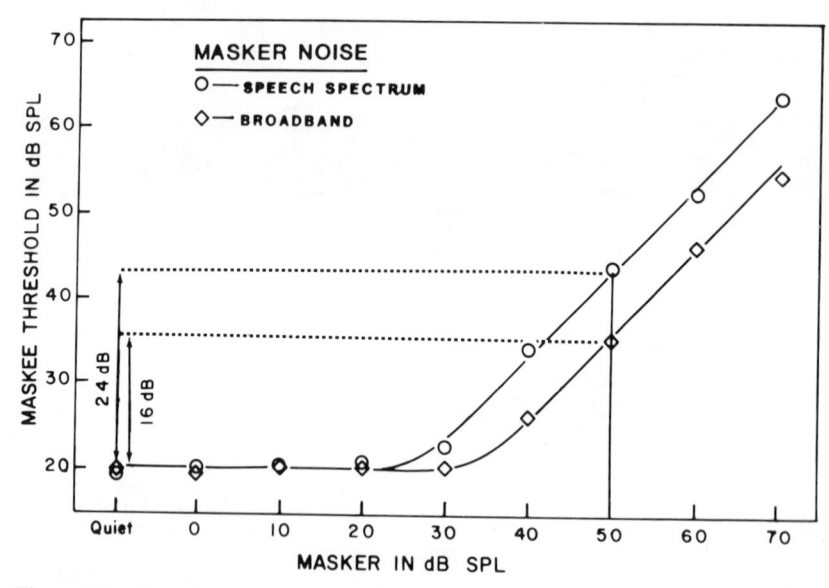

Figure 9-2. Spondee word (maskee) recognition thresholds (in dB SPL) plotted as a function of masker intensity (in dB SPL) for a speech spectrum and a broadband noise masker. Threshold data were obtained using the ipsilateral masking paradigm.

noise with a spectrum that was characterized by the frequency response of the TDH-39 earphone. The other masker was speech spectrum noise that had a 3-dB/octave rise from 250 to 1000 Hz and a 6-dB/octave drop from 1000 to 4000 Hz. Individual data points represent mean threshold values (50 percent correct recognition) for a group of 20 normal-hearing listeners. Note that the intensity of both maskers had to be greater than the intensity of the speech signal before a threshold shift occurred, but that speech spectrum noise caused a threshold shift at a lower intensity compared to the broadband masker (e.g., about 28 dB for the speech spectrum noise and approximately 37 dB for the broadband masker). Specifically, a 5-dB shift in spondee recognition threshold was observed with the speech spectrum noise at 31 dB SPL, whereas the same 5-dB threshold shift was not obtained until the broadband masker was about 39 dB SPL; that is, an 8-dB difference in masker intensity. Once an initial threshold shift was observed, however, the functions of both maskers became linear in that further increases in masker intensity caused similar increases in threshold intensity. Thus, when both maskers were presented at 50 dB SPL, the speech spectrum noise continued to produce approximately 8 dB more masking than the broadband masker. Otherwise stated, the signal-to-noise (S/N) masking ratios at threshold for any given intensity of the spondaic words were about −6 dB and −14 dB for the speech spectrum and broadband noises, respectively.

This "threshold shift" definition of masking and the concepts just explained will be applied throughout this chapter. Although some may argue that other definitions of masking are more appropriate when discussing nonthreshold measures (e.g., suprathreshold speech recognition, or comfortable and uncomfortable loudness levels), the reader should remember that the goal of contralateral masking is to elevate threshold sensitivity in the nontest ear so that it does not perceive the test signal. This basic objective remains unchanged regardless of the audiometric procedure. Finally, defining masking relative to maskee threshold shifts, in conjunction with the following discussion of interaural attenuation, makes it possible to define conveniently several terms that are used to describe various masking levels employed clinically in contralateral masking.

Interaural Attenuation

Recall that under certain conditions it is possible for a monaurally presented signal (i.e., a signal delivered to one ear) to be heard by the opposite ear. This means, of course, that the signal traveled across the listener's head and was present at the other ear with sufficient intensity to be perceived. This does not necessarily mean, however, that the signal was present with equal intensity at each ear. Rather, in most cases the physical properties of the listener's head will cause a reduction in intensity as the signal travels from one ear to the other. The relative difference in the intensities of the signal at each ear is termed interaural attenuation and is one of the most important considerations in developing a rationale for the clinical application of contralateral masking.

Interaural attenuation is important because it defines when masking is necessary and also dictates the maximum intensity of masking that can be used before overmasking results. By way of illustration, if a signal is presented to the right ear at an intensity of 80 dB and the interaural attenuation value is 35 dB, the signal will be present in the left ear at an intensity of 45 dB (i.e., 80 dB − 35 dB = 45 dB). Given this example, and assuming the signal is a test stimulus, it will be necessary to mask the left ear (i.e., the nontest ear) when its threshold for that signal is 45 dB or better. Conversely, if the 80-dB signal presented to the right ear is a masking noise, this masker also will be present in the left ear at a level of 45 dB. If this level (45 dB) is sufficient to cause a left ear threshold shift, the masker will not only be masking the right ear but also will be masking the left ear. This condition will result in overmasking because both the test and nontest ears are masked. Consequently, it is vitally important that the examiner know the interaural attenuation values for both the test signal and masker stimulus.

Unfortunately, a single interaural attenuation value cannot be used for all speech audiometric procedures. Interaural attenuation will vary depending upon: 1) the method used to transduce the signal; 2) the acoustic spectrum of the signal; and 3) the manner used to specify the intensity of the signal at each ear. The appropriate use of contralateral masking, therefore, requires that interaural attenuation be defined precisely for both the maskee and masker stimuli. Moreover, such definitions will depend upon whether the signal is transduced by an earphone (air conduction) or by a bone vibrator (bone conduction). These two modes of signal delivery and their implications for interaural attenuation and contralateral masking are discussed in the following section.

Air Conduction Speech audiologic measurements commonly are made for air conduction stimuli transduced by an earphone mounted in a MX-41/AR cushion. The American National Standards Institute (ANSI) has specified that "For tests by air conduction, the subject's ear which is not under test shall be covered either by a dummy earphone or by an operable earphone" (ANSI S3.6-1969, R-1973; p. 8). This means that during air conduction testing both ears of the listener are covered by an earphone. Interaural attenuation for air conduction signals thus is determined by the combination of earphones, earphone cushions, and the listener's head. Given these circumstances, Studebaker (1979) recommended that interaural attenuation for air conduction signals be defined as "The difference (in dB) between the level of the signal in the ear canal of one ear and its level at the opposite cochlea . . ." (p. 53). Otherwise stated, if a signal is presented by an earphone and both ears are covered by earphones, interaural attenuation is computed by taking the intensity at which the signal is presented and subtracting the intensity of that signal at the cochlea of the opposite ear. For clinical practice, the intensity of the signal in the ear canal can be expressed in the same units used to define the presentation level (i.e., hearing level, SPL, etc.).

It is important to define interaural attenuation for air-conducted stimuli precisely in this manner in order to avoid the influences of conductive hearing loss. Note that defining interaural attenuation simply as the decibel difference between the signal intensities of the two cochleae is inappropriate because the signal is actually transduced to each cochlea in a different manner. Specifically, when the signal is presented by an earphone it reaches the ipsilateral cochlea via the external and middle ear conducting mechanism, whereas it is transmitted to the contralateral cochlea primarily by bone conduction (Sanders, 1978; Studebaker, 1967; Zwislocki, 1953).

The implications associated with these modes of transmission are illustrated in Figure 9-3. Figure 9-3A is a schematic representation of both the ipsilateral and contralateral transmission modes when the external and middle ear conducting mechanisms are functioning normally. When a signal is presented at an intensity of 50 dB it also reaches the ipsilateral cochlea with an intensity of 50 dB (by definition, air conduction sensitivity equals bone conduction sensitivity in the absence of conductive hearing loss) because the normally functioning external and middle ears do not cause a transmission loss. Conversely, the signal arrives at the contralateral cochlea at an intensity of only 10 dB because there is a 40 dB transmission loss as the signal travels

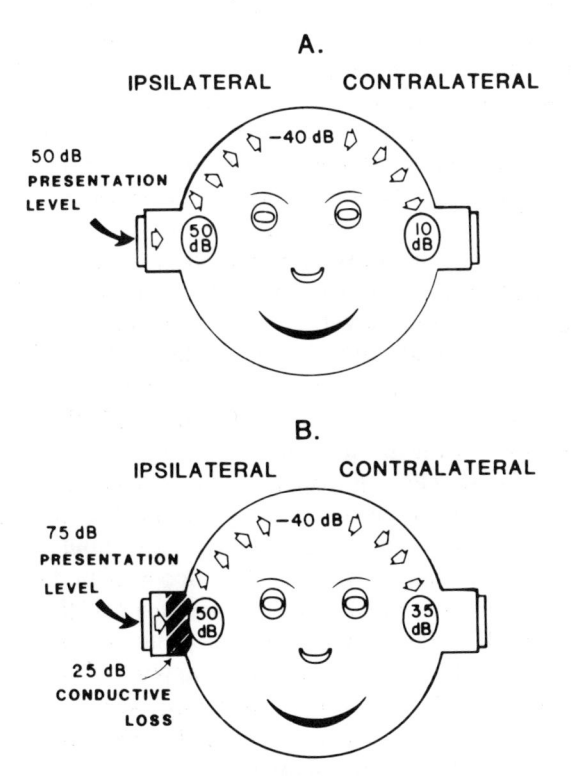

Figure 9-3. Schematic representation of the intensity present at the ipsilateral and contralateral cochleae for stimuli presented monaurally by an earphone when the external and middle ear conducting mechanisms of the ipsilateral ear function normally (3A) and when the ipsilateral ear has a conductive hearing loss (3B). See text for an explanation of the ipsilateral and contralateral transmission modes and the influence of conductive hearing loss.

from the ipsilateral to contralateral ear. This transmission loss results primarily from the poor impedance match that occurs when the cranial bones are forced into vibration (bone conduction) by an air conduction signal. Interaural attenuation in this example is 40 dB (i.e., 50-dB presentation level minus 10-dB signal intensity at contralateral cochlea equals 40-dB of interaural attenuation). The reader should note that this interaural attenuation value remains unchanged when computed as the intensity difference between cochleae. This is true for situations in which the external and middle ears function normally and probably accounts, in part, for the practice of some writers who define interaural attenuation for air-conducted stimuli as the difference in cochlear sensitivity between ears. In the absence of a conductive hearing loss in the presentation ear, therefore, presentation level and ipsilateral cochlear sensitivity are defined as equal. This relationship, however, does not hold when a conductive hearing loss exists in the presentation ear. This is illustrated by Figure 9-3B, in which the same values for interaural attenuation and presentation ear cochlear sensitivity are used, for comparison, as were employed in Figure 9-3A. The situation depicted in Figure 9-3B, however, is confounded by a 25-dB conductive hearing loss in the presentation ear. In order to maintain the same signal intensity at the ipsilateral cochlea it thus is necessary to increase the presentation level by 25 dB to overcome the conductive hearing loss. This means that the presentation level of the signal is 75 dB, and that it is present at the contralateral cochlea at an intensity of 35 dB (i.e., 75-dB presentation level minus 40-dB interaural attenuation equals 35-dB intensity at contralateral cochlea). Given this example, interaural attenuation would only be 15 dB if computed as the difference in cochlear intensities (i.e., 50 dB − 35 dB = 15 dB). Clearly, this value is not appropriate because it fails to include the magnitude of the conductive hearing loss. Recall, that whereas the signal is presented via air conduction, it travels to the opposite cochlea via bone conduction. Because this bone conduction pathway essentially is unaffected by conductive impairment, it follows that increases in the presentation intensity will result in similar intensity increases at the contralateral cochlea. The 40-dB interaural attenuation value used in the examples of Figures 9-3A and B does not necessarily apply to all types of stimuli. Indeed, the interaural attenuation value may vary from as little as 40 dB to as much as 80 dB, depending upon the spectral components of the signal. Also, interaural attenuation will vary greatly as a function of individual listener differences. For clinical purposes, therefore, it is best to use the minimum expected amount of interaural attenuation rather than some measure of central tendency such as the mean or median. The manner used to determine interaural attenuation for speech audiometry is discussed fully in subsequent sections of this chapter.

Finally, it should be stressed that the well documented occlusion effect, whereby the intensity of bone conduction signals presented at the cochlea is enhanced for the frequencies below approximately 1000 Hz when the external auditory meatus is occluded, does not alter the intensity at the contralateral cochlea during air conduction testing. The reason for this, as noted previously, is that the contralateral ear already is occluded by an earphone. In air conduction testing, therefore, the occlusion effect can be ignored so long as both ears are covered by earphones.

In summary, it is both appropriate and convenient to define interaural attenuation for air conduction signals as the difference in intensity of the signal at the ear canal (i.e., presentation level) of the presentation ear and the cochlea of the opposite ear. Such a definition avoids the influences of conductive hearing loss in the presentation ear and is applicable to both threshold and suprathreshold audiological measures.

Bone Conduction Although speech audiometric measurements for bone conduction stimuli are not obtained in most hearing centers, some clinicians use this technique with very young children or when confronted with a severe, mixed-type hearing loss (Martin and Forbis, 1978). In such cases, the speech signal is transduced by a bone vibrator usually placed in contact with the mastoid bone on the side of the test ear, or occasionally on the frontal bone at the midline of the forehead. Regardless of vibrator placement, bone conduction signals are transmitted directly to both cochleae. Hence, interaural attenuation for bone conduction speech stimuli is defined as the difference in intensity of the signal at the two cochleae.

Masking Functions

The foregoing discussions on terminology, masking, and interaural attenuation provide a basis for the following consideration of masking functions. Because the overall intent of this chapter is centered on the practice of contralateral masking in speech audiometry, the content of this section is structured toward clinical applications. Recall that the purpose of contralateral masking is to elevate (make poorer) the threshold sensitivity of the nontest ear to such an extent that cross hearing does not influence the listener's responses. At the same time, the amount of masking must be controlled in order to avoid "cross masking"; i.e., masking the test ear with a contralaterally presented masker. These concepts are best illustrated by consideration of ipsilateral and contralateral masking functions.

Ipsilateral Masking Functions The ipsilateral masking paradigm (see Figure 9-1) was defined as a listening condition in which both the maskee and masker are directed to the same ear. Typical ipsilateral masking functions were presented in Figure 9-2, in which it was observed that: 1) introduction of the masker did not necessarily cause masking to occur; 2) the amount of masking caused by the masker depended upon the maskee threshold shift rather than simply the intensity of the masker; and 3) once masking occurred there was a linear relationship between increases in the intensity of the masker and subsequent threshold shifts (i.e., masking) of the maskee. These relationships make it possible to equate different maskee/masker combinations on a relative basis and conveniently allow various levels of masking to be expressed in terms of the measurement unit used to define maskee threshold. Brief consideration needs to be given to three such masking levels before further discussion of ipsilateral masking functions.

Effective Masking Level Perhaps the most useful term used in conjunction with contralateral masking is *effective masking level* (EML). Similar to the concept of masking, EML is defined relative to maskee rather than masker intensity. Specifically, EML is the threshold intensity of the maskee when it just barely is masked by the masker. It thus follows that EML can be expressed in the same units of measurement as the maskee. The convenience of using this notation for EML is illustrated by examining the ipsilateral masking data presented in Figure 9-2. Note that the unit of measurement for the spondee word (maskee) thresholds in this figure is dB SPL; thus, EML for both the speech spectrum and broadband noise maskers also can be expressed as dB SPL. Consider, for example, that a maskee threshold of 30 dB SPL was obtained when each masker was at a different intensity (i.e., 36 dB SPL for the speech spectrum and 44 dB for the broadband noise), but an additional 1- or 2-dB increase in either masker would be sufficient to just mask the 30 dB SPL threshold. Consequently, a 30 dB EML in SPL for speech spectrum noise would result when this masker was at an intensity of 37 to 38 dB SPL; whereas the broadband noise masker would have to be at 45 to 46 dB SPL to create the same EML. In order to express the level of masking in terms of masker intensity, therefore, it would be necessary to use two units (i.e., the intensity of the masker and the maskee) because different amounts of masking result with various maskee/masker combinations. Conversely, expressing EML relative to maskee intensity requires using only one unit (i.e., the intensity of the maskee) to adequately denote the magnitude of the masker. Moreover, the above definition allows the data in Figure 9-2 to be replotted as a function of EML. Figure 9-4 presents the same ipsilateral masking functions depicted in Figure 9-2, but the data are

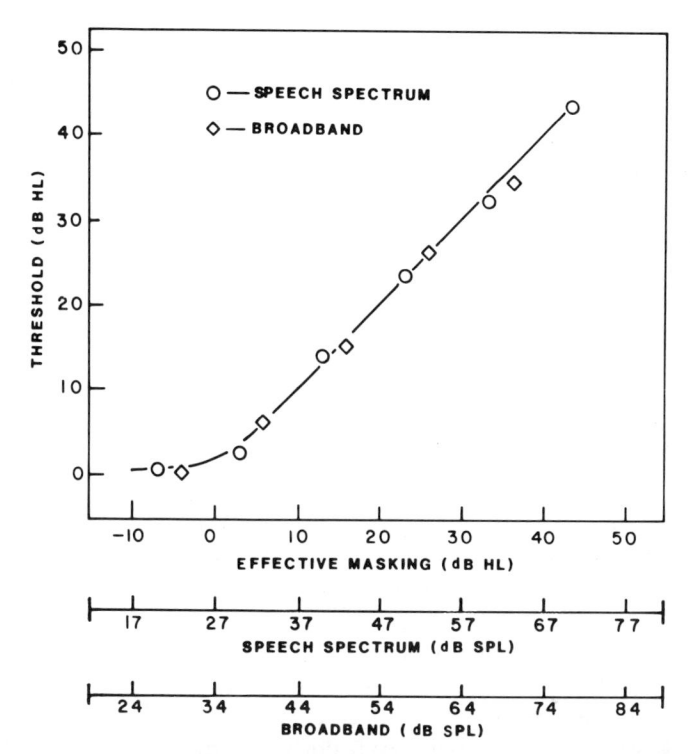

Figure 9-4. Spondee word (maskee) recognition thresholds (in dB HL) plotted as a function of effective masking level (EML in dB HL) for speech spectrum and broadband noise maskers. The SPL for each masker type also is depicted for comparison. The threshold data are the same as shown in Figure 9-2. See text for an explanation of relationship between SPL and EML.

cast as EML rather than dB SPL. Also, the unit of measurement for the maskee has been altered to reflect decibel hearing level (dB HL) (see Chapter 5 for a detailed discussion of HL), because this unit typically is used in clinical settings for threshold-type measures. Finally, the dB SPL values for each masker type are plotted for comparison purposes. It is seen in Figure 9-4 that when ipsilateral masking functions are plotted as dB EML, each function will be superimposed because a single reference (i.e., maskee intensity) is used as a unit of measurement. It is this relationship that makes EML such a useful criterion in the practice of contralateral masking.

Minimum and Maximum Masking Levels In addition to EML, there are two other levels of masking that are useful descriptors in discussing the practice of contralateral masking. Minimum masking level is defined simply as 0 dB EML, although in clinical applications this term is defined more conveniently as the EML at the nontest ear that equals the intensity of the maskee at the nontest ear cochlea plus any air/bone gap (in decibels) of the nontest ear. Maximum masking level, however, requires a definition that relates more to the contralateral masking paradigm (see Figure 9-1) than the ipsilateral condition currently under discussion. Furthermore, the definition of maximum masking level is based on the concepts of interaural attenuation and the intensity level of the test signal (maskee) present at the test ear cochlea. Nevertheless, because maximum masking level can be expressed as an EML, it will be defined here as the EML equal to the interaural attenuation value of the masker plus the intensity level of the maskee at the test ear cochlea. Further consideration and explanation of minimum and maximum masking is provided in the discussion of contralateral masking functions.

The ipsilateral masking paradigm used to gather the data presented in Figures 9-2 and 9-4 is used in clinical settings primarily to define EML. Although this paradigm requires that the maskee and masker both be transduced by the same earphone to a single ear in order to generate an ipsilateral masking function, it also is possible to obtain ipsilateral functions using the contralateral paradigm. Recall from Figure 9-1 that the contralateral paradigm, whereby the test signal is presented to the test ear with the masker directed to the nontest ear, is the strategy most commonly used during contralateral masking procedures. Given this paradigm, it is possible to obtain an ipsilateral masking function for either the nontest or test ear whenever the maskee or masker is present in the opposite ear, respectively. Otherwise stated, when a test signal is presented to the test ear with sufficient intensity to be perceived by the nontest ear, the introduction of effective masking to the nontest ear will result in ipsilateral masking because both the maskee and masker are present in the same ear. Conversely, a masker delivered to the nontest ear at an intensity sufficient to cause effective masking in the test ear (i.e., because of inadequate interaural attenuation) also will result in ipsilateral masking at the test ear. This is so because by definition ipsilateral masking can result only when both the masker and maskee are present simultaneously in the same ear. Ipsilateral masking does not depend upon the manner in which either the maskee or masker reaches the cochlea. The reader should note that ipsilateral and contralateral paradigms refer only to modes of signal delivery and do not define masking functions, nor do masking functions necessarily imply a mode of signal delivery.

Contralateral Masking Functions Contralateral masking functions have been discussed in several other publications concerned with clinical masking of the nontest ear (Martin, 1981; Sanders, 1978; Studebaker, 1979). These functions are classified as contralateral because they are obtained under the contralateral paradigm of stimuli presentation that was presented in Figure 9-1. In reality, however, these functions actually consist of two ipsilateral functions—one representing the nontest ear and the other the test ear. The relationship of these ipsilateral functions to the contralateral paradigm is illustrated in the following example. Assume that an examiner wants to assess the air conduction threshold sensitivity for spondaic words for each ear of a listener who has a pure sensorineural hearing loss of 60 dB HL in the left ear and normal hearing of 0 dB HL in the right ear. If the interaural attenuation value for spondees is 45 dB, then the listener will respond at 45 dB HL when the spondees are presented to the left ear because cross hearing will allow the right ear to perceive the words. In order to minimize the right ear influence and establish the true left ear threshold (i.e., 60 dB HL), it would be necessary to introduce contralateral masking to the right ear. If the interaural attenuation value for the masker also is 45 dB, a masking function would be obtained similar to that depicted in Figure 9-5. This figure illustrates the contralateral paradigm with the test signal directed to the left ear (by definition, the

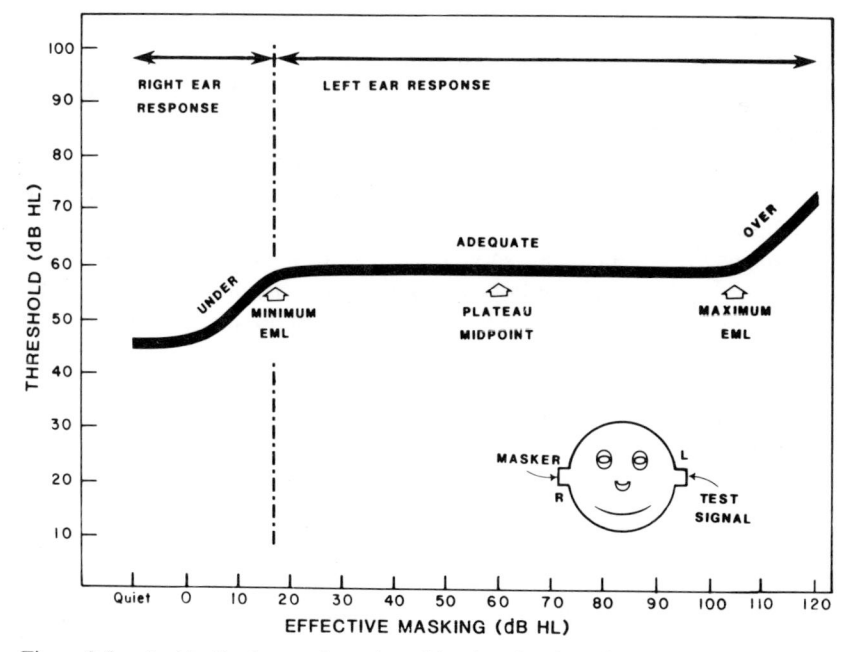

Figure 9-5. An idealized contralateral masking function for a listener with a 60 dB HL hearing loss in the left ear and normal hearing (0 dB HL) in the right ear. See text for a discussion of various aspects associated with the contralateral masking function.

test ear) and the masker presented to the right (nontest) ear. The data in Figure 9-5 represent listener responses consistent with the above example and are plotted as a function of threshold dB HL and EML dB HL. The dashed line distinguishes listener responses referred to the nontest and test ears, respectively. Observe that for the quiet (no masker) condition a threshold of 45 dB HL was measured, but when 5 dB EML was introduced to the nontest ear the threshold shifted to 50 dB HL and continued to shift linearly with each successive 5-dB EML increase until it stabilized for EMLs between 15 and 105 dB HL. When EMLs greater than 105 dB HL were presented, however, the threshold again shifted in a linear manner for each increase in EML. This entire function can be analyzed in terms of three sections: 1) the section labeled *undermasking*; 2) the portion termed *adequate masking* (plateau); and 3) the segment labeled *overmasking*. The section noted as undermasking does not mean an absence of masking; rather this segment represents an ipsilateral masking function of the nontest ear. This was possible since the maskee reaches the nontest ear cochlea by bone conduction because interaural attenuation is inadequate and the masker is transduced directly by air conduction. The *adequate masking* (plateau) portion results because the listener is now responding at threshold (60 dB HL) for the test ear. This results when the EML at the nontest ear (i.e., 15 dB EML) equals the intensity of the maskee at the nontest ear cochlea plus any air/bone gap of the nontest ear. Because there is no air/bone gap in the nontest ear, and the intensity of the maskee at the nontest ear cochlea equals 15 dB (i.e., 60-dB presentation level minus 45-dB interaural attenuation = 15 dB), the minimum masking level can be stated as 15 dB EML, or a 0-dB EML referenced to the portion of the function resulting from test ear responses. The test ear threshold did not shift, however, with additional intensity increases in the contralateral masker (greater than the minimum masking level) because both interaural attenuation for the masker and the 60-dB HL threshold for the test ear precludes masking the test ear. The segment termed overmasking also represents an ipsilateral masking function, but in this case involves the test rather than the nontest ear. This results because the presentation level of the masker is so intense at the nontest ear that interaural attenuation in combination with the test ear threshold are no longer adequate to avoid test ear masking. Note that the maximum EML that could be presented to the nontest ear before overmasking is 105 dB HL. This is consistent with the previous definition of maximum masking level (i.e., 60 dB test stimulus present at the test ear cochlea plus 45 dB interaural attenuation equals 105 dB maximum masking level expressed as EML). The range of the plateau is computed as the difference (in EML) between minimum and maximum masking levels (i.e., 105 dB − 15 dB = 90 dB EML). Observe that the plateau range also is equal to twice the interaural attenuation value (i.e., 45 dB × 2 = 90 dB). The plateau midpoint is defined as an equal distance between the minimum and maximum masking levels, or the minimum level plus the interaural attenuation value (i.e., 15 dB + 45 dB = 60 dB EML). It is stressed that each of these concepts is useful in the clinical application of contralateral masking, especially when deciding upon the appropriate amount of masking necessary to minimize nontest ear influence.

The reader should note that the masking function obtained with the contralateral paradigm just reviewed is illustrative of those situations in which the test signal is presented by air conduction and neither ear has a conductive hearing loss. When the test signal is presented by bone conduction, the characteristics of the contralateral masking function do not change, but the interaural attenuation value for the test stimulus will be greatly reduced because the signal is transduced to both cochleae directly by bone conduction. Hence, the range of the plateau will equal the interaural attenuation value of the masker. During air conduction testing, the influence of conductive hearing loss on the contralateral masking function depends upon whether the test or nontest ear has the conductive component. Regardless of the conductively impaired ear, the characteristics of the contralateral function are not altered. Rather, it will be necessary to present either the test signal or the masker at a higher intensity to overcome the conductive impairment. This will have the effect of reducing the plateau region of the function because presentation levels must be increased in order to maintain equal cochlear intensity. Specifically, when the test ear has a conductive component, the minimum masking level will be increased by the amount of the conductive hearing loss. In situations in which the nontest ear is conductively impaired, the EML must be increased by the amount of the conductive component to obtain the same amount of nontest ear masking that would result without a conductive hearing loss. Thus, the maximum masking level is reached over a restricted range of EML. If both ears have a conductive component, the plateau region during air conduction testing is restricted even further because the maximum masking level is reduced and the EML necessary to mask the nontest ear is increased. Finally, whenever the combined magnitude of the conductive components for each ear equals or exceeds two times the interaural attenuation value for either the test signal or masker, it will not be possible to use contralateral masking to mask the nontest ear and obtain valid test ear responses because a plateau will not occur. Otherwise stated, when the sum of the conductive components is greater than twice the interaural attenuation value, the ipsilateral function for the nontest ear will merge with that of the test ear. Thus, it will not be possible to determine which ear is actually responding to the test stimuli. This situation commonly is termed the *masking dilemma*. Regardless of the magnitude, type, or configuration of hearing loss, however, the examiner can recognize the various segments of the contralateral masking function so long as the definitions for interaural attenuation, EML, and minimum and maximum masking levels are applied as specified in previous sections of this chapter.

CLINICAL APPLICATIONS OF CONTRALATERAL MASKING

The previous sections of this chapter have focused on concepts necessary to provide a rationale for contralateral masking. The intent of those discussions was to develop an understanding of such factors as masking, interaural attenuation and masking levels, and to appreciate the relationships between the ipsilateral and contralateral paradigms of signal delivery and associated masking functions. This information is vitally important because it provides the basis for theoretically sound and clinically efficient procedures for contralateral masking during speech audiometry. Equally important is that the population encountered in most audiologic settings will present a variety of types, magnitudes, and configurations of hearing loss. These impairments may range from mild conductive to profound sensorineural, and be either unilateral or bilaterally symmetrical or asymmetrical in nature. Furthermore, the audiologist uses an array of audiologic procedures and speech stimuli to assess auditory function. Given these factors, it is not too surprising that many clinicians become confused if they attempt to use contralateral masking without a firm understanding of theoretic rationale upon which clinical strategies are based. As stated previously, effective and efficient contralateral masking depends upon the examiner's ability to decide: 1) when to mask; 2) what type of masker to use; and 3) how much masking is necessary. The foregoing discussions of this chapter have provided the background information necessary to answer these questions. Indeed, such answers are not difficult as long as one understands such concepts as interaural attenuation, effective masking level, and under- and overmasking. This understanding, of course, must include an appreciation for the reasons underlying the rather precise definitions that were given to various terms. Failure to develop such an understanding can result only in continued confusion and frustration on the part of both the examiner and the listener, regardless of the specific procedures used during applications of contralateral masking. Conversely, when examiners have a thorough understanding of the rationale for various aspects of contralateral masking they can apply clinical strategies with confidence that the test results accurately reflect the "true" status of the listener's auditory function.

Selection of an Appropriate Masker

There are two types of noise that are appropriate to use in the application of contralateral masking during speech audiometry. These are broadband and speech spectrum noise. The amplitude spectra of these stimuli are shown in Figure 9-6. The broadband masker is produced by a white noise source, but because it is transduced by an earphone it takes on the spectral characteristics associated with the frequency response of the earphone (i.e., the broadband noise spectrum in Figure 9-6 is representative of a TDH-39 earphone). The speech noise masker also is produced by a white noise source, but this signal is band-pass filtered so that its amplitude spectrum approximates the long-term average spectrum of conversational speech. Both broadband and speech noise are appropriate maskers for speech audiometry because their intensity does not fluctuate greatly over time, and thus they provide consistent levels of masking. Moreover, both of these stimuli contain acoustic energy throughout a frequency bandwidth that exceeds the bandwidth of speech. Although either of these signals can be used for contralateral masking of speech stimuli, speech noise is actually the more efficient masker because it provides more effective

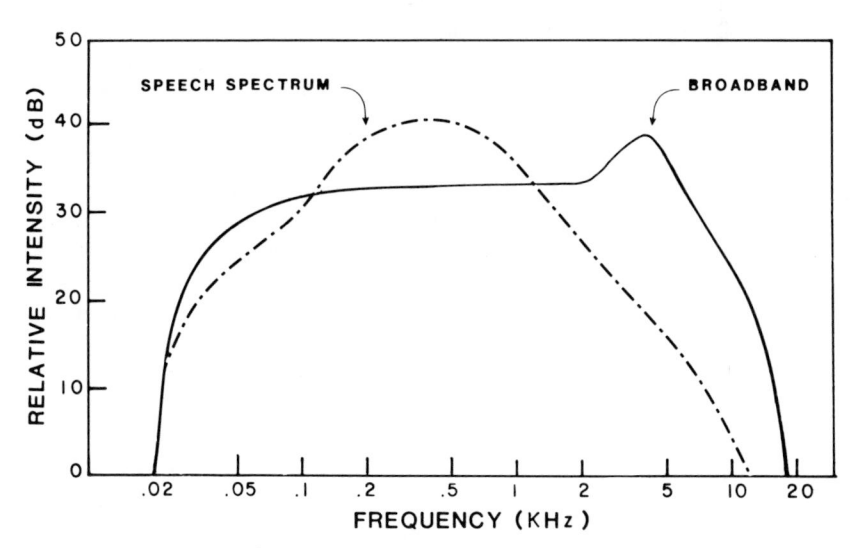

Figure 9-6. The acoustic amplitude spectra for speech spectrum and broadband noise typically used for masking the contralateral ear in speech audiometry. The illustrated spectra are representative of these stimuli when they are transduced by a TDH-39 earphone.

masking for a given SPL than broadband noise (see Figure 9-2). Regardless, either speech or broadband noise can be used as the masker for contralateral masking during speech audiometry.

Once the appropriate masking noise has been determined (i.e., broadband or speech spectrum), it is necessary to calibrate the intensity of the noise as EML. Whereas some clinical audiometers manufactured within the past few years provide a masking source with an attenuator marked in dB HL EML, other clinical audiometers do not provide this designation. Regardless of whether the attenuator is marked as EML or specified in some other manner, the audiologist should determine the EML expected for given settings of the masker attenuator for each audiometer used for speech audiometry.

Perhaps the simplest method of establishing the EML for either broadband or speech noise (or any other masker) is to obtain masking functions for a group of eight-to-ten normally hearing listeners using the ipsilateral paradigm of presenting signals (see Figure 9-1). Because EML is defined relative to threshold of the test signal, one needs to obtain thresholds in the presence of the masking signal presented at several successive intensity levels. Assuming that the attenuators that control the intensity levels of the test signal and the masker are linear (i.e., a change in attenuator dial setting equals the same change in output intensity; see Chapter 4 for a discussion of attenuator linearity), the EML for any given attenuator setting can be computed by taking the average of the differences between the group median thresholds at each setting of the masker attenuator dial. This value is then added to the setting of the masker attenuator, and EML for that attenuator setting is expressed as the next lowest 5 dB increment. This procedure is illustrated in Table 9-1 where the spondee word recognition thresholds in dB HL for eight normal-hearing adult listeners are displayed as a function of masker attenuator dial settings in successive 10 dB steps from 0 through 60. Also presented are the median (Mdn.) threshold values for each masker intensity and the differences between each Mdn. threshold and the respective masker attenuator setting. The EML thus is derived by computing the mean ($\bar{x}$) of the differences between Mdn. scores and dial settings (i.e., 12.5 dB), adjusting the $\bar{x}$ value to the next lowest 5-dB increment (i.e., 10 dB) and adding this value to the masker attenuator dial. For the data shown in Table 9-1, therefore, a 0-dB masker dial setting will equal 10 dB EML, a 10-dB setting equals 20 dB EML, and so on, provided the attenuator of the masking signal is linear.

Spondaic words are a convenient test signal to use when establishing EML. The EML obtained with the spondees not only can be used for threshold procedures, but also can be generalized to other

Table 9-1. Spondee word recognition thresholds (in dB HL) for normal-hearing adults (N = 8) as a function of seven masker attenuator dial settings, the group median threshold for each dial setting, the difference between median values and the masker attenuator setting, the sum (Σ) and mean ($\bar{x}$) of the differences, and the EML associated with each masker dial setting. See text for additional information and explanation.

Listener number[a]	\multicolumn{7}{c}{Masker attenuator dial setting}	Σ	$\bar{x}$
	0	10	20	30	40	50	60		
1	12	24	34	44	54	66	74		
2	8	26	34	42	50	58	70		
3	10	22	34	44	52	62	74		
4	16	26	38	46	56	66	76		
5	10	20	32	42	52	60	70		
6	8	20	30	40	50	60	72		
7	12	24	34	42	50	60	72		
8	14	26	38	46	54	64	73		
Median	11	24	34	43	52	61	73		
Difference	11	14	14	13	12	11	13	88	12.5
EML	10	20	30	40	50	60	70		

[a] N = 8

types of stimuli and measurements. Table 9-2, for example, contains the findings of a series of representative masking studies that used both broadband and speech spectrum maskers with a variety of different test signals. These findings indicate that, in terms of SPL, masking for spondees consistently was obtained at a signal-to-noise (i.e., spondee-to-masker) ratio between -12 and -14.7 dB for broadband maskers (Carhart, Tillman, and Greetis, 1969; Wilson and Carhart, 1969). Johnson and Young (1974), however, reported a S/N ratio of only -8 dB for spondees when using a speech spectrum noise masker. When monosyllables were used as the test stimuli, Dirks et al. (1969) observed S/N masking ratios of -7.5 and -6.0 dB for broadband noise presented at 50 and 90 dB SPL, respectively. This suggests that about 5 to 8 dB more effective masking will result for monosyllables as compared to spondees when the masker is presented at the same intensity level. Thus, about 10 dB should be added to the EML determined for spondees when establishing effective masking for monosyllables. It is convenient to use 10 dB rather than the 5- to 8-dB values because clinical practice usually is conducted with 5-dB steps of the attenuator dial setting. Consequently, the 5 to 8 dB simply is rounded off to the next highest step (i.e., 10 dB). This 10-dB difference between EML for spondees and monosyllables should be remembered because this concept will be considered again under the discussion of appropriate masking levels.

Table 9-2. A summary of findings from representative investigations concerned with masking various types of speech stimuli commonly used in audiometric practice.

Investigation	S/N (dB)	Masker	Masker level (dB SPL)	Maskee	Measure
Hawkins & Stevens (1951)	−8	Broadband noise	50	Continuous discourse	Threshold of intelligibility
	−17	Broadband noise	50	Continuous discourse	Threshold of detectability
Carhart et al. (1969)	−12	Broadband noise	50	Spondees	50% correct
Dirks et al. (1969)	−14.3	Broadband noise	50	Spondees	50% correct
	−12.9	Broadband noise	90	Spondees	50% correct
	−16.4	Broadband noise	50	Sentences	50% correct
	−16.2	Broadband noise	90	Sentences	50% correct
Johnson & Young (1974)	−8.0	Speech spectrum noise	75	Spondees	50% correct
Wilson & Carhart (1969)	−14.7	Broadband noise	90	Spondees	50% correct

A second approach to establishing EML is to calculate such values from the relative differences in the amplitude spectra of the maskee and masker and the physical intensity of the masking noise. Whereas Studebaker (1979) considered these procedures preferable to obtaining actual ipsilateral masking functions, in the practice of speech audiometry it often is difficult to measure the physical parameters of the test signal and masker noise that are necessary to make such calculations. Most hearing clinics do not have the instrumentation required to perform these measurements, especially for acoustically complex speech stimuli. This drawback has been recognized by some authors who have suggested that because it is simpler to measure the acoustic parameters of pure tones, the EML for speech could be calculated from averaged pure tone data (see Studebaker, 1979 for a discussion of this technique). Attempts to generalize the EML for a given speech signal and masker combination from average pure tone EML, however, usually results in a predicted EML for speech that is poorer than the EML measured directly using the ipsilateral paradigm. Recall from Table 9-2 that despite differences in methodology, word lists, and listeners, only an approximate 5-dB range in S/N ratios was observed among three independent investigations on masking speech threshold measures (Carhart et al., 1968; Dirks et al., 1969; Wilson and Carhart, 1969). Thus, it appears that the ipsilateral paradigm of specifying EML for speech directly from masking functions not only is applicable for use in the majority of hearing centers, but also has the advantage of being standardized to the procedures, instrumentation, test materials, and strategies used in each particular center.

When to Mask

The decision of when to mask during speech audiometry depends upon several factors. These include: 1) the presentation intensity level of the test signal at the test ear; 2) the cochlear sensitivity of the nontest ear; 3) the method of presenting the test signal (i.e., air conduction by an earphone or bone conduction via a bone vibrator); 4) the interaural attenuation; and 5) the type of speech measurement (i.e., threshold or suprathreshold measure). Because bone conduction speech audiometry seldom is practiced in most hearing clinics, the following discussion stresses air conduction measurements with only brief attention given to masking of bone conduction test signals. Moreover, the reader should remember that speech audiometric measures can be classified into those that examine threshold listening behavior and those that assess suprathreshold performance. The most common threshold measure is the speech reception threshold (SRT), which is given detailed examination in Chapter 5; suprathreshold testing usually consists of the word recognition measure discussed in Chapter 6. These two assessment strategies, therefore, will be emphasized in the subsequent section.

Air Conduction Threshold Measures It is necessary to use contralateral masking during air conduction speech audiometric threshold measures whenever the presentation level at the test ear equals or exceeds the bone conduction sensitivity of the nontest ear plus the interaural attenuation value of the test signal. This rule is based on the following assumptions that are considered to be valid for clinical applications. First, because the stimuli are transduced by earphones, the presentation level of the test signal at the test ear is taken as the intensity, usually in dB HL, at which the test stimuli are presented. In the case of typical SRT measures, if the spondee words are presented at a level of 30 dB HL, the presentation level of the test signal at the test ear also is 30 dB HL. Second, although the bone conduction sensitivity of the nontest ear could be defined relative to a bone conducted SRT, this practice is awkward and seldom performed clinically. Rather, cochlear sensitivity of the nontest ear is obtained more conveniently from the bone conducted pure tone average (PTA = 500, 1000, and 2000 Hz, or some other combination felt to predict SRT). This is appropriate because of the well-recognized predictive accuracy between the PTA and SRT measures (see Chapter 5 for further information regarding the PTA/SRT relationship). Also, it must be remembered that the test signal reaches the nontest ear cochlea via bone conduction; thus, the sensitivity of this ear is best expressed relative to a bone conduction measurement. Third, the interaural attenuation value for the test signal previously has been defined as the decibel difference between the intensities of the signal in the external ear canal of the test ear and the intensity level at the cochlea of the nontest ear. Although it would be possible to express the intensity level of the test ear (i.e., the presentation level), it would not be possible to measure the intensity of this signal directly at the nontest ear cochlea. Because there are several methods available to compute PTA for the nontest ear cochlea, the method that most accurately predicts SRT should be chosen for this important function (see Chapter 5 for a discussion of the various methods used to compute PTA).

Interaural attenuation usually is determined by presenting the test signal to a group of listeners with unilateral sensorineural hearing loss (i.e., one normal and one profoundly impaired ear) and comparing the difference in thresholds between ears without masking. Several such investigations have been reported using spondaic words as test material (Liden, 1954 and Snyder, 1973, among others). The findings from these studies reveal consistent results; however, the individual scores (interaural attenuation values) typically spanned a range of about 30 dB. Snyder (1973), for example, found interaural attenuation for individual listeners ($N=84$) to range from 48 to 76 dB. Because clinical practice requires masking whenever "cross hearing" influences the test ear response, it appears advisable to use the minimum amount of expected interaural attenuation (Studebaker, 1967; 1979). The interaural attenuation for spondees, therefore, conservatively can be expressed as 45 dB. Based on these observations, the rule for deciding when to mask during threshold assessments can be restated thus: contralateral masking is necessary whenever the presentation level of the test signal (in dB HL) equals or exceeds the bone conduction PTA of the nontest ear (in dB HL) plus 45 dB (interaural attenuation). Stated differently, it is necessary to mask if the test signal is presented at a level of 45 dB or greater above the nontest ear bone conduction PTA.

Air Conduction Suprathreshold Measures It was noted previously that the most common suprathreshold speech audiometric measure is the speech recognition assessment. Recall from Chapter 6 that this procedure consists of presenting a list of stimuli (i.e., nonsense syllables, meaningful monosyllabic words, or sentences, etc.) to the test ear at a constant intensity above threshold to determine the number of items correctly identified by the listener. In this respect the speech recognition procedure differs from threshold measures that typically are defined relative to a 50 percent correct criterion. Essentially, any score between 0 and 100 percent correct can be obtained on the speech recognition measure. This fundamental difference in percent correct criterion makes it necessary to specify nontest ear cochlear sensitivity in a different manner than that used for speech threshold measurements. The bone conduction PTA that is used for threshold assessments cannot be employed to define nontest ear cochlear sensitivity in suprathreshold testing because a small percentage of test items will be perceived correctly when presented at intensity levels equal to, or less than, the SRT (i.e., SRT = bone conduction PTA). Rintelmann et al. (1974), for example, reported mean recognition scores for normal-hearing listeners on the Northwestern University auditory test number 6 (NU #6) of approximately 18 percent when stimuli were presented at intensities equal to SRT, and almost 5 percent correct for presentation intensity levels of -4 dB relative to SRT. This means that if NU #6 words are presented to the test ear at an intensity sufficient to be present at the nontest ear cochlea at a level equal to the bone conduction PTA, approximately 18 percent of the test items could be recognized correctly by participation of the nontest ear. The findings of Rintelmann et al. (1974) with the NU #6 materials are characteristic of those word recognition tests that use monosyllabic words as test stimuli; that is, about 14 to 20 percent of the items will be identified at presentation intensity levels corresponding to the SRT (see Chapter 6 for representative performance-intensity functions for monosyllable word materials, especially Figures 6-2 and 6-3). An even greater percentage of items is identified correctly at SRT intensity levels for sentences compared to monosyllabic word materials. The synthetic sentence identification (SSI) test (Speaks and Jerger, 1965), for example, will result in scores of about 90 percent when presented at an intensity equal to SRT (see Figure 6-4.). Consequently, it is not appropriate to use the nontest ear bone conduction pure tone average as the criterion of cochlear sensitivity to decide when contralateral masking is necessary during suprathreshold speech recognition testing. Specifically, contralateral masking is indicated for suprathreshold measures of speech recognition when test stimuli are present at the nontest ear cochlea at intensity levels lower than those permitted during threshold assessments. The reader should note that this does not change the previous definition of interaural attenuation (i.e., the difference in intensity of the test signal presentation level at the test ear and the cochlea of the nontest ear). Rather, the manner of specifying nontest ear cochlear sensitivity is altered from a threshold criterion to a lower intensity level to reflect the change in percent correct criterion.

Unfortunately, the permissible amount of interaural attenuation for suprathreshold speech recognition measures is not easily obtained by direct assessment of listeners with unilateral hearing loss. Unlike the SRT, repeated measures with speech recognition materials are time consuming and the resultant data are valid only for that particular test material. Examination of the performance-intensity functions for those materials used commonly in suprathreshold speech recognition testing, however, reveals that regardless of whether the stimuli are comprised of nonsense syllables, meaningful monosyllables, or sentences, they either reach 0 percent or chance performance levels at -10 dB relative to the SRT. Based on this observation, the interaural attenuation value for suprathreshold speech recognition measures can be computed as 35 dB. This value is obtained by subtracting 10 dB from the interaural attenuation value (45 dB) used for threshold measurement, thus reducing the permissible intensity allowed at the nontest ear cochlea. Contralateral masking is thus indicated during suprathreshold speech recognition assessments whenever the presentation level at the test ear equals or exceeds the bone conduction PTA of the nontest ear by 35 dB. This rule is both convenient and appropriate because it can be applied to a variety of different stimulus materials and is based on the same pure tone measure (i.e., the bone conduction PTA of the nontest ear) used to determine when to mask for speech threshold measures.

Bone Conduction Measures Although bone conducted speech audiometry seldom is performed in the majority of audiologic centers (Martin and Forbis, 1978), this technique continues to be used by some audiologists. Because this procedure requires that the test signal be presented by a bone vibrator, interaural attenuation for these signals, as defined previously, is the decibel difference of the test signal at the two cochleae. Interaural attenuation is specified in this manner because the pathway of the test signal to each cochlea is by bone conduction. In practice, therefore, interaural attenuation for bone-conducted speech stimuli is essentially nil; that is, interaural attenuation equals 0 dB. It thus is necessary to mask the nontest ear during bone conduction speech threshold assessments when the presentation level to the test ear equals or exceeds the bone conduction PTA of the nontest ear. Suprathreshold speech recognition testing by bone conduction requires contralateral masking when the presentation level to the test ear equals or exceeds the bone conduction PTA of the nontest ear minus 10 dB. Although the authors of this chapter do not necessarily advocate the practice of bone-conducted suprathreshold speech recognition testing, the reader should realize that if such measures are performed it will be necessary to use contralateral masking for essentially every listener.

In summary, the decision of when to mask requires consideration of several factors and an understanding of the rationale for contralateral masking. These factors have been discussed in the preceding sections of this chapter and provide the basis for the following clinical rules for when to mask during speech audiometry:

1. *Air conduction threshold measures* mask the nontest ear when the presentation level of the test signal to the test ear exceeds the nontest ear bone conduction PTA by 45 dB or greater.
2. *Air conduction suprathreshold measures* mask the nontest ear when the presentation level of the test signal to the test ear exceeds the nontest ear bone conduction PTA by 35 dB or greater.
3. *Bone conduction measures* mask the nontest ear for threshold measures when the test signal presentation level equals or exceeds the bone conduction PTA of the nontest ear, or for suprathreshold speech recognition measures when the test signal presentation level equals or exceeds the bone conduction PTA of the nontest ear minus 10 dB.

Application of these masking rules during clinical practice requires first having the results of pure tone testing. In most hearing clinics pure tone audiometry is performed before speech measurements; therefore, such information usually is available for making appropriate decisions regarding masking. This is one of the advantages of obtaining pure tone results before conducting speech audiometry.

Selection of Appropriate Masking Levels

Once the type of masking noise has been selected and the decision to use contralateral masking has been made, the next question that must be answered is how much masking should be presented to the nontest ear. Selection of an appropriate masking level depends upon: 1) the intensity of the test signal estimated to be present at the cochlea of the nontest ear; 2) the relative air and bone conduction threshold sensitivity of each ear; 3) the mode of test signal presentation (i.e., air or bone conduction); and 4) the nature of the measurement (i.e., threshold or suprathreshold). In general, the overall goal is to present enough masking to reach the plateau area that is illustrated in Figure 9-5. Recall from the discussion of contralateral masking functions that the plateau area represented that portion of the function in which increased masker intensity no longer caused a threshold shift because the listener was now responding to test ear rather than nontest ear information. Specifically, the most ideal level of masking would be an amount sufficient to reach the midpoint of the plateau area (see Figure 9-5). There are two procedures that can be used to attain this goal—the threshold shift, or shadowing technique, and the formula approach. It is important to stress that in the following discussion of these two approaches, the EML notation is used to denote various masking levels. Because this notation is expressed relative to the unit of measurement used for the maskee, the EML cited in the following discussions of this chapter refer to dB HL.

The threshold shift or shadowing technique is derived from the procedure made popular by Hood (1957). In essence, this procedure consists of obtaining a masking function by repeatedly establishing thresholds of the test signal for a series of successive 10 dB increases in EML. An unmasked threshold is established initially, and then the threshold is redetermined in the presence of a contralateral masker presented 10 dB EML above the nontest ear air conduction threshold (i.e., an EML of 40 dB HL would be required for a nontest ear the air conduction threshold of which was 30 dB). If a threshold shift is observed between the unmasked and masked conditions, the EML of the masker is increased by another 10 dB and threshold is remeasured. This procedure is continued until the plateau of the masking function is determined. Although Hood (1957) only discussed the use of this technique with pure tone bone conduction measures, others have advocated the application of the threshold shift procedure to air conduction speech threshold measures (Studebaker, 1979) as well as suprathreshold assessment strategies (Priede and Coles, 1975). Although the threshold shift procedure has value for pure tone testing, application of this procedure to speech audiometric measurements is not recommended for three reasons. First, the threshold shift concept does not readily apply to suprathreshold speech recognition measures (i.e., these are not threshold type procedures). Secondly, the threshold shift procedure requires that several different thresholds be established before the plateau area is defined. Such practice is time consuming and thus is not efficient. Furthermore, the repeated measures can add greatly to listener fatigue, especially for young children. Finally, the use of formula approaches to calculate EML for speech measures can be applied equally well to both threshold and suprathreshold speech audiometric procedures. In fact, formula techniques appear more efficient for speech audiometry because their application depends upon prior knowledge of the air/bone gap for both the test and nontest ears. Whereas these criteria are a drawback for pure tone testing, as noted previously, pure tone data usually are available before speech assessments. Hence, the PTA concept can be used to define the air/bone gap for both test and nontest ears.

It was previously noted that the best EML to use during contralateral masking was one that would reach the midpoint of the plateau area. In 1979, Studebaker proposed a formula approach that is consistent with this goal and equally appropriate for all forms of speech audiologic assessments. When masking is necessary, Studebaker (1979) recommended that the examiner "present an effective level (where effective level is defined as that required to produce a 50% score) to the masked ear that is equal to the level of the test signal in the test ear, adjusted for the difference in the air-bone gaps exhibited by the two ears, . . ." (p. 93). Studebaker noted that the decibel difference between the air/bone gaps should be halved and added to the EML when the nontest ear had the larger air/bone gap and deducted from the EML when the air/bone gap was greater for the test ear. This rule is simple and, according to Studebaker, will place accurately the listener's responses at the midplateau point. There are, however, several aspects associated with the rationale underlying this rule that are worthy of further discussion. First, the reader should note that the intensity of the test signal is the presentation level in dB HL, and that EML also is expressed in dB HL as referenced to a 50 percent response criterion. Furthermore, examination of Figure 9-5, in which a typical contralateral masking function is displayed, will reveal that when neither ear has an air/bone gap the presentation of an EML equal to the presentation level of the test signal results in threshold performance at the midplateau point (i.e., 60 dB EML equals the midplateau point in Figure 9-5). This will occur as long as neither ear has an air/bone gap and if the EML is appropriate for the test signal. Whereas it is relatively easy to derive EML for threshold measures by generating ipsilateral masking functions, establishing EML for materials that are used for suprathreshold speech recognition assessment is less direct. The previous discussion of EML, for example, stressed that a constant dB SPL masker would result in about 10 dB more masking for monosyllables as compared to spondee words. Otherwise stated, a masker dial setting that produces an EML of 40 dB HL for spondee words will provide 50 dB HL effective masking for monosyllables.

A second contention of Studebaker's (1979) formula that needs emphasis is that the EML necessary to reach the midplateau point is defined from the 50 percent correct response criterion. This is convenient because the amount of masking necessary to reach the midplateau does not depend upon the listener's response (i.e., 50 percent for threshold measures or any percentage for suprathreshold speech recognition). Rather, the change in response criterion from 50 percent for threshold to 0 percent for speech recognition that was important for determining when to mask only decreases the plateau area, but does not alter the plateau midpoint. This results because of the alteration in the permissible interaural attenuation values between threshold (50 percent) and zero (or chance) performance levels. Recall that the permissible interaural attenuation value for 50 percent correct threshold measures is 45 dB and that the width of the plateau area equals twice this value (i. e., 90 dB). Permissible interaural attenuation for 0 percent or chance performance, however, is 35 dB; thus the plateau width equals 70 dB. Expressed as EML, it is necessary to increase the minimum masking level by 10 dB and decrease the maximum masking level by 10 dB when converting from a 50 percent to zero or chance level. Because each extreme of the plateau is modified by an equal amount, it follows that the plateau midpoint will remain the same regardless of the percent correct criterion. The advantage of using the 50 percent criterion for specifying EML in clinical practice is that it allows the plateau midpoint to be predicted for both threshold and suprathreshold measures by using the same formula. Moreover, because EML is based on the 50 percent response, conversion to a zero or chance performance level (i.e., as in suprathreshold speech recognition testing) is not of concern because the selected EML already is 10 dB more intense than the minimal intensity necessary for correct identification of a few test items. The fact that the plateau midpoint does not change as a function of different listener response criteria is one of the primary advantages of using a formula that is based on the midplateau concept and EML derived from a 50 percent response criterion.

A third consideration is the influence that an air/bone gap in either or both ears has on the selection of appropriate masking levels. The formula to determine adequate masking levels presented by Studebaker (1979) and endorsed by the present authors requires that the selected EML account for conductive components of the nontest or test ears. This is accomplished by computing the difference (in decibels) between the air/bone gaps of each ear and applying one-half of this value to the EML. When the test ear has an air/bone gap the intensity of the test signal reaching the test ear cochlea is reduced by the magnitude of the conductive component. Thus, the intensity of the test signal must be increased (i.e., the presentation level) to overcome the conductive hearing loss (i.e., this concept is illustrated in Figure 9-3). This increase in intensity, however, also results in an intensity increase at the nontest ear. The overall effect is that the maximum masking level of the contralateral function (see Figure 9-5) is shifted downward (i.e., to a lower EML) by an amount equal to the magnitude of the air/bone gap. It follows, therefore, that the midpoint of the plateau also is shifted downward, but only by an amount equal to one-half of the conductive component. The EML thus must be decreased by one-half of the difference in air/bone gaps when the test ear has the larger conductive component. Conversely, when the larger conductive component is present in the nontest ear, the minimum masking level of the contralateral function is shifted upward (i.e., to a higher EML) by the same amount as the air/bone gap, and the midpoint of the plateau shifts upward by one-half of the air/bone gap. Because the conductive component at the nontest ear causes a reduction in the EML reaching the nontest ear cochlea, the EML of masker must be increased (in dB HL) by an amount equal to one-half of the conductive component. When both ears have an air/bone gap the EML should be adjusted according to the ear with the larger conductive involvement. In these situations the EML should be decreased by one-half the difference between air/bone gaps when the test ear has the larger conductive component, and increased when the air/bone gap is larger for the nontest ear. Conductive components of equal magnitude in each ear simply require presenting an EML equal to the test signal presentation level.

Based on the concepts discussed in the preceding paragraphs, the following equation can be used to determine the amount of contralateral masking appropriate during speech audiometry:

$$\mathrm{EML} = \mathrm{PL_{TS}} + \left(\frac{\mathrm{ABG_N} - \mathrm{ABG_T}}{2}\right)$$

where:

EML is the amount of effective masking in dB HL necessary to reach the midplateau point of the contralateral masking function; PL_{TS}, = the presentation level in dB HL of the test signal; ABG_N, the air/bone gap of the nontest ear; and ABG_T, the air/bone gap of the test ear.

This equation can be used for both threshold and suprathreshold measures; however, the EML may become excessively loud during suprathreshold assessments when test signals are presented at intensities well above threshold. In these cases, it is permissible to reduce the EML by one interaural attenuation value, and then add 20 dB as a safety factor plus the air/bone gap (if any) of the nontest ear (Studebaker, 1979). In actual clinical practice this means it is possible to reduce the EML derived from the above equation by 15 dB (i.e., 35 dB interaural attenuation minus a 20 dB safety factor equals 15 dB) when an air/bone gap is not present for the nontest ear.

In this section the use of a formula approach to the selection of appropriate masking levels has been stressed. The advantages to using a formula based on the midplateau concept are especially convenient for use in speech audiometry. The formula presented by Studebaker (1979) is simple, easy to use, applicable to all phases of speech audiometric assessment, and founded on the established rationale for contralateral masking. Consequently, it is recommended that this formula be used to establish appropriate masking levels during the practice of contralateral masking in speech audiometry.

Central Masking

Recall that the primary purpose of contralateral masking is to shift the threshold of the nontest ear without causing a change in sensitivity of the test ear. It is well documented, however, that changes in the threshold sensitivity of the test ear can occur when low intensity masking is delivered to the nontest ear. This effect generally has been referred to as *central masking* and attributed to central rather than peripheral auditory processes. Whereas central masking has been examined in detail for pure tone stimuli (Dirks, 1964; Dirks and Malmquist, 1965; Dirks and Norris, 1966; Ingham, 1959; Sherrick and Mangabeira-Albernaz, 1961; Treisman, 1963; Wegel and Lane, 1924; Zwislocki et al., 1967; Zwislocki, Buining, and Glantz, 1968; Zwislocki, 1953), similar research using speech stimuli has been limited. Martin, Bailey, and Pappas (1965) observed that speech thresholds using a Bekesy tracking technique shifted 5 to 8 dB (i.e., became poorer) when broadband noise maskers were presented to the nontest ear at a sensation level of 75 dB. In a followup study, Martin (1966) examined the effect of a broadband noise contralateral masker on speech thresholds determined with spondee words and on suprathreshold speech recognition scores obtained with meaningful monosyllable word lists. Results of this investigation indicated a shift in speech threshold of approximately 5 dB with essentially no change in speech recognition scores. Martin and DiGiovanni (1979) confirmed these findings, but observed slightly smaller threshold shifts. In 1970, Young and Harbert obtained suprathreshold speech recognition scores with meaningful monosyllabic stimuli in the presence of a broadband contralateral masker in seven normal-hearing subjects, 65 subjects with total hearing loss in one ear and normal hearing in the opposite ear, and 15 listeners with bilaterally symmetrical hearing loss. The results of this study indicated that contralateral masking had little effect on recognition scores until masker intensity levels were reached that were sufficient to cause overmasking. Spencer and Priede (1974), however, suggested that a small percentage of normal-hearing listeners experience an approximate 1 percent decrease in speech recognition for each 3-dB sensation level increase of a broadband contralateral masker. Spencer and Priede attributed this effect to central masking phenomena similar to that observed in speech threshold measures. Thus, it appears that introduction of a contralateral masker will cause speech thresholds to shift by about 5 dB even though the masking intensity level is relatively low. The effect of contralateral maskers on suprathreshold tasks is less clear and the influence of central masking on these measures awaits further research.

CONCLUSION

This chapter has dealt with the topic of contralateral masking in speech audiometry. The reader should be aware that many of the clinical masking techniques presented within this chapter depend upon prior knowledge of pure tone audiometric threshold data. Within this context, therefore, it is equally important that the clinician have a complete understanding of masking procedures associated with pure tone measures. This topic, of course, is beyond the scope of this chapter. There are, however, several excellent sources for this information including Martin (1981), Sanders (1978), and Studebaker (1979). Indeed, the basic rationale for pure tone and speech audiometric masking is essentially the same, but unless the rationale is understood, contralateral masking will continue to be misused by many clinicians. Conversely, an appreciation of the basic psychoacoustic concepts that provide the foundation for contralateral masking procedures will avoid the masking problems that have caused confusion for many audiologists. Given such understanding, the practice of contralateral masking, especially during speech audiometry, becomes a simple and effective procedure.

REFERENCES

American National Standards Institute. 1970. American National Standard Specifications for Audiometers, ANSI-S3.6-1969. American National Standards Institute, New York.

Carhart, R., T. W. Tillman, and E. S. Greetis. 1969. Perceptual masking in multiple sound background. J. Acoust. Soc. Am. 45:694–703.

Dirks, D. 1964. Factors related to bone conduction reliability. Arch. Otolaryngol. 79:551–558.

Dirks, D., and C. Malmquist. 1964. Changes in bone-conduction thresholds produced by masking the nontest ear. J. Speech Hear. Res. 7:271–287.

Dirks, D., and J. Norris. 1966. Shifts in auditory thresholds produced by pulsed and continuous contralateral masking. J. Acoust. Soc. Am. 37:631–637.

Dirks, D. D., R. H. Wilson, and D. R. Bower. 1969. Effects of pulsed masking on selected speech materials. J. Acoust. Soc. Am. 46:898–906.

Hawkins, J. E., and S. S. Stevens. 1950. Masking of pure tones and speech by white noise. J. Acoust. Soc. Am. 22:6–13.

Hood, J. D. 1957. The principles and practice of bone conduction audiometry. Proc. Roy. Soc. Med. pp. 689–697. Reprinted in Laryngoscope 70:1211–1228.

Ingham, J. 1959. Variations in cross-masking with frequency. J. Exp. Psychol. 58:199–205.

Johnson, C., and L. Young. 1974. The masking effectiveness of speech versus speech modulated filtered noise. Paper presented at the convention of the American Speech and Hearing Association, November 4–6, Las Vegas, Nevada.

Liden, G. 1954. Speech audiometry. Acta Otolaryngol. 114(Suppl.):72–76.

Martin, F. 1966. Speech audiometry and clinical masking. J. Aud. Res. 6:199–203.

Martin, F., H. Bailey, and J. Pappas. 1965. The effect of central masking on thresholds for speech. J. Aud. Res. 5:293–296.

Martin, F. N. 1981. Introduction to Audiology, 2nd Ed. Prentice Hall, Englewood Cliffs.

Martin, F. N., and D. DiGiovanni. 1979. Central masking effects on spondee threshold as a function of masker sensation level and masker sound pressure level. J. Am. Aud. Soc. 4:141–146.

Martin, F. N., and N. K. Forbis. 1978. The present status of audiometric practice: A follow-up study. Asha 20:531–541.

Martin, F. N., and C. D. Pennington. 1971. Current trends in audiometric practice. Asha 13:671–677.

Priede, V. M., and R. R. A. Coles. 1975. Masking the nontest ear in tone decay, Bekesy and SISI tests. J. Laryngol. Otol. 89:227–236.

Rintelmann, W. F., and associates. 1974. Six experiments on speech discrimination utilizing CNC monosyllables. J. Aud. Res. 2(suppl.):1–30.

Sanders, J. W. 1978. Masking. In J. Katz (ed.), Handbook of Clinical Audiology, pp. 124–140. 2nd Ed. Williams & Wilkins Company, Baltimore.

Sherrick, G., and P. Mangabeira-Albernaz. 1961. Auditory threshold shifts produced by simultaneous pulsed contralateral stimuli. J. Acoust. Soc. Am. 33:1381–1385.

Snyder, J. M. 1973. Interaural attenuation characteristics in audiometry. Laryngoscope 83:1847–1855.

Speaks, C., and J. Jerger. 1965. Method for measurement of speech identification. J. Speech Hear. Res. 8:185–194.
Spencer, R., and V. Priede. 1974. The effects of contralateral masking on the intelligibility of speech. Unpublished manuscript, Institute of Sound and Vibration Research, Southampton.
Studebaker, G. A. 1967. Clinical masking of the nontest ear. J. Speech Hear. Disord. 32:360–371.
Studebaker, G. A. 1979. Clinical masking. In W. F. Rintelmann (ed.), Hearing Assessment, pp. 51–100. University Park Press, Baltimore.
Treisman, M. 1963. Auditory unmasking. J. Acoust. Soc. Am. 35:1256–1263.
Wegel, R., and C. Lane. 1924. Auditory masking of one pure tone by another and its probable relation to dynamics of the inner ear. Physics Rev. 23:266–285.
Wilson, R. H., and R. Carhart. 1969. Influence of pulsed masking on the threshold for spondees. J. Acoust. Soc. Am. 46:998–1010.
Young, I., and F. Harbert. 1970. Noise effects on speech discrimination score. J. Aud. Res. 10:127–131.
Zwislocki, J. 1953. Acoustic attenuation between ears. J. Acoust. Soc. Am. 25:752–759.
Zwislocki, J., E. Buining, and J. Glantz. 1968. Frequency distribution of central masking. J. Acoust. Soc. Am. 43:1267–1271.
Zwislocki, J., E. Damianopoulous, E. Buining, and J. Glantz. 1967. Central masking, some steady-state and transient effects. Percep. Psychophys. 2:50–64.

CHAPTER 10

SPEECH AUDIOMETRY AND HEARING AID ASSESSMENT: A REAPPRAISAL OF AN OLD PHILOSOPHY

Daniel M. Schwartz and Brian E. Walden

CONTENTS

OVERVIEW OF HEARING AID EVALUATION PROCEDURES 322
   Objective Strategies 322
   Subjective Strategies 331
RELIABILITY OF CURRENT TEST METHODS 337
   Methods Based on Performance Scores 337
   Methods Based on Subjective Judgments 346
AFTERWORD 348
REFERENCES 350

Interest in and use of speech tests to evaluate patient performance with amplification dates back to the early work of Knudsen and Jones (1935). In 1944 Hughson reemphasized the importance of speech tests for evaluating the usefulness of a hearing aid when he stated that ". . . unless the hearing aid provides good speech intelligibility, all other factors related to its performance are essentially irrelevant" (p. 184). Two years later Carhart (1946) proposed a clinical protocol for a comparative evaluation of hearing aid performance based on the results of speech recognition tests. In this procedure, a patient's aided performance as measured by a series of speech recognition tasks was compared for several different amplification systems. The instrument providing the best performance was recommended. Since its development at the Acoustic Clinic, Deshon General Hospital, Butler, Pennsylvania, this time-honored approach to the hearing aid evaluation has been an integral part of clinical audiology.

    It is almost superfluous to note that significant advances in hearing aid technology have been made since 1946. Yet, similar progress in hearing aid evaluation methodology has not occurred. Rather, many audiologists continue to use at least some modification of the comparative hearing aid evaluation for differentiating among amplification systems (Burney, 1972; Chermak, 1977).

    In general, the hearing aid evaluation is founded on three basic assumptions as outlined by Resnick and Becker (1963): 1) significant differences exist among hearing aids as reflected in patient performance on standard speech tests; 2) interactions exist among hearing aids and people; and 3) differences among hearing aids can be measured reliably by speech recognition tests. Because most audiologists continue to select hearing aids on the basis of comparative test results, one must assume that such procedures, as presently used, are justified and support these underlying principals. If, however, there is sufficient evidence to refute these assumptions, then clinical use of the comparative evaluation becomes questionable.

This chapter on hearing aid selection is confined to a review of those evaluative procedures that incorporate speech stimuli. Unlike the so-called "frequency selective amplification" or "prescriptive" methods (i.e., mirroring the audiogram, audiogram bisection, equal loudness methods, or formulae approaches), the comparative hearing aid evaluation does not attempt to prescribe optimum frequency-gain characteristics because these are presumably associated with the preselection process. Rather, comparative procedures use speech tests to assess which of several hearing aids is potentially best suited for a given individual.

The chapter is divided into two parts. The first provides a rather detailed overview of comparative hearing aid evaluation procedures and strategies. The second section focuses on the reliability and validity of evaluative procedures in an effort to determine if their continued use is justified.

OVERVIEW OF HEARING AID EVALUATION PROCEDURES

Objective Strategies

The Carhart Method   In his now classic article, "Tests for the Selection of Hearing Aids," Carhart (1946) stated that, "Obviously, the final criterion of hearing aid excellence is the success with which the instrument functions in everyday situations; thus, selection procedures need to be chosen so as to yield estimates of the future usefulness promised by each hearing aid" (p. 780). Carhart went on to describe a battery of tests that utilized speech as the primary auditory stimulus ". . . both to reduce testing time and because ability to hear speech is the auditory requirement of greatest importance in everyday life" (Carhart, 1946; p. 781). Before testing with amplification, unaided sound-field speech recognition threshold (SRT), tolerance limit, and monosyllabic word recognition at 25 dB sensation level (SL) were measured to permit later comparison between unaided and aided performance. Four dimensions of hearing aid performance were assessed:

1) effective gain, 2) tolerance limit, 3) efficiency in noise, and 4) monosyllabic word recognition.

Test of Effective Gain The effective gain or sensitivity of a hearing aid represents the difference in decibels between the patient's unaided and aided speech recognition threshold in a sound field. Carhart (1946) recommended that the volume control of each hearing aid be adjusted (by the patient) ". . . until speech striking the hearing aid at 40 dB above normal threshold is stimulating the patient in such a manner that he judges the reception most comfortable" (p. 782). This comfort level setting method was advocated because it was thought to yield equivalent volume control settings with different hearing aids and because patients could replicate the same gain setting upon retesting. Empirical evidence has subsequently confirmed this observation (Kopra and Blosser, 1968; Reid, Smiarowski, and McPherson, 1977; Walden, Schuchman, and Sedge, 1977). With the volume control of the hearing aid rotated to a most comfortable level (MCL), aided SRTs were established and from these data Carhart calculated what he called "residual hearing loss for speech" which represented the difference in decibels between normal and aided speech thresholds. A second measure of hearing aid sensitivity was to repeat the aided SRT with the volume control set to full-on gain. Here again, residual loss for speech and effective gain were computed.

Carhart (1946) proposed three criteria for evaluating these test results: 1) SRT differences between instruments of ≤6 dB are insignificant; 2) a hearing aid can be considered sufficiently sensitive for everyday situations if the aided residual loss for speech does not exceed 15 dB; and 3) the significance of sensitivity as a selection criterion increases proportionally to the degree to which residual loss for speech exceeds 15 dB.

Test of Tolerance Limit The threshold of tolerance, often referred to as the loudness discomfort level (LDL), is defined as the sound pressure level above which a listener reports subjectively that an auditory signal is uncomfortably loud. The second dimension of hearing aid performance outlined by Carhart (1946), therefore, was an estimate of tolerance limit which he defined as the input intensity level at which amplified speech becomes intolerable. For this test, the hearing aid volume control was set at MCL and again at full-on gain as was accomplished with the test of aided sensitivity.

Samples of connected speech discourse were presented in a sound field at progressively increasing intensity levels (5- to 10-dB increments) until the listener reported some sensation of discomfort. Accordingly, if the listener's tolerance limit was not reached at an amplified input intensity level of 80 dB above normal threshold, then the

". . . ceiling with the hearing aid is ample for all practical purposes" (Carhart, 1946; p. 784). Carhart went on to state that when all other factors were equal, the hearing aid of choice was the one with the highest tolerance limit.

In essence, this procedure was used to define the patient's dynamic range (i.e., decibel difference between SRT and LDL) for aided hearing. A reduced range between threshold and uncomfortable listening level with amplification suggested that the listener most likely would have difficulty with hearing aid use (Carhart, 1946; Watson, 1944).

Test of Efficiency in Noise In an effort to obtain some estimate of hearing aid performance under adverse listening conditions, Carhart (1946) proposed a third measurement for determining the maximum amount of noise that can be transduced through the hearing aid without affecting the listener's ability to understand speech. With the hearing aid volume control adjusted to a comfort level (re: a 50 dB SL speech signal), spondee words were presented at 50 dB SL in the presence of step-wise increases of background noise. The intensity level of the noise was varied systematically until the patient no longer was able to respond to the spondee materials. Next, the noise level was decreased until speech recognition returned [sic] (Carhart, 1946).

The resulting signal-to-noise (S/N) ratio for each hearing aid was defined as the decibel difference between the fixed sensation level of the speech stimulus (50 dB SL) and the level of the most intense noise at which spondee word recognition was maintained. Unfortunately, Carhart did not provide specific criteria for determining what was an acceptable S/N ratio, or what difference magnitude in decibels between hearing aids constituted clinical significance. He did report, however, that the calculated S/N ratio was dependent, in part, on the type of noise used and suggested that each clinical facility establish its own normative data in order to estimate the significance of individual findings. Carhart (1946) described two noise sources that he found particularly useful for this purpose. One was a combination of a broadband, constant intensity thermal noise with a superimposed acoustic static; this noise was assumed to be analogous to the random fluctuations of environmental noise. The second was a complex or sawtooth noise having a fundamental frequency of 120 Hz. Clearly, neither of these noise sources, nor the concept of establishing individual normative data for the selection of S/N ratio, was ever adopted for routine clinical use.

Test of Monosyllabic Word Discrimination The final and perhaps most universally adopted test in the comparative hearing aid evaluation was the measurement of a listener's aided word recognition ability. This measurement, as originally described, was obtained with the Harvard University Psycho-Acoustic Laboratory Phonetically Balanced (PAL PB-50) word lists presented without background noise (i.e., in quiet). Unquestionably, improvement in speech understanding with amplification is of primary importance to the hearing aid user, and moreover, represents the underlying principal for the Carhart approach to evaluating hearing aid performance.

Carhart's procedure for estimating word discrimination (recognition) was as follows: 1) measure unaided discrimination performance at 25 dB SL (re: the unaided SRT); 2) adjust the volume control of each hearing aid to a comfort level setting; 3) obtain an aided SRT; and 4) assess aided discrimination at a 25 dB SL (re: the aided SRT). An 8 percent criterion for clinical significance was used to differentiate among instruments and to determine which hearing aid yielded the best performance score.

An often overlooked additional measure of word recognition performance described by Carhart was to carry this testing one step further by assessing performance at different input intensity levels. This method was believed to allow the clinician to specify the point of maximum aided discrimination, or the range of intensities across which maximum speech understanding was maintained without saturating either the ear or the hearing aid. A similar adaptation of this method has been advocated by Hood (1970) who administered word recognition tests in both quiet and noise at speech input intensity levels analogous to those of soft, average, and loud conversational speech. Although this approach appears to be rather time-consuming, Hood (1970) maintained that it is more reasonable to evaluate fewer aids definitively, than a greater number of aids with less clinical precision.

To summarize, the comparative hearing aid evaluation procedure described by Carhart (1946) encompassed the measurement of four hearing aid performance dimensions: effective gain; tolerance limit; signal-to-noise ratio; and word discrimination in quiet. The selection of a specific hearing aid was made on the basis of composite results from each of these four measures, although it appears that greater emphasis was given to tolerance limit and signal-to-noise ratio. As is currently found in clinical practice, Carhart also noted that many individuals obtained equivalent performance across different hearing aids on one or more of the seven subtests. Hence, the final decision of which hearing aid to recommend often was based on only one criterion, or on factors not related to test measurement (i.e., cost, size, patient preference).

It is clear from the review of this classic procedure that Carhart promoted the concept of individual specificity and established a fundamental principal for evaluating hearing aids in a clinical setting. He contended that there was a measurable interaction between hearing aids and people and believed, therefore, that comparative testing with different hearing aids was indeed appropriate if the clinician was to extract the necessary information related to the listener's ability to benefit from a given amplification system. During the time that has elapsed since the original protocol, numerous modifications for evaluating patient performance with amplification have been described; however, most of these have continued to assess essentially the same four dimensions of aided performance.

Assessment of effective gain continues to enjoy widespread clinical practice. In most clinical settings, spondee recognition thresholds are obtained both unaided and aided with the decibel difference expressed as effective gain. Unfortunately, the practice has evolved in many audiologic centers whereby the hearing aid providing the best SRT is considered to be the most appropriate system. Decisions based on SRT measures, however, can be misleading because they fail to consider the dynamics of the speech signal. Recall from Chapter 3, for example, that the majority of acoustic energy in a speech signal is comprised of vowel sounds and contained in the frequencies below 1000 Hz. This energy, however, contributes little to the understanding of conversational speech. Conversely, the consonant sounds that contribute greatly to speech intelligibility are comprised primarily of high frequency energy (above 1000 Hz) and are considerably less intense than the vowels. Thus, the expression of effective gain as a single dB value probably places too much emphasis on low-frequency spectral content.

Also, it no longer is common to measure the SRT or the threshold of tolerance with the aid set to full-on gain because these measures provide no practical information relative to the benefits of amplification. If a given patient has to utilize the maximum gain setting for aided speech recognition, then, undoubtedly, one can assume that the particular hearing aid is inappropriate for that person and a more powerful amplification system that provides additional gain is needed.

Without question, the most extensive alteration of the Carhart procedure relates to the assessment of hearing aid efficiency in noise. Recall that Carhart proposed a method for computing signal-to-noise ratio in decibels which was defined as the difference between the fixed sensation level of a speech stimulus (50 dB SL) and the level of the most intense noise at which recognition of spondee materials was maintained. For some reason (perhaps simply by happenstance), which remains unclear at present, the concept of measuring hearing aid performance in noise has been modified drastically to its current form of assessing monosyllabic word recognition performance in the presence of some competing signal at a fixed message-to-competition ratio (MCR).

The rationale for incorporating a competing stimulus in the current hearing aid evaluation is to reduce recognition performance because many individuals with hearing loss often achieve relatively high word recognition scores in quiet. The noise, therefore, serves to increase the range of improvement possible with amplification permitting better differentiation between hearing aids, and helps simulate a more realistic listening situation. This approach to the hearing aid evaluation, however, does not appear to be in any way consistent with the signal-to-noise subtest originally described by Carhart (1946). Furthermore, there still does not exist any accepted clinical procedure relative to the type of competing stimulus, or the most optimal message-to-competition ratio to use. It has been our experience that few clinical programs (if any) actually develop normative data for a specific competing noise source and competition ratio for use in the comparative hearing aid evaluation as recommended by Carhart (1946).

The intensity level at which monosyllabic word recognition lists are administered has also been revised. Whereas Carhart utilized a 25 dB SL (re: the aided SRT), most clinicians today present the word lists at a fixed hearing level (HL), usually 50 or 60 dB, which corresponds to the average intensity of conversational speech.

Finally, as is discussed in detail in Chapter 7, the reliability and validity of the comfort level method for adjusting the optimal acoustic gain of a hearing aid at a constant input intensity, and the loudness discomfort or tolerance level for assessing the input intensity level at which amplified speech becomes intolerable, is subject to considerable criticism. Both of these measures are influenced by such variables as subject response criteria, psychophysical method of measurement, type of stimulus employed, and instructional set. As was noted by Dirks and Morgan (see Chapter 7), ". . . until such time as individuals concerned with hearing aid evaluation procedures resolve the fundamental issues regarding the application of MCL the insight provided by such measures will continue to be severely limited (p. 225).

The Jerger and Hayes Method In pursuit of a more realistic and sensitive test for evaluating differences among amplification systems, Jerger and Hayes (1976) discussed the limitations of using monosyllables and stated that ". . . when only two conditions, PB words presented in quiet and in noise, are used to test the patient's ability to understand speech, substantial differences among hearing aids or aid arrangements (e.g., CROS, BICROS, Binaural) rarely emerge" (p. 214). On the basis of the inherent limitations associated with monosyllabic word lists, Jerger and Hayes described a hearing aid evaluation procedure that incorporated synthetic sentences as the test stimuli. These were the same third-order approximations originally described in 1965 by Speaks and Jerger as the *synthetic sentence identification* (SSI) test (see Chapter 6 for a complete review of these materials). They reasoned that sentential stimuli incorporate more of the parameters of conversational speech and should have greater face validity than that found with monosyllables. Unlike monosyllables, the perception of sentential stimuli approximates more closely that of connected speech because it maintains the multiple overlapping of frequency, temporal, and intensity cues, and thus represents a more appropriate stimulus for evaluating one's ability to understand speech.

Consistent with the early philosophy of Carhart (1946), the Jerger and Hayes (1976) procedure was designed to be part of the total rehabilitative process rather than simply a method for selecting the "best" hearing aid; a point that too often is ignored in audiologic practice. In other words, the application of the SSI technique was not to differentiate among hearing aids per se, but rather, to compare patient performance with different hearing aid arrangements (e.g., monaural versus CROS amplification). Hence, the procedure was designed to meet four specific goals: 1) to determine the most suitable hearing aid arrangement for the individual; 2) to define differences among arrangements in real-life listening conditions; 3) to provide information on realistic expectations of hearing aid use for patient counseling; and 4) to make accountable rehabilitative recommendations to the patient. In addition to these four goals, Jerger and Hayes (1976) considered that an effective hearing aid evaluation technique must achieve face validity by employing test materials that approximate conversational speech, and should be a simple clinical procedure that utilizes standard clinical instrumentation.

For the Jerger and Hayes (1976) test procedure the patient is in a standard sound isolated test suite and is seated equidistant between two loudspeakers placed at 0 degrees and 180 degrees relative to the frontal midline of the listener's head, as illustrated in Figure 10-1. The primary message, 10 synthetic sentences, is delivered from the speaker directly in front of the patient (0°) at a constant input intensity of 60 dB SPL. The competing message, a biographical story of Davy Crockett, is transduced simultaneously from the rear speaker (180°) with the intensity varied between 40 and 80 dB sound pressure level (SPL). Consequently, patient performance is assessed at several message-to-competition ratios representing a range of listening conditions from very easy (+20 dB MCR) to severely adverse (−20 dB MCR).

After a practice session, unaided performance is plotted across

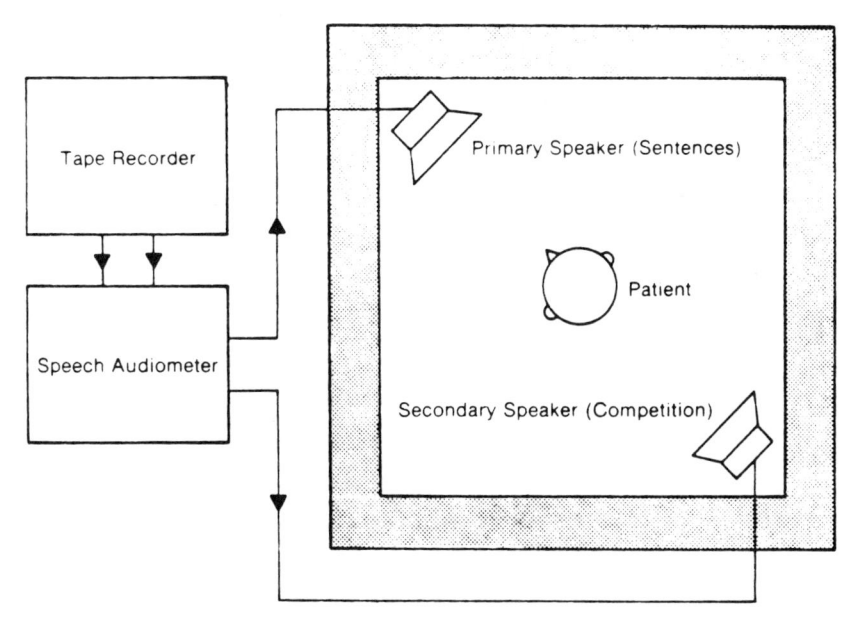

Figure 10-1. Schematic of the seating arrangement used in the Jerger and Hayes (1976) hearing aid evaluation procedure. (From Jerger and Hayes, Archives of Otolaryngology, 1976, 102:214–221; Copyright 1976, American Medical Association.)

MCRs and compared to normative data (shown in Figure 10-2). Next, performance with each hearing aid or aid arrangement is assessed similarly with the gain of the instrument adjusted to MCL. Unaided results are then obtained a second time to control for possible learning effects. According to Jerger and Hayes (1976) the hearing aid yielding a performance function that approximates most closely that of normal hearers is considered to be the most suitable instrument for recommendation. Figure 10-3 exemplifies the type of results obtained from the Jerger and Hayes method. The solid line represents the performance range of normal hearers across MCRs. Observe that for this patient unaided performance was 70 percent in the easy listening condition (+10 dB MCR), 40 percent in the average listening situation (0 dB MCR) and decreased to 0 percent under the more adverse competition ratio (−10 dB MCR). Performance with amplification shows improvement in SSI score across all MCRs. For this patient, the greatest benefit was realized with binaural wide band hearing aids coupled to the ear with exponential horn type occluded earmolds (Killion, 1981; Libby, 1981).

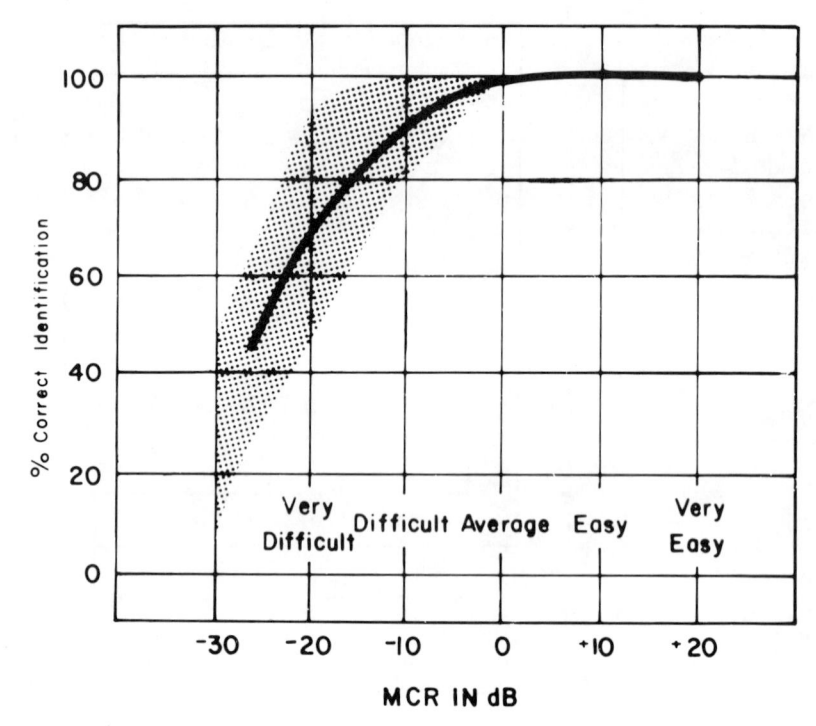

Figure 10-2. Hearing aid evaluation summary form used in Jerger and Hayes (1976) method. The solid line and shaded area represents performance range of normal hearers. (From Jerger and Hayes, Archives of Otolaryngology, 1976, 102:214–221; Copyright 1976, American Medical Association.)

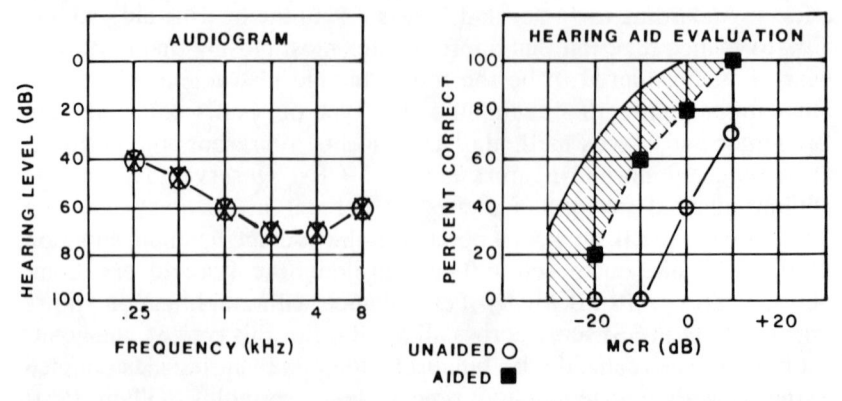

Figure 10-3. Audiogram and hearing aid evaluation summary form illustrating aided improvement for synthetic sentence identification. Hatched area represents the "residual deficit"; i.e., difference between aided improvement and normal performance.

Jerger and Hayes (1976) contended that this method met the stated goals and enabled the clinician to determine the amount of background competition that would not result in marked reduction of speech understanding with amplification. Moreover, the graphic illustration of results assisted in counseling patients relative to expectations for hearing aid improvement, and provided prognostic information as to successful use with the recommended amplification system. The use of several message-to-competition ratios, as well as comparison to normative data for comparing aided performance, appears to represent the closest approximation of the original signal-to-noise subtest outlined by Carhart (1946).

Although the Jerger and Hayes (1976) procedure offers the audiologist a unique method for evaluating differences in patient performance with amplification, it, too, suffers from several procedural problems. Among these is the presence of "acoustic windows" for the competing message on the commercially available recording of the SSI. Because the biographical story is read by a single talker, it is common to perceive pauses in the competing speech stimuli. Such acoustic windows create a brief quiet condition allowing the listener to detect at least one word of the sentence without background competition. Clearly, this can affect the performance scores obtained among various hearing aid systems and listening conditions, and thus reduces the reliability of the test measure. Martin and Mussell (1979) found, for example, that the intelligibility of a single word in the primary sentence as a result of such acoustic windows can lead to complete sentence identification. They suggested, therefore, that speech spectrum noise be mixed acoustically at a level 6 dB below that of the competing story. Martin and Mussell (1979) reported that the addition of this steady-state, speech-shaped noise filled in the momentary natural speech pauses of the connected discourse and created a more difficult listening task. To date, however, there are no published reports on the use of this modification in the Jerger and Hayes (1976) hearing aid evaluation procedure.

Subjective Strategies

In view of the questionable resolving power of most speech recognition tests for distinguishing among hearing aids, individuals concerned with the use of amplification have sought alternative hearing aid evaluation methods. The most common of these alternative techniques is the paired-comparison subjective approach. Here, the listener makes some form of preference judgment based on the perception of either sound quality or the relative intelligibility of hearing-aid-processed speech. The advantage of a paired-comparison paradigm, like other psychophysical tasks, is that the response is one of a simple binary decision based on informing the examiner which hearing aid in a given recorded pair produces either the better sound quality or the more intelligible speech. This can be accomplished verbally, in writing on a simple answer form, or electromechanically by pressing a button on a response panel. Of course, the major advantage of the latter method of recording responses is that the results can be fed directly into a computer for later scoring or as a means of storing responses for future research application.

Judgments of Hearing Aid Sound Quality Jeffers (1960) was one of the first to explore the use of quality judgments for differentiating among hearing aids in a relatively informal clinical setting. Thirty-four subjects with conductive hearing loss were asked to judge the quality of continuous discourse reproduced by four pairs of five vacuum tube hearing aids, three of which were electroacoustically dissimilar. Results revealed a systematic order preference for the various hearing aid comparisons and a preference for one instrument by the majority of subjects. These findings led Jeffers to conclude that judgments of speech quality permitted a simple means of differentiating among instruments with dissimilar electroacoustic characteristics. Unfortunately, Jeffers did not correlate the subjective ratings of sound quality with the actual electroacoustic performance data of the five aids used in her study. Rather, Jeffers relied on the manufacturers specification sheets for the description of the physical properties of the particular make and model of hearing aid. In contrast to the ability of these patients to differentiate clearly among hearing aids on the basis of sound quality, Jeffers reported that no differences among these five hearing aids were achieved for monosyllabic word recognition scores in quiet.

In recent years there have been several formal investigative attempts to assess the reliability of quality judgments for differentiating among hearing aids (Punch, 1978; Punch and Howard, 1978; Witter and Goldstein, 1971). When we examine the results of each of these studies carefully, it becomes apparent that paired-comparison preference judgments of hearing aid sound quality generally yield consistent differences among instruments and that individual listeners tend to produce highly similar rank ordering of hearing aids on the basis of their quality judgments.

Although a recurrent theme among each of these studies is that hearing-impaired listeners evaluate their success with amplification at least partly on the basis of the quality of amplified speech, the relationship between listener perceived sound quality judgments and the electroacoustic characteristics of hearing aids has only recently been clarified (Punch and Beck, 1980; Punch et al., 1980; Schwartz et al., 1979, Yanovitz et al., 1978).

With the aid of *a posteriori* multidimensional scaling these independent investigators reached the same conclusion that low-frequency cutoff (LCO) appeared to be the most dominant feature influencing quality judgments of hearing-aid-processed speech. These findings held true for normal hearers (Gabrielsson and Sjögren, 1979; Punch et al., 1980; Yanovitz et al., 1978), as well as for listeners with sensorineural hearing loss of various configurations (Punch and Beck, 1980; Schwartz et al., in press).

The most obvious implication of the foregoing reports is that improvement in speech quality associated with the extension of the low-cutoff frequency may cause speech intelligibility to be degraded as a possible consequence of the upward spread of masking (Danaher, Osberger and Pickett, 1973; Danaher and Pickett, 1975; French and Steinberg, 1947; Martin and Pickett, 1970). When viewed in light of some more contemporary evidence, however, the long held belief that low-frequency amplification may affect adversely the hearing-impaired listener's ability to understand speech may be open to debate.

Beck, Leatherwood, and Punch (1980) studied the effects of parametric variations in low-cutoff frequency on a master hearing aid for both the perceived quality of hearing-aid-processed speech and phonemic identification on the nonsense syllable test (NST) (Resnick et al., 1976; see Chapter 6 for detailed consideration of the NST). In contrast to previous research findings, Beck et al. (1980) found that phonemic identification in quiet improved with the introduction of a mild degree of low-frequency emphasis and that the addition of speech babble did not degrade phonemic identification substantially when low-frequency information was increased in proportional amounts.

It appears from the available evidence that the concept of a hearing aid-listener interaction is not supported. That is, there is a substantial consistency across listeners in their ability to differentiate among hearing aids on the basis of sound quality preference judgments such that the aid providing the most preferable sound quality to one listener is likely to do the same for others. Because it is highly probable that if the hearing impairments among the patients being evaluated are relatively similar, and if the hearing aids preselected for evaluation are considered to match the auditory characteristics of the impaired ear, then the same amplification system most likely will be preferred by the majority of these patients. Consequently, the value of subjective judgments of hearing aid sound quality is open to serious question.

Finally, the recent findings of Harris and Goldstein (1979) that quality judgments in a reverberent room (reverberation time = 0.50

sec) could not be predicted from similar judgments obtained in an audiometric test suite (mean reverberation time ≤ 0.18 sec), provide additional evidence to question the continued use of quality judgments as the primary method of evaluating hearing aids. The implication here, of course, is that a patient who exhibits preference for a particular hearing aid when evaluated under the "sterility" of an audiometric test suite may not necessarily consider the quality of amplified speech to be equally as good when worn in a more realistic reverberent room. As Harris and Goldstein (1979) recommended, perhaps the patient should be given an opportunity to use the hearing aid in a variety of listening situations prior to making a final recommendation.

Judgments of Relative Speech Intelligibility In 1962 Zerlin described a paired-comparison procedure that required the listener to make judgments about the relative intelligibility of hearing-aid-processed speech. In an anechoic space he presented a 30-second passage of tape-recorded speech to two hearing aids that were connected to individual coupler-microphone assemblies. The resulting output of each aid was then recorded on separate tracks of magnetic tape for later playback. This procedure was repeated until the recorded speech stimuli were processed through successive pairs of six hearing aids. For the clinical protocol, the recorded signal was transduced through a monaural earphone and presented to each of 21 listeners with sensorineural hearing loss. A two-selector push button response box allowed the subject to listen alternately to a given channel of the two-channel tape recorder, thus permitting paired-comparison judgments of the relative intelligibility of hearing-aid-transduced speech. It was assumed that if differences in the electroacoustic characteristics among the six hearing aids resulted in "listenable differences," a preference ranking for the instruments should be achieved. Zerlin (1962) evaluated the success of this procedure by comparing rankings with monosyllabic word recognition scores obtained from half-list recordings of the CID W-22s which were also preprocessed (in quiet) through each of the six aids. He found that this paired-comparison paradigm differentiated effectively between five of six hearing aids for which there were no observable differences in monosyllabic word test score.

Despite the apparent success of Zerlin's approach and the relative ease by which hearing-aid-processed speech could be recorded and played back in a clinical setting, a potential problem exists with his playback procedure. There is a possible discrepancy in the spectrum of the speech signal at the listener's tympanic membrane when transduced through an earphone versus that when the instrument is worn by the listener and coupled to the ear with an earmold. As Cox and Studebaker (1977) have shown, the use of audiometric earphones to transduce hearing-aid-processed speech signals results in a reduction in sound pressure level (SPL) below 500 Hz and an increase in SPL near 3000 Hz. The effect of low-frequency intensity reduction is due to an acoustic leak under the earphone cushion, whereas the high frequency increase is clearly the result of ear canal resonance effects.

Another cause for spectral alteration associated with this technique relates to the spectral differences observed when the signal is presented to the hearing aid microphone in an unoccupied sound field as was done by Zerlin (1962), versus that which is presented to the hearing aid microphone with the aid mounted on a listener's head (Dalsgaard, 1977).

In recent years, investigators involved in research that concerns hearing-aid-processed speech have circumvented these potential confounding variables by utilizing the acoustic manikin KEMAR (Burkhard and Sachs, 1975) and its associated Zwislocki-type occluded ear simulators (Zwislocki, 1970, 1971). Additional methods for correcting spectral alterations include the use of analog or digital spectrum equalization instruments as well as using a flat hearing aid receiver/earmold assembly instead of an audiometric earphone to present the test stimuli (Punch and Howard, 1978; Punch, 1978).

It is also worth noting that, even though the absence of observable differences in speech recognition scores among the six hearing aids shown by Zerlin (1962) is not surprising, the use of 25-word half-lists to assess word recognition under earphones or in a sound field for evaluating hearing aids has since been shown to be unreliable (Edgerton, Klodd, and Beattie, 1978; Schwartz, Bess, and Larson, 1977).

In recent years the concept of listener-assessed intelligibility of hearing-aid-processed speech has gained renewed and mounting interest as a viable method of hearing aid selection. Gray and Speaks (1977) sparked the interest in this measurement procedure by demonstrating that estimates of the intelligibility of unprocessed connected discourse by hearing-impaired listeners was highly reliable at three intensity levels and three message-to-competition ratio conditions. Unfortunately, the relationship between subjective estimates of speech intelligibility and measured scores on a monosyllabic word list (CID W-22) were not encouraging.

In general, however, pairwise judgments of the relative intelligibility of hearing-aid-processed speech has been shown to correlate relatively well with direct measures of speech recognition (Punch and Parker, 1981; Studebaker et al., 1979a), at least for averaged data.

One rather novel paired-comparison approach described recently by White and Studebaker (1978) and Studebaker et al. (1979a, 1979b), is the single elimination (SE) tournament strategy analogous to that used in sporting events. This approach has the advantage over the round robin pairwise design in that the SE strategy requires relatively few pairings of aids, whereas 28 pairings or "matches" would be required in a round robin design to evaluate eight hearing aids [$n(n-1)/2$ pairs of aids]; a SE design requires only seven aid pairings. This reduction in matches played in a single elimination tournament is achieved through a pairwise selection strategy based on winners of preceding rounds as illustrated in Figure 10-4. The eight aids (1–8) are matched in the initial round according to a specific seeding; that is, 1 plays 2 and 2 wins the match, 3 plays 4 and 3 wins the match, and so on. Hearing aids 2 and 3 then advance to the second round where 2 wins the match. 2 and 8 eventually play and 2 emerges as the winner of the single elimination event. An underlying assumption of this strategy is that the winning aid would have emerged as the winner regardless of the particular aid it might have been paired against in any given round (i.e., the seeding arrangement).

In 1979 Studebaker and co-workers reported results of an empirical study to determine the efficacy of the SE tournament as a clinical

SINGLE ELIMINATION
HEARING AID TOURNAMENT

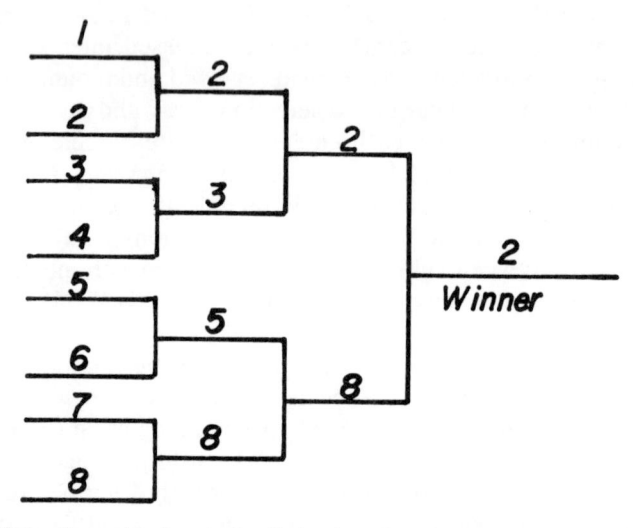

Figure 10-4. Example of a single elimination (SE) tournament event for hearing aid selection.

method for hearing aid selection. Continuous discourse was recorded in the presence of uncorrelated cafeteria noise (0 dB and +7 dB MCR) through eight pairs of binaural hearing aids fitted to the manikin KEMAR. Subjects were asked to listen alternately to recorded pairs of aids through a level equalized playback system and to judge which hearing aid pair delivered the more intelligible speech. A two-out-of-three win rule was used to determine the winner of the match. In addition, Northwestern University Auditory Test No. 6 (NU #6) lists were recorded under identical conditions and presented to each subject. The results at 0 dB MCR showed a test-retest agreement (85 percent) among winners of the SE event. Moreover, the two aids that produced the best word recognition scores were chosen consistently as winners in the tournament. At +7 dB MCR the findings were less encouraging, particularly for the normal-hearing subjects.

The data reported by Studebaker and colleagues led Montgomery, Schwartz, and Punch (in press) to question whether the selection of the winning aid is affected not only by the listening condition (e.g., quiet versus noise) but also by the specific seeding arrangement. Of particular importance was that examination of the insertion responses of the four commercial instruments used by Studebaker et al. (1979a, 1979b) suggested rather disparate frequency ranges and in situ pressure gain across instruments. Hence, these four aids represented a rather heterogeneous sample not likely to be selected for routine clinical evaluation. Consequently, Montgomery et al. (in press) sought to examine the effects of seeding in both single and double elimination hearing aid tournaments on rankings achieved by eight electroacoustically homogeneous hearing aids in a relative intelligibility judgment task using a computer-simulation technique that employed actual data gathered earlier from 12 listeners with high-frequency sensorineural hearing loss (Punch and Parker, 1981). The results indicated that although group performance was reliable and correlated highly with nonsense syllable identification, the distribution of tournament winners was unreliable and was dependent upon the effects of seeding. Based on these data, the overall clinical application of the elimination tournament strategy for hearing aid selection remains to be demonstrated.

RELIABILITY OF CURRENT TEST METHODS

Methods Based on Performance Scores

Perhaps the most fundamental of all assumptions underlying comparative hearing aid evaluation is that the measurement device used to assess each of the instruments has sufficient test-retest reliability. Reliability, of course, is not an absolute that the measure either has or does not have. Rather, it must be evaluated relative to some external criterion or criteria. Most frequently, the reliability of aided test measures has been assessed via statistical criteria. Perhaps an even more important criterion, however, is that the measure must have adequate reliability for the specific purpose for which it is intended. Salient to comparative hearing aid evaluations is that the test employed must show test-retest variability that is less than the interaid differences typically observed in clinical testing. If for a given test the difference between two speech recognition scores with the same aid is comparable to the interaid difference between that aid and another, then any meaningful interpretation of test results is, at best, trial and error.

It is clear that the assumption of adequate test-retest reliability also is highly related to the other two assumptions; that is, significant differences exist among hearing aids as reflected in patient performance on some speech tests, and interactions exist among hearing aids and people. If the test materials employed have relatively poor test-retest reliability, apparent differences among aids may appear in the hearing aid evaluation which are attributable primarily to test variability. It is interesting in this regard that test variability may have the effect of obscuring possible real differences among instruments for group data and creating what appear to be real differences among instruments for individual data. Insufficient test-retest reliability also will have a similarly confusing effect on the detection of interactions between aids and patients. Such interactions may appear in the results of the hearing aid evaluation where none actually exist. Likewise, real interactions may be obliterated by insufficient test reliability. In short, the error (i.e., noise) introduced by test variability will have only a negative effect on meaningful interpretations of hearing aid evaluation results.

In 1960, more than a decade after the published description on hearing aid selection by Carhart (1946), two studies addressed the issue of the reliability of word recognition tests in the hearing aid evaluation. One of these (Shore, Bilger, and Hirsch, 1960) concluded that speech recognition tests were not sufficiently reliable to differentiate among hearing aids, whereas the second (McConnell, Silber, and McDonald, 1960) reached the opposite conclusion. Hence, the evidence available to the practicing clinician at that time was both sparse and conflicting and certainly did not offer overwhelming support for change. Moreover, each of these two studies was found to have several design weaknesses. For example, Shore et al. (1960) used 25-word half-lists and not 50-word full lists to assess word recognition, thus reducing the reliability of their test results (Edgerton et al., 1978; Schwartz et al., 1977; Thornton and Raffin, 1978). Also, they used an unconventional method of adjusting the hearing aid gain control. Despite the high test-retest reliability ($r = 0.83$) reported by McConnell et al. (1960), they presented results from group data only. Because individual data were not reported, it is difficult to determine the actual magnitude of performance score variability on test and retest among the 40 subjects in that study.

Recall that Carhart (1946) suggested that "Whenever discrimination scores (between aids) differed by 8% or more, the discrepancies were generally taken as indicating sufficient distinction in instrument performance" (p. 788). Since that time, clinicians have worked under the assumption that an 8%, or even a 6% (Jerger, Speaks, and Malmquist, 1966) difference in performance score between aids represented a clinically significant difference. Not often considered, however, is that interaid differences in performance can be clinically meaningful only in relation to the magnitude of typical intraaid differences. If the difference between two word recognition test scores with the same hearing aid is comparable to score differences observed between that aid and another, then apparent differences among instruments noted in the hearing aid evaluation are most likely related to test-retest variability; therefore, they do not reflect "true" performance differences between hearing aids.

Beattie and Edgerton (1976) examined the test-retest reliability of the NU #6 test with a competing white noise at 0 dB MCR for differentiating among hearing aids. Their results with four electroacoustically dissimilar instruments revealed a standard deviation of the test-retest differences for all aids combined of only 6.2 percent with a range from 0 to 26 percent. Stated differently, 95 percent of the time test-retest differences were within 12.4 percent. From these data Beattie and Edgerton (1976) recommended that a 14 percent criterion be used for differentiating among instruments. In addition, they concluded that the use of white noise did not assist in the selection of the "best" aid, but did tend to identify an "inferior" amplification system.

In a similar investigation using the Jerger and Hayes (1976) procedure, Madory (1978) reported an inability for the SSI method to distinguish among four hearing aids with different frequency/gain characteristics. Like Beattie and Edgerton (1976), Madory found a standard deviation of test-retest difference scores of 7.8 percent across five MCRs ($+20, +10, 0, -10, -20$ dB). Using the two standard deviation criteria for significant difference as recommended by Beattie and Edgerton, Madory (1978) was unable to distinguish among any of the four instruments for both the test and retest sessions.

In a most enlightening clinical study, McDonald, Crowley, and Jerome (1978) examined the variability associated with the comparative hearing aid evaluation for repeated speech measures. A "traditional" Carhart (1946) procedure was performed in quiet and under adverse listening conditions with 24 sensorineural-hearing-loss subjects who had no prior experience with amplification. The test procedure was replicated three times except that the same aid was used throughout, without the subjects' knowledge. The data from McDonald et al. (1978) are shown in Figure 10-5 in the form of a cumulative frequency distribution based on the mean differences in aided word recognition score between trials. If an 8 percent criterion is used to define a clinically significant difference, as suggested by Carhart (1946), then these data indicate that the performance score differences on three repeated trials with the same hearing aid exceeded the 8 percent criterion about 30 percent of the time, even though the same hearing aid was used for all testing. Thus, the often used 6 or 8 percent rule for choosing the "best" hearing aid often is based simply on test-retest error and does not reflect any real differences in performance between hearing aids. McDonald et al. (1978) went one step further by asking each patient to rate which of the three hearing aids sounded the "best." Interestingly, the results for group data revealed that the majority of subjects

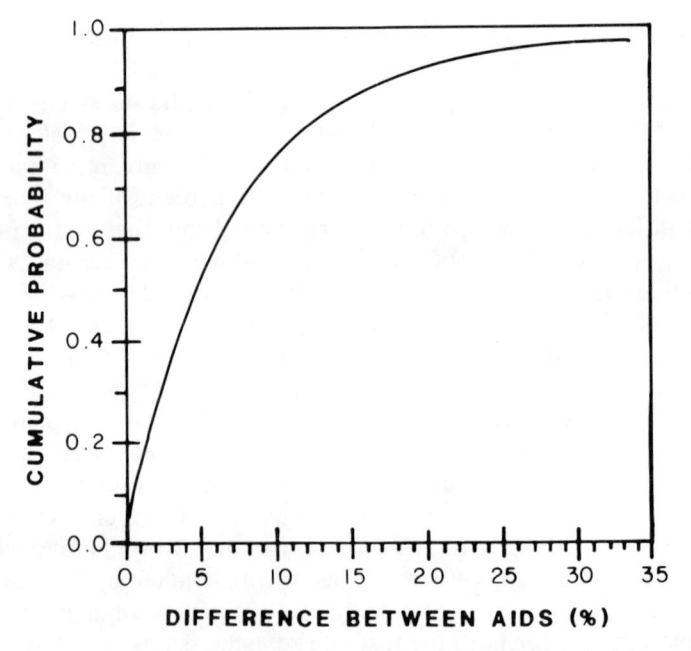

Figure 10-5. Cumulative frequency distribution showing the differences in monosyllabic word recognition obtained for one hearing aid across three trials. (From McDonald et al. (1978); reproduced with permission.)

Hearing Aid Assessment 341

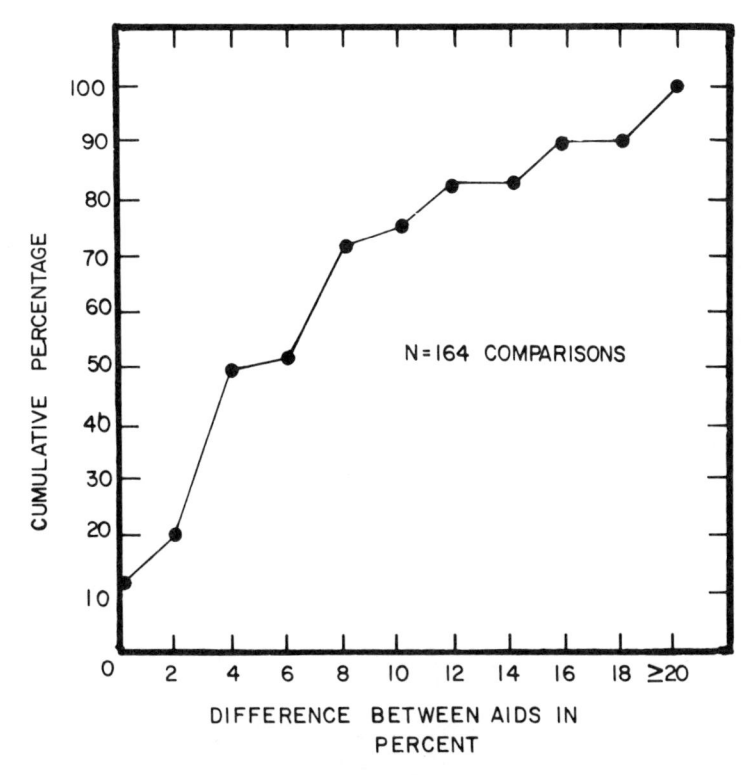

Figure 10-6. Cumulative frequency distribution showing differences in word recognition obtained for 164 interaid comparisons. (From Schwartz and Walden, 1980)

reported a preference for hearing aid 2, even though the same aid was used for all trials.

Data obtained by Schwartz and Walden (1980) are presented in Figures 10-6 and 10-7 and lend additional support as to the unreliability of the "traditional" hearing aid evaluation. Figure 10-6 represents a cumulative frequency distribution depicting the magnitude of differences in monosyllabic word recognition scores (NU #6 at +6 dB MCR) observed between hearing aids for 164 interaid comparisons. Here again, if one uses an 8 percent rule for clinically significant differences, then reference to the figure shows that 70 percent of the 164 interaid comparisons yielded score differences among three to four hearing aids of 8 percent or less. This suggests, therefore, that most hearing aid comparisons typically do not show performance score differences much greater than 8 percent, thus making it rather difficult to delineate among hearing aids on the basis of speech test results. Of course, this is not entirely unexpected because the majority of hearing

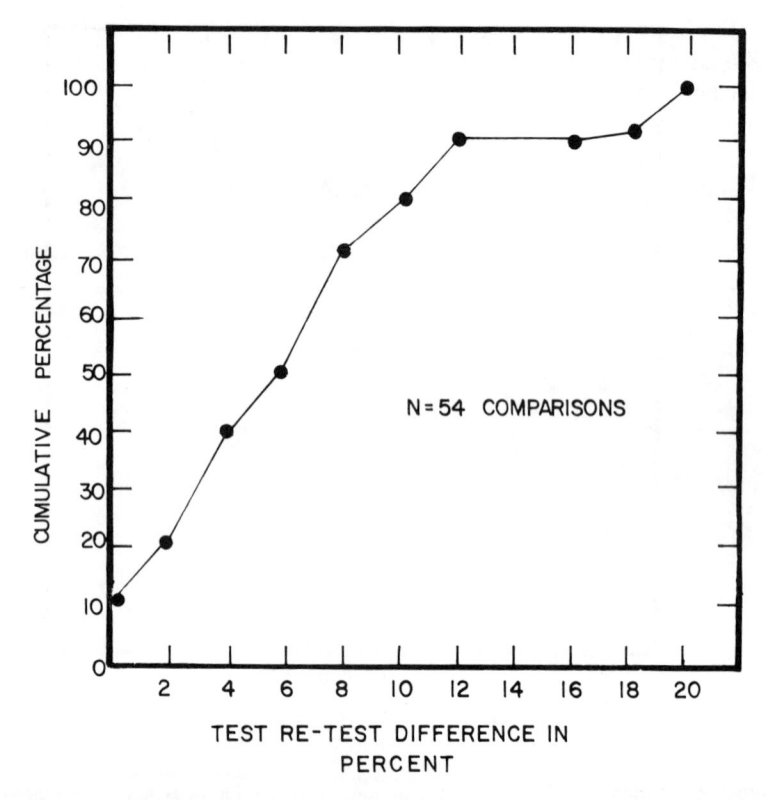

Figure 10-7. Cumulative frequency distribution showing test-retest differences in word recognition performance for 54 intraaid comparisons. (From Schwartz and Walden, 1980)

aid evaluations are performed in most clinical settings with a homogeneous set of hearing aids; that is, similar electroacoustic characteristics carefully preselected by the clinician as being appropriate to the listener's hearing loss. Although these data show that an 8 percent criterion for significant difference was indeed met in approximately 30 percent of the comparisons, recall that meaningful interpretation of these results is dependent on the test-retest reliability of the procedure under the same conditions; that is, test-retest differences with a single aid must be considerably less than that observed between aids if an aid is to be selected on the basis of some difference score criterion. Reference to the data of McDonald et al. (1978) shown in Figure 10-5 leads us to conclude that test-retest differences with a single instrument are not less than typical interaid differences.

The data presented in Figure 10-7 from Schwartz and Walden (1980) also do not support that assumption. Here, the results of 54 test-retest hearing aid comparisons are also depicted as a cumulative frequency plot. The abscissa represents the mean difference in monosyllabic word recognition (NU #6 at +6 dB MCR) obtained between test and retest sessions for the same amplification system averaged across 54 hearing aid comparisons. The mean intraaid difference was 7.3 percent. As was seen in Figure 10-5 (McDonald et al., 1978), an 8 percent or greater difference in test versus retest was obtained in 30 percent of the cases. Comparatively, if Figures 10-5 to 10-7 are superimposed on one another, it becomes readily apparent that the data from these two studies are remarkably similar.

Clearly, the independent clinical data lead to the conclusion that differences in word recognition often observed between hearing aids are most likely the result of test-retest variability of the measuring device and are not necessarily related to "true" performance differences between the instruments being evaluated.

Perhaps the most convincing evidence to demonstrate the variability associated with speech recognition testing was proffered in a seminal paper by Thornton and Raffin (1978). They considered performance on a speech recognition test (CID W-22) as a binomial variable in that a listener's response was scored either "correct" or "incorrect." According to this mathematical model, test variability is dependent upon the subject's "true" performance level as well as the test sample size (i.e., number of test items). Assuming a sampling distribution with known characteristics, a confidence interval was determined from the sample mean to make inferences about the subject's "true" score. From this, Thornton and Raffin (1978) went on to develop tables of "critical differences" at the 95 percent level of confidence for test lists of 10, 25, 50, and 100 items, respectively (see Table 10-1). The table depicts a range of scores within which there is a 95 percent probability that the subject's score would not exceed the upper and lower limits of the interval upon repeated testing, or with a different hearing aid. Review of the table illustrates clearly that the reliability of a given test score is dependent on the number of test items, as well as the actual performance of the listener. If, for example, a patient scores 70 percent with one hearing aid on a 50-item test, then the score with a second instrument would have to exceed 86 percent or be poorer than 52 percent before performance differences with these two hearing aids achieves statistical significance. Of course, if the examiner elects to have less confidence (e.g., 90 or 80 percent level) that score differences are statistically significant, then the "critical difference" range will be restricted further; for example, for a similar score of 70 percent with one aid, a score with a second aid would have to be less than 58 percent or greater than 80 percent (12 percent difference) to achieve significance at the 80 percent level of confidence.

Recall from Table 10-1 that the magnitude of difference scores necessary to exceed a given confidence level also is dependent on the subject's actual performance score and the number of test items. Hence, if the clinician presents only 25 items, as in the studies by Zerlin (1962) and Shore et al. (1960), then the variability associated with the measurement will become greater, particularly for scores that approach 50 percent (Schwartz et al., 1977; Edgerton et al., 1978). Note, for instance, the 95 percent "critical difference" for a score of 60 percent and word lists of 50, 25, and 10 items (see Table 10-2). As the number of items decrease, the "critical difference" range increases. If, therefore, one wanted to delineate between two hearing aids using only a 10-item test, such as the SSI (Jerger and Hayes, 1976), and the score with the first aid was 60 percent, then the score with another

Table 10-1. Lower and upper limits of the 95% critical differences for percentage scores

% Score	$N = 50$	$N = 25$	$N = 10$	% Score	$N = 100$[a]
0	0–4	0–8	0–20	50	37–63
2	0–10			51	38–64
4	0–14	0–20		52	39–65
6	2–18			53	40–66
8	2–22	0–28		54	41–67
10	2–24		0–50	55	42–68
12	4–26	4–32		56	43–69
14	4–30			57	44–70
16	6–32	4–40		58	45–71
18	6–34			59	46–72
20	8–36	4–44	0–60	60	47–73
22	8–40			61	48–74
24	10–42	8–48		62	49–74
26	12–44			63	50–75
28	14–46	8–52		64	51–76
30	14–48		10–70	65	52–77
32	16–50	12–56		66	53–78
34	18–52			67	54–79
36	20–54	16–60		68	55–80
38	22–56			69	56–81
40	22–58	16–64	10–80	70	57–81
42	24–60			71	58–82
44	26–62	20–68		72	59–83
46	28–64			73	60–84
48	30–66	24–72		74	61–85
50	32–68		10–90	75	63–86

Table 10-1. (Continued)

% Score	N = 50	N = 25	N = 10	% Score	N = 100[a]
52	34–70	28–76		76	64–86
54	36–72			77	65–87
56	38–74	32–80		78	66–88
58	40–76			79	67–89
60	42–78	36–84	20–90	80	68–89
62	44–78			81	69–90
64	46–80	40–84		82	71–91
66	48–82			83	72–92
68	50–84	44–88		84	73–92
70	52–86		30–90	85	74–93
72	54–86	48–92		86	75–94
74	56–88			87	77–94
76	58–90	52–92		88	78–95
78	60–92			89	79–96
80	64–92	56–96	40–100	90	81–96
82	66–94			91	82–97
84	68–94	60–96		92	83–98
86	70–96			93	85–98
88	74–96	68–96		94	86–99
90	76–98		50–100	95	88–99
92	78–98	72–100		96	89–99
94	82–98			97	91–100
96	86–100	80–100		98	92–100
98	90–100			99	94–100
100	96–100	92–100	80–100	100	97–100

Values within the range shown are not significantly different from the value shown in the percentage Score columns ($P > 0.05$). (From Thornton and Raffin, 1978, with permission)

[a] If score is less than 50%, find % Score = 100-observed score and subtract each critical difference limit from 100.

instrument would have to be 0 percent (identification of no sentences) or 100 percent (all 10 items correct) before assuming that the probability of this change will occur by chance only 5 percent of the time.

Clearly, the foregoing clinical data (Figures 10-5 to 10-7), as well as the discussion of the binomial model, indicate that the application

Table 10-2. Lower and upper limits of the 95% critical differences for three word recognition scores as a function of test length. Only scores falling outside of these ranges are considered to be significantly different based on a 95% decision rule.

Performance score (%)	Number test items (%)			
	100	50	25	10
80	68–89	64–92	56–96	40–100
70	57–81	52–86	54–86	30–90
60	47–73	42–78	36–84	10–90

of a 6 or 8 percent criterion for significant difference is inappropriate for use in the hearing aid evaluation unless one is willing to compromise clinical confidence. In essence, these data suggest that most performance score differences observed in the comparative hearing aid evaluation between a homogeneous set of hearing aids most likely are related to test-retest variability and do not represent real differences between amplification systems.

Despite the inherent variability of most commonly used speech testing materials and, hence, the unreliability of this measure for differentiating among amplification systems that are preselected to meet the auditory needs of the individual to be fitted, there is considerable value in using speech tests to demonstrate relative improvement with amplification via a comparison of unaided and aided performance scores (Orchik and Roddy, 1980). It is not uncommon, for example, to observe aided improvements in monosyllabic word recognition performance in excess of 30 percent for some listeners. Consequently, the unaided-to-aided difference score plays an important role in patient counseling by allowing the prospective user to experience an immediate increase in speech understanding when the hearing aid is first used. By quantifying patient performance, both unaided and aided, relative to the performance of normal listeners under identical test conditions, this measure can assist the practitioner in counseling patients as to possible expectations of hearing aid use.

Methods Based on Subjective Judgments

It is evident from the preceding discussion that speech recognition tests may not be sufficiently reliable, or sensitive, to differentiate among hearing aids. Because of the questionable resolving power of speech tests, clinicians have sought the use of subjective patient judgments relative to the perceived sound quality or intelligibility of hearing-aid-processed speech. Indeed, there can be little argument that the successful use of a hearing aid depends to some extent on the listener's subjective impressions of the quality of amplified speech. There is ample data to suggest that listeners perceive the quality or intelligibility of hearing-aid-processed speech as distinctively different when various hearing aids (different electroacoustic characteristics) are compared. Furthermore, intrasubject reliability of paired-comparison quality/intelligibility preference judgments of aided speech has been shown to be acceptably high (Punch, 1978; Punch et al., 1978; Schwartz et al., in press; Studebaker et al., 1979a, 1979b). Although subjective judgments of hearing aid sound quality appear attractive as an alternative method for hearing aid selection, it is important to consider that judgments of quality do not necessarily equate to speech intelligibility (Punch and Parker, 1981). Moreover, the relatively high reliability of this procedure has been demonstrated only under laboratory conditions. Nevertheless, the solicitation of a patient's subjective opinion always has been an integral part of the hearing aid selection process and most clinicians probably would agree that considerable weight is placed on such judgments in the decision making process. Yet, little is known about the consistency or stability of such "informal" subjective measures over time. Recall, for example, the study of McDonald et al. (1978) who examined the variability associated with the hearing aid evaluation for repeated speech measures by testing subjects three times with the same aid. An additional finding of that study was that the results of a "preference" questionnaire indicated that the majority of listeners preferred "the second hearing aid" even though the same instrument was used for all three test sessions. Importantly, only 12.5 percent of the subjects reported no difference among the three instruments.

The authors of this chapter recently asked eight new hearing aid users enrolled in an extensive aural rehabilitation program to rate subjectively which of the three hearing aids used in their initial evaluation provided the best sound quality across five separate test days. Of the eight subjects, only one reported a consistent preference for the aid that was recommended as a result of the initial hearing aid selection. The remaining seven subjects varied in their preference judgments sporadically across the five days. The clinical implication here, of course, like that of Harris and Goldstein (1979) and Barford (1979) is that the evaluation of the performance of an aid when first fitted is a poor predictor of long-term performance. What the patient prefers in the way of sound quality on the day of the initial evaluation, may not be the same after a period of adjustment to amplification. Consequently, the value of such informal tests of sound quality preference judgments should not attract the notice that it has enjoyed since 1949 when Hedgecock suggested that quality judgments were useful in the selection of hearing aids.

Although judgments of the relative intelligibility of hearing-aid-processed speech relate more closely to objective measures of speech recognition, the use of this approach for differentiating among amplification systems probably is no better than any of the other methods described. As Montgomery et al. (in press) have shown, paired-comparison intelligibility judgments suffer from the same problems of variability inherent in most other procedures.

As long as the patient is being evaluated with a series of hearing aids having similar electroacoustic response characteristics, there is little reason to believe that significant differences among these "homogeneous" instruments should emerge on any clinical measure.

AFTERWORD

It is clear that hearing aid evaluation methods that utilize speech as the primary acoustic stimulus have been resistant to change and, hence, progress has been painfully slow. Most clinicians continue to use at least some modification of the original protocol advocated by Carhart (1946) which focuses on differentiating between hearing aids on the basis of a percent correct performance score. Indeed, Carhart's method represented a solution to a real problem encountered at that time; however, the available contemporary research leads one to question the continued use of the procedure that has been an integral part of audiology for almost half a century. In fact, Schwartz (in press) recently wrote a critical essay on all hearing aid selection/evaluation methods and indicated that in reality, no single procedure meets all of the criteria for effectiveness. That is, no method meets all of the assumptions that underlie the hearing aid evaluation. These include:

1. Significant differences exist among instruments as reflected in patient performance.
2. Observed differences among aids vary across patients; that is, hearing aid-patient interaction.
3. Differences among aids can be measured reliably by the test that is used to compare the amplification systems (e.g., words, sentences, functional gain, etc.).
4. Relative performance of a group of hearing aids remains stable over time.
5. Patient performance with a given hearing aid or set of aids on the clinical test(s) is indicative or prognostic of the patient's relative performance with those same instruments in the real world.

Implicit in this chapter is the underlying need to define a "clinically significant difference" between aided test scores, and to relate this to typical test-retest variability and inter-aid differences. That test scores for two different hearing aids are significantly different from a statistical model does not in any way guarantee that this difference is clinically important. If, for example, we were to develop a test that would reliably detect differences between aids of less than 1 percent, this would be of minimal value because such insignificant differences are unlikely to be clinically relevant. The reliability of current test materials used in the hearing aid evaluation are under attack and probably rightly so. Until a clinically significant difference is defined through appropriate validation studies (i.e., relating differences in test scores to listener performance differences in realistic communicative situations), we will not have a precise definition of what is acceptable test variability.

For those clinicians who choose to continue with the traditional Carhart (1946) approach to hearing aid evaluation using some speech recognition test, evaluation of clinical decisions as to differences in performance between aids should be considered in light of the Thornton and Raffin (1978) data. (*Caveat:* Although this will not indicate the clinical importance of a difference, it will suggest whether there is any basis for concluding that a meaningful numerical difference exists.) Of course, the data presented in Figures 10-5 to 10-7 tend to suggest that differences between carefully preselected hearing aids often will not exceed even 8 percent. Most likely, the value of speech testing in the hearing aid evaluation, therefore, lies within a comparison of unaided to aided performance as well as permitting the patient to listen to hearing-aid-processed speech. In contrast to the inability to demonstrate relatively large differences in speech recognition between hearing aids, often it is common to show improvements in excess of 30 percent (for a 50-word list) from an unaided to aided condition. In fact, a retrospective analysis of 100 clinical files demonstrated an average aided improvement in monosyllabic word recognition of 20 percent with a range from 0 to 64 percent.

It is unlikely that this chapter will revolutionize hearing aid evaluation procedures because a suitable alternative justified by research findings is not available at this time. Hence, most audiologists will still be faced with the daily necessity of selecting amplification for the hearing-impaired patient. Yet, we find it difficult to justify the enormous amount of clinical time spent on the "traditional" hearing aid evaluation with the (false) assumption that speech recognition test scores or subjective judgments of quality or intelligibility can indeed delineate among carefully preselected instruments.

As a final point, hearing aid technology is far ahead of the hearing aid evaluation. What is lacking is not the hearing aid engineer's ability to produce the required electroacoustic characteristics, but rather the audiologist's ability to specify what is needed. Perhaps the time has come for researchers and practitioners to expend more of their time in the habilitative arena in an effort to develop improved methods for predicting success with amplification. (For a discussion on validating measures for hearing aid success see Walden, in press.) Unquestionably, every person experienced in the art of hearing aid selection gradually develops certain concepts as to which hearing aids are most successful with a specific type of hearing loss; however, unless these conclusions are validated through clinical follow-up, they will remain untested assumptions.

REFERENCES

Beattie, R. C., and B. J. Edgerton. 1976. Reliability of monosyllabic discrimination tests in white noise for differentiating among hearing aids. J. Speech Hear. Disord 41:464–476.

Beck, L. B., R. W. Leatherwood, and J. L. Punch. 1980. Aided low-frequency response: Speech quality and speech intelligibility. Paper presented at the Annual Convention of the American Speech-Language-Hearing Association, Detroit, Michigan.

Burkhard, M. D., and R. M. Sachs. 1975. Anthropometric manikin for acoustic research. J. Acoust. Soc. Am. 58:214–222.

Burney, P. A. 1972. A survey of hearing aid evaluation procedures. Asha 14:439–444.

Carhart, R. 1946. Selection of hearing aids. Arch. Otolaryngol. 44:1–18.

Chermack, G. 1977. Hearing aid evaluation procedures and theoretical assumptions of Illinois audiologists. J. Illinois Speech Hear. Assoc. 9–18.

Cox, R. M., and G. A. Studebaker. 1977. Spectral changes produced by earphone-cushion reproduction of hearing-aid-processed signals. J. Am. Aud. Soc. 3:26–33.

Dalsgaard, S. C. 1977. The influence of diffraction on the performance of hearing aids. Paper presented at the Ninth International Congress on Acoustics, Madrid.

Danaher, E. M., M. J. Osberger, and J. M. Pickett. 1973. Discrimination of formant frequency transitions in synthetic vowels. J. Speech Hear. Res. 16:439–451.

Danaher, E. M., and J. M. Pickett. 1975. Some masking effects produced by low-frequency vowel formants in persons with sensorineural hearing loss. J. Speech Hear. Res. 18:261–271.

Edgerton, B. J., D. A. Klodd, and R. C. Beattie. 1978. Half-list discrimination measures in hearing aid evaluations. Arch. Otolaryngol. 104:669–672.

French, N. R., and J. C. Steinberg. 1947. Factors governing the intelligibility of speech sound. J. Acoust. Soc. Am. 19:90–119.

Gabrielsson, A., and H. Sjögren. 1979. Perceived sound quality of hearing aids. Scand. Audiol. 8:159–169.

Gray, T. F., and C. E. Speaks. 1977. Ability of hearing-impaired listeners to understand connected discourse. J. Am. Aud. Soc. 3:159–166.

Harris, R. W., and D. P. Goldstein. 1979. Effects of room reverberation upon hearing aid quality judgments. Audiology 18:253–262.

Hedgecock, L. D. 1949. Prediction of the efficiency of hearing aids from the audiograms. Doctoral dissertation. University of Wisconsin. Cited in L. A. Watson, and T. Tolan. Hearing Tests and Hearing Instruments. 1949. Williams & Wilkins Company, Baltimore.

Hood, R. B. 1970. Modifications in hearing aid selection procedures. Acad. Rehabil. Audiol. Newsl. 3:7–10.

Hughson, W. 1944. Hearing aids. Trans. Am. Acad. Ophthalmol. Otolaryngol. 48:180–190.

Jeffers, J. 1960. Quality judgment in hearing aid selection. J. Speech Hear. Disord. 25:259–266.

Jerger, J., and D. Hayes. 1976. Hearing aid evaluation: Clinical experience with a new philosophy. Arch. Otolaryngol. 102:214–221.

Jerger, J., C. Speaks, and C. Malmquist. 1966. Hearing-aid performance and hearing aid selection. J. Speech Hear. Res. 9:136–149.

Killion, M. C. 1981. Earmold options for wideband hearing aids. J. Speech Hear. Disord. 46:10–20.

Knudsen, V. O., and J. H. Jones. 1935. Artificial aids to hearing. Laryngoscope 45:48–69.

Kopra, L. L. and D. Blosser. 1968. Effects of method of measurement on most comfortable loudness level for speech. J. Speech Hear. Res. 11:497–508.

Libby, E. R. 1981. Achievement of transparent smooth wideband hearing aid responses. Hearing Instruments (in press).

Madory, R. D. 1978. The test-retest reliability of the synthetic sentence identification hearing aid evaluation procedure. Master's thesis, Central Michigan University, Mount Pleasant, Mich.

Martin, E. S., and J. M. Pickett. 1970. Sensorineural hearing loss and upward spread of masking. J. Speech Hear. Res. 13:426–437.

Martin, F. N., and S. A. Mussell. 1979. The influence of pauses in the competing signal on synthetic sentence identification scores. J. Speech Hear. Disord. 44:282–292.

McConnell, F., E. F. Silber, and D. McDonald. 1960. Test-retest consistency of clinical hearing aid tests. J. Speech Hear. Disord. 25:273–280.

McDonald, V. B., A. L. Crowley, and J. J. Jerome. 1978. Determinants in hearing aid selection. Paper presented at the Annual Convention of the American Speech-Language-Hearing Association, San Francisco, California.

Montgomery, A. A., D. M. Schwartz, and J. L. Punch. Tournament strategies in hearing aid selection. J. Speech Hear. Disord. In press.

Orchik, D. J., and N. Roddy. 1980. The SSI and NU6 in clinical hearing aid evaluation. J. Speech Hear. Disord. 45:401–407.

Punch, J. L. 1978. Quality judgments of hearing-aid-processed-speech and music by normal and otopathologic listeners. J. Am. Aud. Soc. 3:179–188.

Punch, J. L., and E. L. Beck. 1980. Low-frequency response of hearing aids and judgments of aided speech quality. J. Speech Hear. Disord. 45:325–335.

Punch, J. L., and M. T. Howard. 1978. Listener-assessed intelligibility of hearing-aid-processed speech. J. Am. Aud. Soc. 4:69–76.

Punch, J. L., A. A. Montgomery, D. M. Schwartz, B. E. Walden, R. A. Prosek, and M. T. Howard. 1980. Multidimensional scaling of quality judgments of speech signals processed by hearing aids. J. Acoust. Soc. Am. 68:458–466.

Punch, J. L., and C. Parker. 1981. Pairwise listener preferences in hearing aid evaluation. J. Speech Hear. Res. 24:366–374.

Resnick, D. M., and M. Becker. 1963. Hearing aid evaluation—a new approach. Asha 5:695–699.

Resnick, S. B., J. R. Dubno, D. G. Howie, S. Hoffnung, J. Freeman, and R. M. Slosberg. 1976. Phoneme identification on a closed-response nonsense syllable test. Paper presented at the Annual Convention of the American Speech-Language-Hearing Association, Houston, Texas.

Reid, L., R. A. Smiarowski, and L. T. McPherson. 1977. Hearing aid gain—setting performance of experienced users. Arch. Otolaryngol. 103:203–205.

Schwartz, D. M. Hearing aid selection methods: An enigma. In G. Studebaker and F. Bess (eds.) The Vanderbilt Hearing Aid Report. Monographs in Contemporary Audiology, Education Services Division, Instrumentation Associates, Inc., Upper Darby, Pa. In press.

Schwartz, D. M., F. H. Bess, and V. D. Larson. 1977. Split-half reliability of two word discrimination tests as a function of primary-to-secondary ratio. J. Speech Hear. Disord. 42:440–445.

Schwartz, D. M., A. A. Montgomery, J. L. Punch, B. E. Walden, R. A. Prosek. 1979. Quality judgments of hearing-aid-processed speech by hearing impaired listeners. Paper presented at the Annual Convention of the American Speech-Language-Hearing Association, Atlanta.

Schwartz, D. M., and Walden, B. E. 1980. Current status of the clinical hearing aid evaluation. In Studies in the use of amplification for the hearing impaired: Proceedings of a symposium. Excerpta Med. 15–28.

Shore, I., R. C. Bilger, and I. J. Hirsh. 1960. Hearing aid evaluation: reliability of repeated measurements. J. Speech Hear. Res. 25:152–170.

Speaks, C., and J. Jerger. 1965. Method for measurement of speech identification. J. Speech Hear. Res. 8:185–194.

Studebaker, G. A., R. E. C. White, S. Hoffnung, and R. M. Cox. 1979a. Studies of a paired-comparison hearing aid selection procedure. Paper presented at the Annual Convention of the American Speech-Language-Hearing Association, Atlanta, Georgia.

Studebaker, G. A., R. E. C. White, and S. Hoffnung. 1979b. Paper presented at the 97th Meeting of the Acoustical Society of America. Cambridge, Mass.

Thornton, A. R., and M. J. M. Raffin. 1978. Speech discrimination modeled as a binomial variable. J. Speech Hear. Res. 21:507–518.

Walden, B. E. Validating measures for hearing aid success. In G. Studebaker and F. Bess (eds.) The Vanderbilt Hearing Aid Report. Monographs in Contemporary Audiology, Education Services Division, Instrumentation Associates, Inc., Upper Darby, Pa. In press.

Walden, B. E., G. I. Schuchman, and R. K. Sedge. 1977. The reliability and validity of the comfort level method of setting hearing aid gain. J. Speech Hear. Disord. 42:456–461.

Watson, L. A. 1944. Certain fundamental principles in prescribing and fitting hearing aids. Laryngoscope 54:531–558.

White, R. E. C., and G. A. Studebaker. 1978. An evaluation of elimination tournament strategies for hearing aid selection. Paper presented at the Annual Convention of the American Speech-Language-Hearing Association, San Francisco, California.

Witter, H. L., and D. P. Goldstein. 1971. Quality judgments of hearing aid transduced speech. J. Speech Hear. Res. 14:312–322.

Yanovitz, A., B. J. Bickford, J. Lozar, and D. R. Farrell. 1978. Electroacoustic distortions: Multidimensional analysis of hearing aid transduced speech and music. IEEE International Conference on Acoustics, Speech and Signal Processing.

Zerlin, S. 1962. A new approach to hearing aid selection. J. Speech Hear. Res. 5:370–376.

Zwislocki, J. 1970. An acoustic coupler for earphone calibration. Report LSC-S-7, Laboratory of Sensory Communication, Syracuse University.

Zwislocki, J. 1971. An ear-like coupler for earphone calibration. Report LSC-S-9, Laboratory of Sensory Communication, Syracuse University.

CHAPTER 11

SPEECH RECOGNITION AND AURAL REHABILITATION

Elmer Owens

CONTENTS

SPEECH RECOGNITION	354
Word Recognition	354
Phoneme Recognition (Nonsense Syllables)	355
Phoneme Recognition Within Words	357
Sentence Tests	359
Self-Report Scales	362
AURAL REHABILITATION	363
Phoneme Recognition	364
Auditory and Visual Modalities in Phoneme Recognition	365
Sentence Materials	367
NEW PROCEDURES AND DIRECTIONS	367
Tracking	367
The Use of Context in Sentences	367
Continuous Speech	368
EQUIPMENT INNOVATIONS	368
AUDITORY TRAINING FOR CHILDREN	369
CONCLUSIONS	370
REFERENCES	370

The purpose of this chapter is to review the relationship between clinical tests of speech recognition and the aural rehabilitation process. Ideally, speech recognition performance should serve both to indicate an individual's need for an aural rehabilitation program and to assess improvement in communication as a result of the program. Of the several facets of aural rehabilitation, major attention is directed to auditory training because of its unique relation to speech recognition measures.

The material of this chapter is oriented to persons with postlingual hearing impairment, and the problem under consideration is the reduction in clarity of speech at suprathreshold levels. It will be assumed that hearing aids are being used to compensate for decrements in the loudness domain.

At the outset of the chapter an account of speech recognition measures is presented as they may relate to aural rehabilitation. Next is a review of some aural rehabilitation procedures that may employ these same measures along with others as indicators of improvement.

The preparation of this chapter was supported in part by National Institutes of Health Research Grant no. NS12998.

SPEECH RECOGNITION

The term *speech recognition* will be used generally in referring to the clarity of speech at comfortable loudness levels. The reader is referred to Chapters 1, 5, and 6 of this book for a discussion of terminology. Comprehensive accounts of the history, development, and uses of speech recognition tests and procedures are readily available (Chapter 6, this volume; Goetzinger, 1978; Olsen and Matkin, 1979). This account centers on the aspects relating primarily to rehabilitative procedures.

Word Recognition

Three series of test lists for word recognition are in common clinical use, namely, the Harvard PB-50 (Egan, 1948); the Central Institute for the Deaf (CID) W-22 (Hirsh et al., 1952); and the Northwestern University (NU) #6 (Tillman and Carhart, 1966). Each list of all three tests is phonemically balanced in the sense that the sounds of American English are represented in proportion to their occurrence in everyday speech. According to Egan (1948) the proportional representation of speech sounds stems from a consideration of the problem of validity.

Except for a general indication of speech perception difficulty based on the overall score, these word tests are somewhat limited in their relevance to aural rehabilitative considerations. One limitation is that the open response form, in which the patient says or writes the word he heard, prevents accurate assessment of the phoneme errors associated with the word errors. Schubert and Schultz (1960), for example, reported that a tabulation of erroneous responses for the CID W-22 lists failed to permit any straightforward interpretation of the acoustic nature of test errors. On the one hand, a word error might result from misidentification of one, two, or three phonemes in a consonant-vowel-consonant word. Conversely, auditory cues from two of the phonemes, supplemented by linguistic constraints, might enable a person to "guess" the test word without actually having recognized the third phoneme. It should be noted, however, that Boothroyd (1968) has found advantages in the use of phonemic scoring for specially constructed monosyllabic word lists. He required the patient to repeat the consonant-vowel-consonant words, but the responses were scored in terms of the number of phonemes correct.

Another limitation of the monosyllabic word lists is that, despite their phonemic balance, the overall scores fail to predict consistently the amount of difficulty experienced with everyday speech. Pertinent to this poor predictive value is the disappointment in the Social Adequacy Index (SAI), discussed by Davis (1978). The SAI for a given individual was derived from a combination of the PB-50 word recognition score and the speech recognition threshold. Observations over several years showed frequent discrepancies in a person's SAI and the amount of difficulty experienced in real life situations. In commenting on the demise of the SAI as a predictor of handicap, Davis (1978) pointed out that we do not yet know enough about the relations of connected speech to its component frequencies, phonemes, and syllables. It may be added that differences among patients in factors such as language background, verbal ability, motivation, general intelligence, and speechreading ability also contribute in varying amounts to the everyday handicap presented by a given hearing loss.

Other evidence regarding the predictive limitations of word lists lies in the finding of Giolas and Epstein (1963) that CID W-22 and PB-50 scores do not correlate well with a sample of connected speech.

Finally, a word recognition score may be misleading in some instances. For example, it is common clinical experience to obtain a word recognition score closely approaching 100 percent for a person with a high-frequency loss who complains of difficulty hearing in certain situations. Documentation is provided by Walden, Prosek, and Worthington (1975) who noted NU #6 scores averaging 97.5 percent for Army personnel with high-frequency losses, the majority of whom complained of difficulty in daily communication. Findings reported for some phoneme tests (Schwartz and Surr, 1979; Sher and Owens, 1974) and some sentence tests (Lacroix and Harris, 1979) have indicated that such materials provide results more consistent with such complaints.

Given the limitations of monosyllable word recognition tests in predicting either specific phonemic errors or the amount of everyday difficulty experienced by the individual, information with respect to aural rehabilitation must be gleaned from other kinds of speech recognition measures. These include phoneme recognition tests, sentence tests, and self-report scales.

Phoneme Recognition (Nonsense Syllables)

The use of nonsense syllables in phoneme recognition eliminates the influence of linguistic cues and also permits easy compilation of equivalent lists. Nonsense syllables have been used infrequently in clinical applications because of difficulty in eliciting appropriate responses from patients. Hirsh (1952) suggested that the obtaining of accurate responses would require that the observers (that is, the listeners) write down the syllables in phonetic transcription using the International Phonetic Alphabet. Hirsh (1952) further stated: "If we attempt to avoid the difficulties of written repetition by using oral repetition, we find ourselves doing a double test: we are testing the ability of the observer to hear the phonetic elements and at the same time the ability of the tester to hear the phonetic elements as they are repeated by the observer" (p. 129). On the other hand, Levitt (1978) has reported successful use of nonsense syllables in hearing aid evaluations and Edgerton and Danhauer (1979) have developed lists of nonsense syllables that they feel show much promise for clinical use. Most recently, Dubno and Dirks (1982) introduced a closed-set nonsense syllable test which they found to be highly reliable. In another study (Dubno, Dirks, and Langhofer, 1982), it was suggested that the test might be useful in the evaluation of an aural rehabilitation program.

Miller and Nicely (1955) reported on phonemic confusion of normal hearers listening to nonsense syllables under various conditions of frequency filtering and signal-to-noise ratios. They divided the phonemes into five distinctive features: voicing, nasality, affrication, duration, and place of articulation. The voicing and nasality features were much less affected by distortion than the other features. Several other investigators also used nonsense syllables to study distinctive features of consonant sounds in hearing-impaired patients as well as normal hearers. Walden and Montgomery (1975) found that sonorance (in which they included /m/, /n/, /r/, /l/, /w/, /j/) was the dominant feature in sloping loss and sibilance was the dominant feature in flat configurations. In the sloping loss group the sonorance feature was further divided into a nasal dimension and a liquid-glide dimension. Voicing did not emerge as a feature. Bilger and Wang (1976) reported that sibilance, duration, and voicing were prominent for flat or rising pure tone loss configurations—but not nasality. For high-frequency loss, nasality and voicing were well perceived—but not sibilance. Danhauer and Lawarre (1979) reported that sibilance was a clearly perceived feature by both flat and sloping hearing loss groups. Sonorance was prominent for both groups, but in the flat loss group the nasals (/m/, /n/) were distinguishable from the liquid glides (/r/, /l/, /w/, /j/). It is difficult to summarize these studies because of differences in procedure, in the consonants studied, and in the distinctive feature groupings. Obviously, there are some discrepancies among them with respect to the relation between distinctive features and pure tone configurations. There seems to be good agreement, however, that nasality is generally easy to distinguish, as is the group variously called *liquid glides* or *sonorants* (/r/, /l/, /w/, /j/). Sibilance is a distinguishable feature mainly with flat hearing loss configurations. Voicing varies from a strong feature by Miller and Nicely (1955) to an inconspicuous feature in the Walden and Montgomery (1975) study.

Phoneme Recognition within Words

The rhyme test developed by Fairbanks (1958) was a means of identifying phonemic errors in a word context. Only the vowel-consonant (VC) portions of the words appeared on the answer sheet, so that the response depended on the initial consonant and the consonant-vowel (CV) transition. The subject's task was to fill in the letter corresponding to the initial phoneme upon hearing the word. Fairbanks listed the phonemes in order of difficulty for eight normal listeners who received the stimuli in the presence of background noise. In general, nasal sounds and sonorants ranked high in recognizability and fricatives and stop plosives, low.

The modified rhyme test (MRT), introduced by House et al. (1965), employed a closed set (or multiple choice) format in which six alternative word responses were presented for each test item. All response choices, one of which was the test word, had the same VC or CV stems. The use of complete words permitted the testing of phonemes spelled with two letters (i.e. th, ch, sh) that could not be tested in the Fairbanks format. The main purpose of the test was to evaluate the performance level of speech communications systems by the use of relatively naive (untrained) talkers and listeners, as opposed to the common practice at that time of using only a few highly trained personnel. Among the advantages mentioned for the closed set format were (1) a probable reduction in word familiarity effects and (2) a simple response task. House et al. also ranked the phonemes in order of difficulty according to the errors of normal hearers listening in noise, but the order of ranking was noticeably different from that of Fairbanks. The authors attributed the ranking differences to differences in the characteristics of the noise used in the two studies. A later version of the MRT by Kreul et al. (1968), the modified rhyme hearing test (MRHT), was proposed in an attempt to make the MRT more appropriate for clinical testing of hearing-impaired patients. Changes were made in the carrier phrase, timing sequences, speakers, instructions, and test format. Reports on this test to date have dealt more with overall scores than with specific phoneme errors and confusions.

Other tests (Griffiths, 1967; Pederson and Studebaker, 1972) have used the multiple choice format, but no data on hearing-impaired patients have been published to date. Griffiths' aim was to modify the MRT for research. The modification was mainly in choosing alternative responses so that each differed from the stimulus word in only one distinctive feature. Pederson and Studebaker presented test lists that included vowel items as well as initial and final consonant items to normal hearers in a background of broadband noise. The authors reported that their results for recognition of consonants (voiced plosives, voiceless plosives, voiced fricatives, voiceless fricatives) were consistent with Miller and Nicely's (1955) findings.

Two tests have provided rhyming pairs of words in which only one phoneme varies. One of these two-choice response tests (Larson, 1950) includes consonants in both the initial and final positions. There seems to be no published data on the usefulness of this test, although the items themselves have been used for practice since the early days of aural rehabilitation. Both Sanders (1982) and Alpiner (1978) discuss this test and the reader is referred to these sources for additional information. The other test (Voiers, 1977) has been directed to the testing of communication systems. The test is designed for initial consonants only; the consonants in each pair vary by a single feature. Six distinctive features are involved in the pairings.

Vowel items by themselves have also been tested in a multiple choice format. Findings for items such as hit-heat-hurt-hate or bead-bed-bid-bird, one of the four choices being the test word, indicated that the confusion of one vowel with another occurred at an extremely low rate for hearing-impaired persons (Owens, Talbott, and Schubert, 1968; Owens, Benedict, and Schubert, 1971). The latter authors stated, however, that ". . . the results should not be interpreted to mean that vowel sounds are not contributing to the testing of speech discrimination. The more reasonable interpretation is that, despite the convenience of speaking as though we test the discrimination of individual sounds, the smallest unit operating except in rare circumstances is a syllabic combination of sounds" (p. 847).

These results on vowel recognition are in disagreement with those of Oyer and Doudna (1959) and Schultz (1964). Oyer and Doudna reported that the probability of vowel error on CID W-22 lists was greater than the probability of consonant error for hearing-impaired patients. Schultz also used the CID W-22 words on a sample consisting of several groups of hearing-impaired patients and stated that vowel errors occurred with sufficient frequency to merit more attention in speech recognition testing. Because of the free-choice response method of the CID W-22, however, the errors in both studies must be viewed as word substitutions. That is, the adjacent consonants presumably have greater influence on recognition of the vowel than in a closed-set that permits relatively greater focus on one phoneme—the vowel in this instance, as in bit-bat-beet-boot. Thus, distortion of the consonants in the open response mode might lead to word errors that could not rightly be called vowel errors. Moreover, the published data of Oyer and Doudna seem to contain an error. A recomputation of their published data is in agreement with their probability of error for the vowel sounds (0.016), but there appears to be an inaccuracy involving the consonant error probability. They do not state the N used for obtaining their consonant error probability, but assuming two consonants sounds per word on the 50-word list (an overestimate for the CID W-22) the probability for consonant error would be 0.030. This probability, in contrast to their reported 0.009, is higher than the vowel error probability. In order to obtain their consonant error probability of 0.009, one would have to assume more than six consonant sounds per word.

A series of six successive multiple choice test lists for the study of consonant recognition in hearing-impaired patients has culminated in a suggested 100-item test, the California consonant test (CCT) by Owens and Schubert (1977). Items were of the kind pin-tin-kin-fin and had-hag-have-has, one of the four choices being the stimulus (test) word. Although there was no attempt at phonemic balance, certain language constraints seemed to be operating in the process of item elimination from an initial pool of over 400 items. Results from the first few test limits showed that phonemes of opposite voicing were seldom confused, nasal phonemes were seldom confused with non-nasals, and errors rarely occurred for sonorants /r/, /l/, /w/, /j/. These sounds were discontinued on subsequent lists along with other sounds that were unsatisfactory because the language provided only one or two confusable alternative responses. Thus, the CCT is comprised primarily of phonemes that are (1) difficult for hearing-impaired persons to hear clearly and (2) easily confused auditorily with at least two or three other phonemes. These two characteristics would probably cause the most difficulty for hearing-impaired persons in their understanding of everyday speech. An analysis was made of substitution errors for the stimulus phonemes as shown in Tables 11-1 and 11-2 (Owens, 1978). It may be noted that major substitutions were usually, but definitely not always, in the same distinctive feature group as the stimulus.

Sentence Tests

Sentence test materials are important not only because they are closer to everyday speech, but because they permit the investigation of factors such as rate, intonation, semantic context, and syntax in speech perception. Unfortunately, however, there are several obstacles to constructing a satisfactory sentence test. Because of sequential patterning and other language constraints, some sentences can be identified by recognition of perhaps only one or two words, rendering them much too easy for test purposes. Also, once a sentence is known, even fewer cues may suffice for recognition; accordingly, it cannot be repeated as a test item. Another problem is that some items in the form of questions may involve a patient's knowledge rather than speech rec-

Table 11-1. Sounds frequently substituted for the test sound, final position from CCT (Form 7) test results of 550 patients

Stimulus	N_{Items}[a]	Responses[a]
p	10	t_{30} f_{20} k_{16} (θ, tʃ, ʃ, s)
t	5	p_{20} k_{13} f_{11} (ʃ, tʃ)
k	6	t_{30} p_{16} $θ_{10}$ (f, tʃ, s, d)
tʃ	8	t_{24} k_{13} $θ_{12}$ s_{10} (f, p, ʃ)
s	10	$θ_{45}$ f_{31} t_{17} p_{14} (ʃ, k, tʃ)
ʃ	3	f_{12} $tʃ_{12}$ s_{11}
f	4	p_{19} t_{18} s_{17} (k, ʃ)
θ[b]	3	p_{23} t_{21} k_{17} (s)
b	2	$ð_{46}$ d_{25} (v, z, l)
d[b]	5	b_{37} v_{14} (n, g, z, dʒ)
dʒ	5	d_{21} b_{20} v_{10} (z, g, m)
z	4	v_{33} d_{13} (dʒ, m, n)
v	5	z_{18} d_{12} b_{11} (m, dʒ, n, g)

From Owens, 1978.
[a] Subscript numbers indicate percentage of times that sound was substituted for test sound. Symbols in parentheses denote sounds that were substituted less than 10% of the time, in decreasing order of frequency.
[b] Results from previous experiment.

Table 11-2. Sounds frequently substituted for the test sound, initial position from CCT (Form 7) test results of 550 patients

Stimulus	N_{Items}	Responses[a]
p	4	t_{27} k_{12} $θ_{12}$ (f, s)
t	6	p_{18} k_{14} (θ, f, s)
k	6	t_{24} p_{11} (θ, tʃ, f, s)
tʃ	4	t_{13} (p, θ, ʃ, s, h, k)
s	6	$θ_{29}$ f_{24} $ʃ_{11}$ $tʃ_{10}$ (t, h, p)
ʃ	3	$tʃ_{18}$ s_{11} (k, θ, f)
f[b]	2	(p, s, t, ʃ)
θ	2	s_{28} (t, ʃ, tʃ)
b[b]	2	v_{26} (ð, d, b, g)
d	2	b_{21} g_{21} (v, dʒ, w)

From Owens, 1978.
[a] Subscript numbers indicate percentage of times that sound was substituted for test sound. Symbols in parentheses denote sounds that were substituted less than 10% of the time, in decreasing order of frequency.
[b] Results from previous experiment.

ognition ability, per se. Finally, the scoring of responses poses a problem: should all words be heard, or just a few key words, or should a general sense of the meaning be an acceptable response?

The Kent State University (KSU) test (Berger, 1969) constituted an attempt to test phonemic confusion within a sentence context. For example, in the item "They had a (pact, pan, pass, pack, pad) between them," the listener's task was to choose which of the five words the announcer used for the sentence. Berger, Keating, and Rose (1971) found that the mean score for a group of sensorineural hearing loss patients on the KSU test was 83.4 percent in contrast to a mean of 69.3 percent on a CID W-22 list, suggesting that the KSU, as it was used in this investigation, may be too easy for clinical applications.

Owens and Schubert (unpublished) also experimented with sentences in a format similar to the KSU test—for example, "All enjoyed the (sun, pun, fun)" or "Did she (pack, patch, pass) it?" The number of foils had been reduced from four to three, but it was difficult to find even two foils confusable acoustically that would at the same time fit a sentence with equal appropriateness. That is, it could not be ascertained that meaning effects had been completely controlled unless the sentences became extremely concrete and virtually meaningless, as in the two examples above.

Harris, Haines, and Myers (1960) constructed a series of sentences that might be useful in aural rehabilitation. Based on the Harvard Psycho-Acoustic Laboratory (PAL-8) sentences, the test items took the form of statements or questions with multiple choice answers related to key words. The authors used the sentences effectively in a study of speech rate. Lacroix, Harris, and Randolph (1979) used the same items to explore the effects of multiple distortion on speech comprehension.

Another sentence test, synthetic sentence identification (Speaks and Jerger, 1965), has received increasing clinical use, both in hearing assessment and in the selection of hearing aids; but its value for aural rehabilitation remains to be determined. Each sentence in a set of 10 was constructed according to conditional probabilities of word sequences. The 10 sentences constitute a closed-set response, and the patient's task is one of identification.

Sentences already receiving use in aural rehabilitation, notably at the National Technical Institute for the Deaf, are commonly called the *everyday speech* sentences. They were prepared at the Central Institute for the Deaf according to specifications laid down by a Working Group of the Armed Forces-National Research Council Committee on Hearing and Bio-Acoustics (CHABA) (Silverman and Hirsh, 1955). There are 10 sentences in each of 10 sets, and scoring is on the basis of 50 key words in a set. Giolas (1966) has reported a high correlation between responses on these sentences and responses to a sample of conversational speech. It is widely known that the sentences are much too easy for ordinary clinical use unless various kinds of distortion are introduced.

A promising new sentence test with respect to aural rehabilitation is the speech perception in noise (SPIN) test (Kalikow, Stevens, and Elliot, 1977), which provides 10 lists of sentences that measure the extent to which an individual benefits by context. An open response is used in which the listener must repeat or write the last word of the sentence. In general, the higher the degree of context related to the last word, the higher the probability of a correct response. Both high and low context sentences are presented within a list, and an overall score is obtained from the difference between the low-context score and the high-context score. Presumably, patients vary in the benefit they obtain from context. Bilger et al. (1979) reported on the responses of 128 subjects with sensorineural hearing loss to all 10 forms of the test. Although reliabilities were high (0.91 for high-context and 0.85 for low-context items), large differences among the low-context items made it difficult to identify a subset of equivalent forms. Other orderings were suggested for greater inter-form equivalence.

Self-Report Scales

In a self-report scale individuals judge their own hearing abilities. Alpiner (1978) has described a number of self-report scales in present use. The hearing performance inventory (HPI) (Giolas et al., 1979), which was introduced after the Alpiner publication, seems to be the most comprehensive of all, especially with respect to word recognition. Moreover, it is statistically based on a large population of hearing-impaired patients. The purpose of the HPI is to provide a profile of hearing performance in everyday situations according to an individual's own evaluations. The items fall into six sections: 1) understanding of speech, 2) intensity, 3) response, 4) social, 5) personal, and 6) occupational. Each item places the respondent in a specific situation or activity and asks the individual to rate his or her usual behavior by choosing one of the five possible answers: 1) practically always, 2) frequently, 3) about half the time, 4) occasionally, or 5) almost never. A recently completed revision of the HPI (Lamb, Owens, and Schubert, in preparation) was undertaken because of patient complaints that the first published version was too long and too repetitious. The revision, based on responses of 156 hearing-impaired patients, consists of 90 items that can be completed in about 20 minutes. Items concerning understanding of speech (speech recognition) with and without visual cues constitute the largest single section. A typical item for understanding speech is: "You are with a female friend or family member and several people are talking nearby. Can you understand her when her voice is loud enough for you and you can see her face?"

AURAL REHABILITATION

An organized approach to aural rehabilitation was first undertaken early in the 1940s to help persons who incurred hearing impairment during World War II. During the 1950s and 1960s, however, the research and clinical interest in audiology was directed primarily toward measurement of hearing, particularly to specialized tests in the evaluation of hearing in young children, in the localization of lesion within the auditory system, in the selection of hearing aids, and in the detection of functional hearing loss (pseudohypacusis). A resurgence of interest in rehabilitative considerations is reflected by several recent reviews—Alpiner, 1978; Berg, 1976; O'Neill and Oyer, 1973; Oyer and Frankmann, 1975; Sanders, 1982. These writers have stressed the dire need for research concerning aural rehabilitation, especially regarding objective measurements of changes that may occur in communication skills. Consequently, particular attention will be given here to procedures that are amenable to objective measurement.

The aural rehabilitation process is one of remediation directed to all aspects of an individual's communication problem. Insofar as the process can be broken down, it includes counseling, speech conservation, speechreading, and auditory training. Because of the emphasis on speech recognition in this chapter, the first two are not included and speechreading is mentioned only briefly. New terms have been suggested for aural rehabilitation, but it appears that a consensus will not be reached for some time.

Auditory training refers to the process in which hearing-impaired persons learn to take full advantage of sound cues still available to them (Carhart, 1960). The patient may be asked, for example, to identify a word in a group of words, or to determine whether pairs of words are the same or different, or to identify which word has a particular sound in it.[1] An impetus has been given to such training by the incorporation of programmed instruction. Holland and Matthews (1963) outlined the procedures and Costello (1977) has reviewed the principles and components. Basically, a wide range of recognition tasks are em-

---

[1] Although *recognition* is preferred generally, other terms may seem more appropriate in specific instances; for example, *discrimination* for a same/different response and "identification" in the selection of a given (stimulus) consonant from among a number of alternate choices.

ployed, and programming techniques including reinforcement, shaping, fading, and branching lead to increasingly difficult judgments by listeners. Applied to identification of phonemes by patients with hearing impairment, improvement might result from a sharpening in awareness of the barest "remnants" of phonemes, or to an alertness for transitional cues, or to both factors.

Sanders (1971) has expressed the desirability of broadening the definition of auditory training as follows: "Auditory training constitutes a systematic procedure designed to increase the amount of information that a person's hearing contributes to his total perception" (p. 205). Sanders's definition will be used in this chapter. One advantage is that this definition incorporates work in the comprehension of connected speech, whereas earlier definitions have come to refer primarily to phoneme and word recognition activities.

Phoneme Recognition

The studies of phoneme recognition provide a good indication of the phonemes most apt to be misperceived. Primary attention in a relearning program would best be directed to the consonant sounds rather than to the vowels, except possibly in cases of severe to profound hearing loss. Regarding the consonant sounds, research findings have been consistent in showing that nasality, sonorance, and voicing differences facilitate recognition.

The assumption is that items for relearning can be varied in difficulty by manipulating the response foils. Support comes from Owens and Schubert (1977), who found that listeners often seemed to respond by a process of elimination. On a four-choice item, for example, the response process was one of narrowing the choice to the two or three consonants that sounded most like the stimulus and "guessing" between them when uncertain of the correct response.

For each stimulus (target) consonant there are usually about two others that cause the most confusion, as shown in Tables 11-1 and 11-2. These sounds are most apt to produce programmed instruction "ceilings," that is, consonant comparisons that cannot be differentiated by the listener even with training. The consonants of opposite voicing, the nasals, and the sonorants serve for comparisons that are fairly easy. Therefore, the target consonant is paired with one of these consonants for "same/different" judgments that are relatively easy and thus would be placed in the early part of a program or in parts of a program in which the subject might be in need of a successful experience. A correct response is followed by reinforcement, usually a pulse of light. Comparisons graduated in difficulty are then introduced. For example, in a program requiring "same" or "different" responses, items such as pass-pan, pal-pass, or pad-pass would be easier than pat-pass or pass-path. If the required task is to identify the word with /s/, the programmer might want to use three- or four-choice responses. Items such as lease-lean-lead-leave would occur early in the program and items such as leaf-leak-lease-leap would be introduced later on. The learning criterion either for the same/different response or for the identification of /s/ task might be a 90 percent correct response rate before going to a new program. According to the findings of Reed (1975), the discrimination (same/different) of phonemes requires a different auditory process than the identification (labeling) of phonemes. Ability on one task does not imply ability on the other. In the same study, Reed also observed reaction time in responding, which might be a helpful measuring device in programmed instruction sequences. Formulations of programs can follow the suggestions of Green (1962) and Thiagarajan (1971). It is conceivable that the clinician may have to work face to face presenting live-voice stimuli for patients with severe phoneme recognition problems. That is, the process may require visual cues and more flexibility in activities such as stressing certain phonemes, increasing the intensity selectively, and overarticulating at the start of the program to prevent a series of early failures. Improvement in this work is signaled by meeting the success criterion on each learning sequence. In short, it will be observed that phonemes not identified successfully at the beginning of a program are identified consistently at the end.

Thus, programmed instruction provides a basis for objective evaluation of improvement in phoneme recognition. The measuring process is inherent in each program, although a pre- and posttraining scale is often desirable. The aim of the testing would be first to determine which consonants are being confused and then to see if improvement is shown after programmed instruction on these sounds. For severe or profound hearing losses, the nasal, sonorant, and voicing features would need to be included in the test and training items. Evidence of recognition improvement through programmed instruction is abundant (see Berg, 1976 for a listing of several pertinent experiments and demonstrations).

Auditory and Visual Modalities in Phoneme Recognition

A seemingly complementary relationship exists between auditory and visual modalities in phoneme recognition. Miller and Nicely (1955) found five groups of phonemes that were seldom confused auditorily by normal-hearing listeners: /p,t,k/, /f,θ,s,ʃ/, /b,d,g/, /v,z,ʒ/, and /m,n/; that is, confusions occurred not between but within these groups. The authors stated that the addition of speechreading should facilitate recognition of consonants within the groups. Walden, Prosek, and Worthington (1974) have pointed out the redundancy between the auditory and visual modalities in recognition of consonants by hearing-impaired subjects, supporting Miller and Nicely's findings for normal hearers. In the visual modality, consonant groupings seldom confused are called *visemes*. Several investigators have agreed in general with viseme groupings presented by Woodward and Barber (1960). Using these groupings, Binnie, Montgomery, and Jackson (1974) have shown that normal hearers on speechreading tests (with no sound and no practice) make errors only within visemes, not between them. Their viseme groups consisted of /p,b,m/, /t,d,n,s,z,k,g/, /f,v/, /θ,ð/, and /ʃ,ʒ/. These investigators suggested, as a result of their findings, that auditory training and the use of contextual cues should receive major emphasis in aural rehabilitation rather than speechreading.

Except for a few pairs of consonants like /t-k/ and /d-g/ that tend to be confused both auditorily and visually, the underlying phonemic structure seems distinctly favorable to the hearing impaired. That is, visual confusions within the viseme groups are reduced by auditory cues, and auditory confusions within auditory distinctive feature groups are reduced by visual cues. Complementary relations between the auditory and visual modalities seem to indicate that, when both are operating, phoneme recognition in the so-called analytic tasks described above is virtually assured in most instances. Verification by appropriate tests would, of course, be necessary in the individual case. Accordingly, the major emphasis in aural rehabilitation would be away from phoneme recognition, per se, and toward listening and watching expressly for the meaning of connected speech materials.

On the other hand, Walden et al. (1977) demonstrated that directed-learning approaches can improve visual consonant recognition even within viseme groups. In a more extensive study, of hearing-impaired subjects, Walden et al. (1981) demonstrated that: 1) subjects trained in auditory recognition of consonant phonemes improved significantly on an auditory test of consonant identification; 2) subjects trained in visual recognition of phonemes improved significantly on a visual test of consonant phonemes; and 3) both groups improved significantly in an auditory-visual test of sentence recognition. Assuming that understanding of speech is impeded when certain phonemes cannot be recognized, and that some everyday situations preclude speechreading, logic would suggest that an aural rehabilitation program provide phoneme recognition work, at least in the auditory modality, until ceilings are demonstrated. This logic is supported strongly by the work of Walden et al. (1981).

Sentence Materials

The aural rehabilitation program for young adults at the National Technical Institute for the Deaf (NTID) attests to the important role that can be played by sentence materials (Sims, 1978). CHABA everyday sentence lists are used as part of a profile for each student. For those students who show some ability in understanding these sentences, instruction is given on other sentence materials in technical, social, and survival communication subject areas. Sims (1978) has reported that pre- and post-training tests on these materials for 55 students indicated that an average of 30 percent improvement occurred after 20 hours of training. Moreover, the improvement was maintained on retest at 5, 10, and 15 weeks after the initial posttraining test. Moore (1975) has described the programmed self-instruction procedures that were used to obtain these results.

NEW PROCEDURES AND DIRECTIONS

Tracking

A procedure that emphasizes watching and listening for meaning is called "tracking" (DeFilippo and Scott, 1978; Owens and Telleen, 1981). Applied to aural rehabilitation, it is a process in which a hearing-impaired person repeats short segments of connected speech after a talker. The talker and receiver sit face to face in the manner of a typical two-person communicative situation. The procedure offers concomitant auditory, visual, and kinesthetic cues to the receiver and also affords practice in different ways of resolving communication blockages that occur with hearing loss. Improvement is directly measurable in terms of an increase in speed (words per minute) with practice. If a before-and-after measure is needed, the hearing performance inventory (Giolas, et al., 1979) would likely be applicable.

The Use of Context in Sentences

Another aural rehabilitation approach with sentence materials involves the use of context in facilitating sentence understanding. Several studies in psycholinguistics have indicated that contextual cues evoked by the meanings of certain words and by word order facilitate the identification of other words by restricting the number of possible responses (Leventhal, 1973; Lieberman, 1963; Miller and Isard, 1963; Pollack and Pickett, 1964; Rosenberg and Lambert, 1974; Stowe, Harris, and Hampton, 1963; Treisman, 1965; Winitz, LaRiviere, and Harriman, 1973). For example, in the sentence, "The tent was blown over by the

_____", the listener grasps the meaning of the context and is able to assign the word *wind* to the last position of the sentence even though it is not heard. Similarly, with sentences of the kind, "The little dog has a (pail, tail)," Stinson (1978) has shown that context facilitates hearing-impaired childrens' discrimination of acoustically similar words in sentences. He has also observed (personal communication) the effects of context on six adult subjects with profound postlingual hearing loss. Materials were Morton's (1967) norms for sentence completion and Rosenberg and Koen's (1968) norms of sequential associative dependencies. Morton's data are 64 sentences presented to 526 respondents who were in the British military. Rosenberg and Koen's data are 71 sentences presented to 120 university undergraduates. Subjects were simply asked to fill in the last word. Both sets of norms yield sentences in which the most frequently given last word for the sentence has strong semantic links with earlier words in the sentence. Stinson varied the contextual information in these sentences, usually by adding or deleting key words, and presented them to the six subjects so that each sentence would be heard with and without the change in context. The final word was deleted in the presentation of the sentences. Context was shown to be a strong facilitator in the identification of the final word. Sentences of this kind can be ranked in order from easy to difficult and, accordingly, can be directed to programmed instruction in listening for context. Evidence of improvement again would lie in the patient's meeting predetermined criteria.

Continuous Speech

Some evidence indicates that continuous speech at first unintelligible to normal-hearing listeners may become increasingly more intelligible with repeated listening as cues to understanding develop (Blesser, 1972; Tobias and Irons, 1972). This kind of listening has not been tried with hearing-impaired persons in any organized manner. A research approach would require continuous speech materials of varying difficulty in terms of parameters such as rate, phonologic structure, and redundancy. For example, a paragraph of four or five sentences would be repeated several times. The patient might understand only a fragment the first time, and the response would be reinforced if correct. Understanding of one fragment might facilitate the understanding of an additional fragment the second time, and so on until the whole passage is understood.

EQUIPMENT INNOVATIONS

Microprocessors that are relatively inexpensive can provide increased efficiency in programmed instruction. A major advantage is the immediacy with which any part of a program on tape or disc can be found and played back. Rapid retrieval is invaluable for branching sequences and, in general, for ensuring that the subject is always at his appropriate level of difficulty. The microprocessor also directs the reinforcement (reward) signals, counts correct and incorrect responses, and provides for an ongoing and final readout of progress.

Another recent innovation, namely, digitized speech,[2] requires a certain level of computer capacity. Speech in its ordinary analogue form can be changed by a computer into digital form, after which it becomes readily amenable to computer processing. In other words, various parameters of the speech signal can be changed to test the effects on the speech perception of hearing-impaired listeners. For example, different rates of speed can be presented until the one providing the best speech perception is found.

AUDITORY TRAINING FOR CHILDREN

For hard-of-hearing children, *habilitation* is a more appropriate term than *rehabilitation*. That is, the work must involve acquisition of language rather than a relearning process. There are several reviews of programs that have included auditory training in the habilitation process (Berg, 1976; Erber and Hirsh, 1978; Rodel, 1978; Sanders, 1971).

This section is limited simply to mentioning some of the approaches to auditory training that have been advocated for hard-of-hearing children. Berg (1976), for example, has provided summaries of several programs, materials, and methods, including: Project SKI-HI for infants and pre-schoolers (Clark, 1975); the contributions of Wedenberg (1954); programs at the Institute of Logopedics (Wait, 1975) and the Bill Wilkerson facility (Horton, 1973); a program by Pollack (1973); an approach based on the ideas of Guberina (Asp et al., 1973); and other programs by individual practitioners.

A program published more recently is the Auditory Skills Instructional Planning System, developed by the Audiologic Services of the Los Angeles County Schools (Trammell et al., 1976). It is designed for children of ages 4 through 12 years with moderate to profound hearing losses. One major component, the test of auditory comprehension (TAC), assesses with the use of pictured material the auditory functioning of the child. The results of the TAC provide for: 1) a measure of a variety of skills inherent in the auditory processing of speech; 2)

---

[2] The computer samples the incoming speech wave form at a rapid rate and converts the voltages to numbers (analogue to digital). These numbers can then be manipulated by the computer to produce any desired changes in the digitized wave form. The numbers can then be changed back to voltages (digital to analogue).

a basis for selection of appropriate auditory skills objectives; 3) an evaluation of growth in the acquisition of auditory abilities; and 4) an indication for educational placement decisions. All test materials are recorded on audio cassettes. Another major component, the Auditory Skills Curriculum, provides the actual training materials. This curriculum comprises a large number of individual and group activities based on criteria developed in the areas of discrimination, memory-sequencing, auditory feedback, and figure-ground. Programmed instruction methods are utilized; and training proceeds from messages that have high redundancy and acoustic dissimilarity to messages progressively decreasing in redundancy and increasing in acoustic similarity. All stimuli are presented in meaningful linguistic contexts.

CONCLUSIONS

The monosyllable word tests commonly used for audiologic assessment of word recognition seem of limited relevance to aural rehabilitative considerations. Newer tests provide greater information regarding phoneme confusions and auditory comprehension of connected speech. Self-report scales offer another dimension of measurement in that they are based on an individual's own appraisal of communication difficulty in everyday situations.

Programmed instruction has lent impetus to auditory training by permitting both greater efficiency in the relearning process and an objective measurement of change. A new procedure called "tracking" helps the hearing-impaired individual to take advantage of auditory, visual, and kinesthetic cues; changes in skill can be measured directly in words per minute of successful tracking.

Although the relearning of skills at the phoneme and word levels continues as an important aspect of auditory training, the more recently introduced materials and methods seem to be emphasizing comprehension of connected speech. These materials and methods are being introduced at a time coinciding with the advent of microprocessors for controlling the training sequences and digitized speech for enhancing aspects of speech that provide easier understanding. The combination permits an optimistic outlook for aural rehabilitation.

REFERENCES

Alpiner, J. G. (ed.). 1978. Handbook of Adult Rehabilitative Audiology. Williams & Wilkins Company, Baltimore.

Asp, C. J., J. Berry, and C. Berry. 1973. Auditory Training Procedures for Children and Adults. University of Tennessee, Knoxville.

Berg, F. S. 1976. Educational Audiology: Hearing and Speech Management. Grune & Stratton, New York.

Berger, K. N., L. W. Keating, and D. E. Rose. 1971. An evaluation of the Kent State University speech discrimination test on subjects with sensorineural loss. J. Aud. Res. 11:140–143.

Berger, K. W. 1969. A speech discrimination task using multiple choice key words in sentences. J. Aud. Res. 3:247–262.

Bilger, R. C., C. Rzcezkowski, J. M. Nuetzel, and W. P. Rabinowitz. 1979. Evaluation of a test of speech perception in noise (SPIN). Paper presented at the American Speech and Hearing Association Convention, Atlanta.

Bilger, R. C., and M. C. Wang. 1976. Consonant confusion in patients with sensorineural hearing loss. J. Speech Hear. Res. 19:718–748.

Binnie, C. A., A. A. Montgomery, and P. L. Jackson. 1974. Auditory and visual contributions to the perception of consonants. J. Speech Hear. Res. 17:619–630.

Blesser, B. 1972. Speech perception under conditions of spectral transformation. J. Speech Hear. Res. 15:5–41.

Boothroyd, A. 1968. Developments in speech audiometry. Sound 2:3–10.

Carhart, R. 1960. Auditory training. In H. Davis and S. R. Silverman (eds.), Hearing and Deafness, pp. 360–369. 3rd Ed. Holt, Rinehart & Winston, New York.

Clark, T. (ed.). 1975. Programming for Hearing Impaired Infants Through Amplification and Home Intervention. Utah State University, Logan.

Costello, J. M. 1977. Programmed instruction. J. Speech Hear. Disord. 42:3–28.

Danhauer, J. L., and R. M. Lawarre. 1979. Dissimilarity ratings of English consonants by normally-hearing and hearing-impaired individuals. J. Speech Hear. Res. 22:236–246.

Davis, H. 1978. Hearing handicap, standards for hearing, and medicolegal rules. In H. Davis and S. R. Silverman (eds.), Hearing and Deafness, pp. 253–279. 4th Ed. Holt, Rinehart & Winston, New York.

DeFilippo, C. L. and B. L. Scott. 1978. A method for training and evaluating the reception of ongoing speech. J. Acoust. Soc. Am. 63:1186–1192.

Dubno, J. R., and D. D. Dirks. 1982. Evaluation of hearing-impaired listeners using a nonsense-syllable test. I. Test reliability. J. Speech Hear. Res. 25:135–141.

Dubno, J. R., D. D. Dirks, and L. R. Langhofer. 1982. Evaluation of hearing-impaired listeners using a nonsense-syllable test. II. Syllable recognition and consonant confusion patterns. J. Speech Hear. Res. 25:141–148.

Edgerton, B. J., and J. L. Danhauer. 1979. Clinical Implications of Speech Discrimination Testing Using Nonsense Stimuli. University Park Press, Baltimore.

Egan, J. 1948. Articulation testing methods. Laryngoscope 58:955–991.

Erber, N. P., and I. J. Hirsh. 1978. Auditory Training. In H. Davis and S. R. Silverman (eds.), Hearing and Deafness, pp. 358–374. 4th Ed. Holt, Rinehart & Winston, New York.

Fairbanks, G. 1958. A test of phonemic differentiation: The rhyme test. J. Acoust. Soc. Am. 30:590–600.

Giolas, T. G. 1966. Comparative intelligibility scores of sentence lists and continuous discourse. J. Aud. Res. 6:31–38.

Giolas, T. G., and A. Epstein, 1963. Comparative intelligibility of word lists and continuous discourse. J. Speech Hear. Res. 6:349–358.

Giolas, T. G., E. Owens, S. H. Lamb, and E. D. Schubert. 1979. Hearing performance inventory. J. Speech Hear. Disord. 44:169–195.

Goetzinger, C. P. 1978. Word discrimination testing. In J. Katz (ed.) Handbook of Clinical Audiology, pp. 149–158. 2nd Ed. Williams & Wilkins Company, Baltimore.

Green, E. J. 1962. The Learning Process and Programmed Instruction. Holt, Rinehart & Winston, Inc., New York.

Griffiths, J. D. 1967. Rhyming minimal contrasts: A simplified diagnostic articulation test. J. Acoust. Soc. Am. 42:235–241.

Harris, J. D., H. Haines, and C. Myers, 1960. The importance of hearing at 3,000 Hz for understanding speeded speech. Laryngoscope 70:131–146.

Hirsh, I. J. 1952. The Measurement of Hearing. McGraw-Hill Book Company, New York.

Hirsh, I. J., H. Davis, S. R. Silverman, E. G. Reynolds, E. Eldert, and R. W. Benson. 1952. Development of materials for speech audiometry. J. Speech Hear. Disord. 17:321–337.

Holland, A. L., and J. Matthews. 1963. Applications of teaching machine concepts to speech pathology and audiology. Asha 5:474–482.

Horton, K. 1973. Every child should be given a chance to benefit from acoustic input. Volta Rev. 75:348–350.

House, A. S., C. E. Williams, M. H. L. Hecker, and K. D. Kryter. 1965. Articulation testing methods: Consonantal differentiation with a closed-response set. J. Acoust. Soc. Am. 37:158–166.

Kalikow, D. N., K. N. Stevens, and L. L. Elliot. 1977. Development of a test of speech intelligibility in noise using sentence materials with controlled word predictability. J. Acoust. Soc. Am. 61:1337–1351.

Kreul, E. J., J. C. Nixon, K. D. Kryter, D. W. Bell, J. S. Lang, and E. D. Schubert. 1968. A proposed clinical test of speech discrimination. J. Speech Hear. Res. 11:536–552.

Lacroix, P. G., and J. D. Harris. 1979. Effects of high-frequency cue reduction on the comprehension of distorted speech. J. Speech Hear. Disord. 44:236–246.

Lacroix, P. G., J. D. Harris, and K. J. Randolph. 1979. Multiplicative effects on sentence comprehension for combined acoustic distortions. J. Speech Hear. Res. 22:259–269.

Lamb, S. H., E. Owens, and E. D. Schubert. A revision of the hearing performance inventory. In preparation.

Larson, L. L. 1950. Consonant Sound Discrimination. Indiana University Press, Bloomington.

Leventhal, G. 1973. Effect of sentence context on word perception. J. Exp. Psychol. 101:318–323.

Levitt, H. 1978. Hearing aid evaluation: A suggested new approach. Paper presented at the Annual Convention of the American Speech and Hearing Association, November, San Francisco.

Lieberman, P. 1963. Some effects of semantic and grammatical context on the production and perception of speech. Lang. Speech 6:172–187.

Miller, G. A., and S. Isard. 1963. Some perceptual consequences of linguistic rules. J. Verb. Learn. Verb. Behav. 2:217–228.

Miller, G. A., and P. Nicely. 1955. An analysis of perceptual confusions among some English consonants. J. Acoust. Soc. Am. 27:338–352.

Moore, E. 1975. Programmed self-instruction in auditory training. J. Acad. Rehab. Aud. 8:90–94.

Morton, J. 1967. Population Norms for Sentence Completion. Applied Psychology Unit, Cambridge, England.

Olsen, W. O., and N. D. Matkin. 1979. Speech Audiometry. In W. F. Rintelmann (ed.) Hearing Assessment, pp. 133–206. University Park Press, Baltimore.

O'Neill, J. J., and H. J. Oyer. 1973. Aural rehabilitation. In J. Jerger (ed.), Modern Developments in Audiology, pp. 212–247. Academic Press, Inc., New York.

Owens, E. 1978. Consonant errors and remediation of sensorineural hearing loss. J. Speech Hear. Disord. 43:331–374.

Owens, E., M. Benedict, and E. D. Schubert. 1971. Further investigation of vowel items in multiple choice speech discrimination testing. J. Speech Hear. Res. 4:841–847.

Owens, E., and E. D. Schubert. 1977. Development of the California Consonant Test. J. Speech Hear. Res. 20:463–474.

Owens, E., and E. D. Schubert (unpublished). p. 11.

Owens, E., C. B. Talbott, and E. D. Schubert. 1968. Vowel discrimination of hearing impaired listeners. J. Speech Hear. Res. 11:648–655.

Owens, E., and C. C. Telleen. 1981. Tracking as an aural rehabilitative process. J. Acad. Rehab. Audiol. 14:259–273.

Oyer, H. J., and M. Doudna. 1959. Structural analysis of word responses made by hard of hearing subjects on a discrimination test. Arch. Otolaryngol. 70:357–363.

Oyer, H. J., and J. P. Frankmann. 1975. The Aural Rehabilitation Process. Holt, Rinehart & Winston, Inc., New York.

Pedersen, O. T., and G. A. Studebaker. 1972. A new minimal contrasts closed response-set speech test. J. Aud. Res. 12:187–195.

Pollack, D. 1973. Learning to listen in an integrated preschool. Volta Rev. 75:359–367.

Pollack, I., and J. M. Pickett. 1964. Intelligibility of excerpts from fluent speech: Auditory vs. structural context. J. Verb. Learn. Verb. Behav. 3:79–84.

Reed, C. 1975. Identification and discrimination of vowel-consonant syllables in listeners with sensorineural hearing loss. J. Speech Hear. Res. 18:773–794.

Rodel, M. A. T. 1978. Visual and auditory training for children. In J. Katz (ed.), Handbook of Clinical Audiology. pp. 581–588. 2nd Ed. Williams & Wilkins Company, Baltimore.

Rosenberg, S., and M. Koen. 1968. Norms of Sequential Associative Dependencies in Active Declarative Sentences. (Studies in language and language behavior, Supplement, Vol. 6). Center for Research on Language and Language Behavior, University of Michigan.

Rosenberg, S., and W. E. Lambert. 1974. Contextual constraints and auditory perception of speech. J. Exp. Psychol. 102:178–180.

Sanders, D. A. 1982. Aural Rehabilitation. 2nd Ed. Prentice-Hall, Inc., Englewood Cliffs, New Jersey.

Schubert, E. D., and M. C. Schultz. 1960. Item analysis of discrimination. Office of Vocational Rehabilitation Project, Dec. 1958–March, 1960.

Schultz, M. C. 1964. Suggested improvements in speech discrimination testing. J. Aud. Res. 4:1–14.

Schwartz, D. M., and R. K. Surr. 1979. Three experiments on the California Consonant Test. J. Speech Hear. Disord. 44:61–72.

Sher, A. E., and E. Owens. 1974. Consonant confusions associated with hearing loss above 2,000 Hz. J. Speech Hear. Res. 17:669–681.

Silverman, R. S., and I. J. Hirsh. 1955. Problems related to the use of speech in clinical audiometry. Ann. Otol. Rhinol. Laryngol. 64:1234–1244.

Sims, D. G. 1978. Visual and auditory training for adults. In J. Katz (ed.)

Handbook of Clinical Audiology, pp. 565–582, 2nd Ed. Williams & Wilkins Company, Baltimore.

Speaks, C., and J. Jerger. 1965. Method for measurement of speech identification. J. Speech Hear. Res. 8:185–194.

Stinson, M. 1978. Use of contextual cues in spoken sentences by hearing impaired children and adolescents. Paper presented at the Model Secondary Schools for the Deaf Research Conference. September, Washington, D.C.

Stowe, A. N., W. D. Harris, and D. B. Hampton. 1963. Signal and context components of word recognition behavior. J. Acoust. Soc. Am. 35:639–644.

Thiagarajan, S. 1971. The Programming Process: A Practical Guide, Charles A. Jones Publishing, Worthington, Ohio.

Tillman, T. W., and R. Carhart. 1966. An expanded test for speech discrimination utilizing CNC monosyllabic words. Northwestern University Auditory Test No. 6. USAF School of Aerospace Medicine Technical Report, Brooks Air Force Base, Texas.

Tobias, J., and F. Irons. 1972. Learned intelligibility—improvement for distorted speech. Asha (abstract) 14:464.

Trammell, J. L., C. Favor, S. L. Francis, S. L. Owens, D. E. Shepard, R. P. Witlen, and L. H. Faist. 1976. Auditory skills instructional planning system. Foreworks, North Hollywood, California.

Treisman, A. M. 1965. Verbal responses and contextual constraints in sentences. J. Verb. Learn. Verb. Behav. 4:118–128.

Voiers, W. D. 1977. Diagnostic evaluation of speech intelligibility. In M. E. Hawley (ed.) Speech Intelligibility and Speaker Recognition (Benchmark Papers in Acoustics, II), Hutchinson and Ross, Strausberg, Penn.

Wait, D. 1975. Pulsatone. Predoncini Oral/Aural Program. Wichita State University, Wichita, Kansas.

Walden, B. E., S. A. Erdman, A. A. Montgomery, D. M. Schwartz, and R. A. Prosek. 1981. Some effects of training on speech recognition by hearing-impaired adults. J. Speech Hear. Res. 24:207–216.

Walden, B. E., and A. A. Montgomery. 1975. Dimensions of consonant perception in normal and hearing impaired listeners. J. Speech Hear. Res. 18:444–456.

Walden, B. E., R. A. Prosek, A. A. Montgomery, C. K. Scherr, and C. I. Jones. 1977. Effects of training of visual recognition of consonants. J. Speech Hear. Res. 20:130–145.

Walden, B. E., R. A. Prosek, and D. W. Worthington. 1974. Predicting audiovisual consonant recognition performance of hearing impaired adults. J. Speech Hear. Res. 17:270–278.

Walden, B. E., R. A. Prosek, and D. W. Worthington. 1975. The prevalence of hearing loss within the selected U.S. Army branches. Final Report, Medical Research and Development Command. Washington, D.C.

Wedenberg, E. 1954. Auditory training of severely hard of hearing preschool children. Acta Otolaryngol. (Stockh.) 94(Suppl):129.

Winitz, H., C. LaRiviere, and E. Harriman. 1973. Perception of word boundaries under conditions of lexical bias. Phonetica 27:193–213.

Woodward, M. F., and C. G. Barber. 1960. Phoneme perception in lip reading. J. Speech Hear. Res. 3:212–222.

CHAPTER 12

RESEARCH TRENDS AND CLINICAL NEEDS IN SPEECH AUDIOMETRY

Wayne O. Olsen

CONTENTS

MATERIALS	375
Variability in Performance	376
Error Analyses	376
Acoustic Analyses	379
Single Words, Sentences, Noise	380
OTHER PSYCHOACOUSTIC DATA AND SPEECH UNDERSTANDING	382
Frequency Resolution	383
Temporal Resolution	384
Reaction Time	385
NEURAL CODING OF SPEECH	386
ASSESSMENT OF CENTRAL AUDITORY NERVOUS SYSTEM FUNCTION	387
SUMMARY	392
REFERENCES	392

It is not the intent of this chapter to reiterate research or clinical needs for improved speech audiometry stated in other chapters of this text. Rather, the goal is to mention several recent (or relatively recent) developments and methods which, in the opinion of this writer, hold promise for providing information for more clinically useful speech audiometry. Not all areas will be covered, nor will all possible references be cited; however, it is hoped that the bibliography can serve as a useful starting point for readers wishing to study specific topics more thoroughly.

The chapter is divided into three areas without any intended rank ordering of topics. The different sections deal with materials, relationship of speech understanding to other aspects of measured auditory behavior, and assessment of the central auditory nervous system using speech test materials.

MATERIALS

Over the years a plethora of lists of test words and a few lists of sentences have been described for the purpose of assessing speech intelligibility rendered by transducers, speech transmission systems, auditoria, and the speech understanding capabilities of normal hearers and hearing-impaired listeners in various quiet or noisy situations (see Webster, 1972). Lists for test materials have varied in length from 10 items to 100 or more items per list. Variability in performance for a single listener or among listeners on any given test of word recognition or word identification is a problem common to all test materials.

Variability in Performance

The problem of variability in performance among listeners on various tests of word recognition and word identification and for individuals on a test-retest basis has been well recognized but not dealt with effectively until recently. The work of Hagerman (1976), Thornton and Raffin (1978), Raffin and Thornton (1980), and Raffin and Schafer (1980) in applying the statistical model of the binomial distribution to word recognition scores represents, in the view of this writer, a major development. This model clearly demonstrates the relationship between variability in performance on repeated measures and the number of test items used. Hence, this model allows the examiner to determine how many test items are necessary to reflect a "real" difference in performance dependent upon whether the expected (or "significant") differences are large or small. For smaller expected differences, more items must be presented to demonstrate the difference to be real. Similarly, use of this model and tables derived from it published by Raffin and Thornton (1980) allow the clinician or researcher to determine, on an individual basis, whether two-word recognition scores for a given listener differ from one another by more or less than would be expected on the basis of chance alone at a given statistical confidence level. Such applications should be of value to clinicians and researchers alike dealing with repeated measurements of word recognition.

Error Analyses

Results obtained from presentation of a given set of test materials to a listener (or groups of listeners) generally have been considered in terms of quantitative scores. Information relative to types of errors largely has been ignored. To be sure, there are notable exceptions (particularly in evaluating the influence of reverberation on speech understanding (e.g., Nabalek and Mason, 1981) but error analyses in clinical settings appear to be the exception rather than the rule. Nevertheless, a number of studies (Bilger and Wang, 1976; Owens, 1978; Owens, Benedict, and Schubert, 1972; Sher and Owens, 1974; Wang, Reed, and Bilger, 1978) have demonstrated some relatively consistent relationships between types of errors and configurations of hearing loss even though different types of test materials (consonant-vowel and vowel-consonant nonsense syllables, and monosyllables) have been used. It is also worth noting that these investigators (Sher and Owens, 1974; Wang et al., 1978) have observed similar patterns of errors when their test materials were presented to normal hearers after being filtered externally to resemble the internal filtering action imposed by the hearing losses of their hearing-impaired subjects.

Walden et al. (1981), on the other hand, observed differences in the performance of the two ears of unilateral hearing loss subjects when the signal presented to the normal ear was shaped to match the hearing loss and loudness experience of the impaired ear. Performance was considerably poorer for the hearing-impaired ear for five of eight subjects. Contrary to this observation, LaCroix and Harris (1979) obtained better performance for patients having high-frequency losses than for normal hearers responding to sentences in a noise background. The materials presented to the normal hearing subjects were low-pass filtered to simulate the hearing losses of the hearing-impaired subjects. This observation led LaCroix and Harris to conclude that individuals having hearing losses ". . . of long standing may learn to use residual cues more effectively. Whether they use more efficiently the lower frequency cues for feature extraction or learn to use more efficiently prosodic or other cues to word prediction/intelligibility cannot be determined from these results. At least it is clear that in experimental situations where a population of persons with high frequency sensorineural losses is required, it is not altogether permissible to simulate hearing losses by frequency-filtering in normals" (p. 244). Obviously, unlike test materials and dissimilar test conditions yield different results. It still remains to be determined which test materials and test conditions best reflect communication problems encountered in typical noisy listening situations outside the test environment.

Although Gengel (1973) and Owens and Schubert (1977) have noted that errors made by hearing-impaired subjects are not necessarily the same upon repeated presentation of a given closed set of test materials, it was Owens' (1978) contention that knowledge of errors is useful in the design and implementation of remediation programs for hearing-impaired individuals (see Chapter 11, this text). Parenthetically, it might be noted that closed-response sets restrict the choices of the listener. It might be that none of the given items resemble what the individual hears (Nixon, 1973). Oyer and Doudna (1959) also reported inconsistency of errors for an open-ended set of test materials, but in the view of this writer, further investigation in this area seems warranted.

Error analyses of responses to test materials currently in use can provide data about patterns of errors, or lack of any systematic pattern of errors observed for individual subjects, or for different groups of hearing-impaired listeners. Such data can be gathered readily with closed nonsense syllable test materials such as described by Resnick et al. (1975) and by Edgerton and Danhauer (1979), closed-set monosyllabic test materials such as the modified rhyme test (House et al., 1965; Kruel et al., 1968), rhyming minimal contrasts (Griffiths, 1967), multiple choice discrimination test (Schultz and Schubert, 1969), University of Oklahoma closed response speech test (Pederson and Studebaker, 1972), or California consonant test (Owens and Schubert, 1977). Griffiths' rhyming minimal contrasts test lists may be of particular interest. It appears that this test has received little if any clinical application even though it would seem ideally suited for error analysis. Its design is such that each item in a given set of five items differs from each other item in the set by only one of the distinctive features characterizing speech sounds, that is, manner of articulation, place of articulation, or voicing. It is worth noting that Sergeant, Atkinson and LaCroix (1979) and Harris (1980) recently have described a test procedure in which Griffiths' test items are presented as three-word utterances rather than as single words. This procedure continues to allow single word scoring, error analysis, and so on, but also is sentence-like for the listener. Test time is approximately 7 minutes for 150 items compared to about 5 minutes per 50-word list when items are presented singly. In the opinion of this writer, procedures using these materials with the words presented singly or in triplets, or other like materials, warrant further study and development.

Phoneme and whole word scoring (Markides, 1978) of open-ended sets of test materials such as CID W-22, Northwestern University Auditory Test No. 6, or isophonemic word lists also could yield useful information as to whether errors made by an individual (or group) appear to be random or systematic. Of particular interest here may be Boothroyd's (1968) isophonemic word lists. Fifteen lists of 10 consonant-nucleus-consonant (CNC) words per list contain the same 10 vowels and 20 consonants. Because the same 30 phonemes occur in each list, presentation of more than one isophonemic word list for a given listening condition probably could yield interesting data relative to consistency or lack of consistency in types of errors. However, the observation of Dubno and Levitt (1981) that identification of different consonant-vowel combinations required different sets of acoustic information must be kept in mind.

Plotting the data in graph form in the manner of Stevenson (1975) with the phonemes indicated in terms of place of articulation on the abscissa and manner of articulation on the ordinate yields a clearer representation of error patterns than do confusion matrices (Olsen, 1981).

Acoustic Analyses

Based on acoustic analyses of test stimuli and test results obtained from normal-hearing subjects responding to nonsense syllable test items, Dubno and Levitt (1981) stated that the ". . . confusion matrices show complex idiosyncratic patterns, specific to procedures and experimental conditions employed . . . (Nevertheless) certain variables did stand out as being particularly important for each condition . . . The variables selected for the quiet condition were consonant energy, consonant duration, and the origin frequency of the second formant transition. For the noise condition the isolated variables were consonant-to-noise ratio, consonant spectral peak frequency, and consonant duration. It appears that differences in consonant duration provide discriminating information which is not affected by the presence of noise" (p. 258).

Identification functions for nonsense syllables using natural voice or synthetic (computer generated) stimuli (usually with voiced and voiceless plosive consonants) have begun to delineate acoustic variables that influence the correct and incorrect identification of these consonants (e.g., Blumstein and Stevens, 1980; Dorman, Studdert-Kennedy, and Raphael, 1977; Van Tassell and Crump, 1981). Computer generation of the stimuli allows the experimenter to vary systematically and independently temporal and spectral characteristics, such as, duration, voice onset time, formant frequencies, formant transitions, and so on. Such investigations already have provided vital information regarding the importance of various acoustic cues such as voice onset time for the correct identification of nonsense syllables.

Similarly, as indicated by Kamm et al. (1980), computer storage of naturally spoken test items facilitates not only storage of test materials, but also their presentation in randomized orders, manipulation of presentation level, and so on. Computer storage also allows precise description of the time, frequency, and intensity features of a given sound, word, or group of words. Application of this technology should not only facilitate research in speech audiometry, but also can lend itself to clinical application in test administration, scoring, and analysis of responses. Additional investigations testing a variety of hearing-impaired subjects with computer-generated or computer-stored stimuli will provide important information relative to the speech cues being used correctly as well as erroneously by these individuals. Such information should have important implications for modification of speech stimuli necessary for improved understanding of speech by hearing-impaired individuals and for developing remediation programs.

Following the lead of Walden et al. (1981) in comparing the performance of the normal and impaired ear of unilateral hearing loss patients, it seems to this writer that it would be of particular interest to present synthetic speech stimuli to subjects having unilateral hearing losses. Such individuals can serve as their own controls to compare overall performance and error patterns when various features of the speech signal are varied systematically. For such subjects one might also attempt to modify the speech signal presented to the impaired ear such that it more closely resembled a normal signal delivered to the normal ear and vice versa. Hopefully, such efforts might lead to a better understanding of the manner in which speech stimuli are processed by impaired ears.

Another area in which there appropriately seems to be rekindled interest is the concept of the articulation index (American National Standards Institute, 1969; French and Steinberg, 1947; Kryter, 1962).

> The articulation index (AI) is based on . . . the effective proportion of the normal speech signal that is available to a listener for conveying speech intelligibility.
> AI is computed from acoustical measurements or estimates of the speech spectrum and of the effective masking spectrum of any noise which may be present along with the speech at the ear of a listener . . . The AI presumes to predict the relative performance of communication systems operating under given conditions when tested with a given group of typical talkers and listeners and when training and other listener-talker proficiency factors are kept constant or controlled for different tests by proper experimental procedures (American National Standards Institute, 1969; pp. 6, 23).

It is worth noting that Aniansson (1974) applied the concept of the AI to predict performance for his normal-hearing and hearing-impaired subjects responding to Swedish monosyllables presented in a noise background. Predicted and observed average scores agreed reasonably well. Aniansson cautioned, however, that scores were not predicted well for each individual because of individual variability. Dugal, Braida, and Durlach (1978) also found that predictions based on the articulation index agreed relatively well with data obtained independently by another investigator for six hearing-impaired subjects in a variety of listening conditions. Similarly, Dirks (1982) observed that the articulation index predicted the relative performance of hearing-impaired subjects for a nonsense syllable identification task. Given these observations for hearing-impaired subjects, the articulation index merits further investigation relative to the ability of hearing-impaired persons to use the speech spectra available to them.

Single Words, Sentences, Noise

Although the use of lists of monosyllabic words is most common for assessing speech understanding in speech audiometry, it is recognized that word recognition tests using open-ended word lists, or word identification tests using closed-set lists, does not represent everyday speech. However, Niemeyer's (1965) strategy of using the same words in meaningful sentences and randomized in lists of single words might be considered a means of assessing an individual's ability to use context and to recognize single words. Comparisons of performance for words heard in meaningful sentences and words heard in isolation should provide additional information of value for understanding problems in communication encountered by hearing-impaired individuals.

Similarly, addition of background noise to the test situation renders the test more difficult and more representative of communication problems encountered in noisy environments. Some tape recordings of test materials incorporate filtered noise mixed with the test items (Kruel et al., 1968) or competing speech on a second channel of the tape recording (e.g., Kalikow, Stevens, and Elliot, 1977).

A different approach utilizing meaningful prose presented in a noise background has been described by Speaks et al. (1972) and Gray and Speaks (1978). Rather than repeat (or write) words or sentences, Speaks et al. instructed their subjects to adjust the level of the speech to achieve 75, 50, or 25 percent understanding of the sentences or phrases heard from a tape-recorded short story. As a separate task these investigators also instructed their listeners to estimate in percent how much they understood of the prose passage for a given condition. Comparison of signal-to-noise ratios at which subjects estimated understanding a given percentage of the message in noise and signal-to-noise ratios at which key words in CID sentences were understood revealed a reasonably linear relationship. Gray and Speaks (1978) followed a similar strategy when instructing hearing-impaired subjects to estimate how well they understood connected discourse in quiet and in noise. Their observations indicated that all but three of 36 subjects repeated their estimates within ± 10 percent of the individual mean estimate for a given condition for at least ⅔ of the repeated measurements. Gray and Speaks suggested that this procedure ". . . should be useful when attempting to predict how well a patient will understand speech in various noise situations . . ." (p. 165). They cautioned that ". . . estimation of percentage of understanding is not a procedure that is appropriate to measure hearing handicap for all hearing impaired individuals. However, it appears to be a reasonable approach that could be used with a large segment of the hearing impaired population . . ." (p. 165). This approach appears to merit further investigation. Might such an approach be used in an attempt to validate other measures of word recognition, word identification, sentence identification, and so on as indicators of communicative difficulties experienced by normal hearers and hearing-impaired listeners in various listening situations?

Rather than instructing listeners to estimate percentage of speech understood, Dirks, Morgan, and Dubno (1982) used a procedure in which a preselected performance level is determined via an adaptive procedure (Levitt, 1971; Levitt and Rabiner, 1967). While spondees or monosyllables were maintained at three specific levels between 60 and 96 dB sound pressure level (SPL) the intensity of the competing speech babble was increased or decreased after each correct or incorrect response, respectively, to determine the signal-to-competition ratio required for 50 percent correct response. For a 29.3 percent correct response level the intensity of the competition was increased after an incorrect response, but decreased after two consecutive correct responses; the 70.7 percent performance point on the psychometric function was obtained by decreasing the level of the competition after an incorrect response and increasing the intensity of the competition after two consecutive correct responses. It was their observation that virtually all of their hearing-impaired subjects required a more advantageous signal-to-competition ratio to achieve the preselected performance level than did their normal-hearing subjects. They also observed that as the intensity of the test materials was increased, some hearing-impaired listeners required a less favorable signal-to-competition ratio for a given performance level than had been necessary when the test items were presented at lower intensities; however, for other hearing-impaired individuals the signal-to-noise ratio for a selected performance level remained constant in spite of increases in sound pressure level of the test materials. The authors suggested that such information might prove useful in assessing potential benefit of amplification for hearing-impaired individuals. They concluded that the adaptive procedure may provide a practical method for evaluating the relative effects of competition on speech recognition for individual listeners. Certainly, further work incorporating adaptive strategies for assessing speech understanding in a variety of conditions is indicated. Comparison of results obtained for the same subjects using the procedures described by Speaks et al. (1972) and Gray and Speaks (1978) and the adaptive procedure utilized by Dirks et al. (1982) is one area warranting further study.

OTHER PSYCHOACOUSTIC DATA AND SPEECH UNDERSTANDING

Just as there has been new (or renewed) interest in the features of the speech signal vital to correct perception, there is developing interest in the parameters of auditory function, other than hearing sensitivity, that are abnormal for hearing-impaired individuals. Particularly, what are the psychoacoustic phenomena that relate to the ability or inability of a hearing-impaired individual to understand speech in noise?

Frequency Resolution

Importantly, many of the careful psychoacoustic procedures developed and used to describe fine details of auditory function of normal-hearing individuals now are being applied to hearing-impaired subjects in an effort to describe their behavior in terms of differences from "normal" auditory function (e.g., Dreschler and Plomp, 1980; Florentine et al., 1980; Humes, 1982; Scharf, 1978). However, as carefully pointed out by Humes (1982), it is critical that comparisons of psychoacoustic performance of hearing-impaired subjects and normal hearers be made at equal sound pressure levels rather than equal sensation levels. For example, Humes noted that some reports of excess masking or excess spread of masking for hearing-impaired subjects have failed to consider the unmasked thresholds of the hearing-impaired individuals. Actually, the masked and unmasked thresholds may have been the same for some of the hearing-impaired subjects in frequency regions where no masker was present; but, because their masked thresholds were poorer than for the normal-hearing subjects, the results were interpreted as reflecting abnormal spread of masking, wider critical bandwidths, or poorer frequency resolution, and, hence, as an explanation for poorer speech understanding by the hearing-impaired subjects. Nelson and Bilger (1974), however, observed that the masked threshold for a signal one octave above a tonal masker was the same for normal and hearing-impaired subjects when the masked threshold of the normal hearers exceeded the unmasked threshold of the hearing-impaired subjects.

Similar cautions about interpretations of psychophysical tuning curves obtained for normal and for hearing-impaired subjects (e.g., Florentine et al., 1980) are indicated according to Humes (1982). When a tonal signal at $\simeq 10$ dB sensation level is masked by a pure tone masker varying in frequency and level to generate a psychophysical tuning curve, the signal and maskers are necessarily at higher sound pressure levels for hearing-impaired individuals than for normal hearers. The result is that at equal sensation levels the tuning curves are broader for the hearing-impaired subjects. It must be remembered that tuning curves become broader for normal listeners also at more intense signal levels.

Based on data from a study investigating speech understanding and frequency resolution as measured by pure tone thresholds in broad band noise, pure tone thresholds in the presence of a pure tone masker, and psychophysical tuning curves with normal-hearing and hearing-impaired individuals, Tyler, Wood, and Fernandes (1982) also noted many problems associated with measurements of frequency resolution. They stated that the "Three main areas of concern in measurement of frequency resolution in normals and hearing impaired subjects are: (1) interactions between the signal and masker; (2) off-frequency listening; and (3) the comparison of data at equal SPL or equal SL" (Tyler et al., 1982, p. 58). Use of psychophysical tuning curves was suggested by them as the method of choice, however, because it provided more specific information and was more applicable to individuals having more severe hearing losses. In statistical analysis of their data, these investigators noted the relationships between the degree of hearing loss, frequency resolution, and speech understanding; generally, the greater the hearing loss, the poorer the frequency resolution and the poorer the speech understanding. On the basis of correlational analysis of their results, they stated, "Partialing out threshold effects generally reduces the correlation between frequency resolution and speech intelligibility. This does not suggest that frequency resolution is unrelated to speech intelligibility; only that both are correlated highly with pure-tone threshold loss" (Tyler et al., 1982, p. 60). Tyler et al. completed their frequency resolution measurements in the 500- and 4000-Hz frequency regions. Hopefully, they and other investigators will continue to pursue such studies utilizing similar low and high frequencies and also other frequencies in the 1000- to 3000-Hz frequency region.

Temporal Resolution

Although frequency resolution capabilities of normal hearers and hearing-impaired subjects may be relatively similar at least for masked tones at high intensity levels, it appears that temporal resolution is poorer for individuals having sensorineural hearing losses than for normal hearers at all intensity levels. Irwin, Hinchcliff, and Kemp (1981) conducted gap detection experiments, which assess temporal resolution by requiring the listener to detect a brief interruption in a noise stimulus, testing normal-hearing and hearing-impaired subjects. Normal hearers could detect gaps on the order of 3 msec for stimuli presented at 50 to 90 dB SPL. Gap detection for the sensorineural hearing loss subjects was considerably poorer even at high sound pressure levels. Data are needed that compare temporal resolution, for example, gap detection or other experimental paradigms, to assess temporal resolution of normal and hearing-impaired ears and speech understanding. It remains to be determined if it is the speech spectra available to the listener, frequency resolution capabilities, temporal resolution capabilities, or some other feature(s) of auditory performance that are most important, or equally important, for normal-hearing and hearing-impaired individuals in hearing and understanding speech in quiet, and especially in noise.

Reaction Time

Another temporal parameter that merits further investigation in the opinion of this writer is the reaction time required for responses to speech stimuli. Hecker, Stevens, and Williams (1966) observed a consistent relationship between word identification scores for the modified rhyme test and reaction time, that is, the higher the score, the shorter the latency between presentation of the stimulus and the response. In comparing performance of three different microphones on the basis of percent correct and reaction times for two-word identification tests, Pratt (1981) found that only one of six comparisons reached statistical significance for the identification scores; however, three of six differences in reaction times were statistically significant. He suggested ". . . that a consideration of the subject's reaction time may increase the sensitivity of the test and permit finer distinctions to be made" (p. 255).

Using a different experimental paradigm, Reed (1975) compared nonsense syllable identification and reaction times for discriminating two nonsense syllables as "same" or "different" for normal-hearing and sensorineural hearing loss subjects. She found that not only did the identification scores for the two groups differ (as would be expected), but they seemed to process "same" and "different" responses differently also. Normal hearers generally provided "same" responses more quickly than "different" responses; whereas the reverse was observed for some of the hearing-impaired subjects. Reed interpreted these findings as indicating that the normal-hearing subjects processed the phonemes as codeable stimuli whereas the hearing-impaired listeners processed the signals as noncodeable stimuli. Performance on the discrimination task did not necessarily relate to performance on the identification task. Reed cautioned ". . . that the ability to discriminate between two sounds does not necessarily imply the ability to identify each of the two sounds. The processing demands on the auditory system are different for recognition and discrimination; and a person with hearing loss may be able to discriminate two sounds without being able to extract information from the auditory waveform necessary for labeling the phonemes" (p. 790).

Whether the interest is in speech spectra available to the listener, frequency resolution, temporal resolution, reaction time, or some other psychoacoustically measurable parameter, it seems to this writer that here too individuals having unilateral hearing losses could serve as useful research subjects for such investigations. As pointed out by many investigators, variability in performance among individuals is large for many of these tasks, especially for those having hearing losses. Unilateral hearing loss subjects can serve as their own controls and also could describe to the investigator how the stimulus differs for each ear, or how they approach the tasks using different strategies dependent upon whether the stimuli are heard via the normal ear or the impaired ear.

NEURAL CODING OF SPEECH

Electrophysiologic recording of response to speech stimuli from single units in the auditory nerve of animals provides exciting insights to neural transmission of speech information. Kiang and Moxon (1974) and Kiang (1980) have reported such data. As part of experiments investigating tuning curves for single units of the auditory nerve of cats, a tape loop of "shoo cat" was presented also for electrophysiologic recording of responses from the same nerve fibers. Tuning curves obtained with pure tone stimuli revealed best response to a particular frequency (characteristic frequency) with a sharp diminution in response to higher frequencies, but a more gradual decrease in response to frequencies below the characteristic frequency of each fiber. Introduction of masking noise centered at a frequency well below the characteristic frequency of a given nerve fiber revealed that responsiveness at its characteristic frequency was decreased considerably more than was the response at other frequencies. Kiang and Moxon (1974) interpreted these findings as indicating that nerve fibers having high characteristic frequencies also can carry considerable low-frequency information. Recordings of responses to "shoo cat" revealed considerable activity from low-frequency units (characteristic frequencies of 200 and 500 Hz), midfrequency fibers (1.5 kHz, characteristic frequency), and high frequency units (16 kHz and 30 kHz, characteristic frequencies). Addition of noise (low-pass filtered at 3000 Hz) soon "covered" the responses of the midfrequency units, but not the low-frequency units (noise level too low, according to Kiang and Moxon) nor the high-frequency units well above the low-pass noise band. For these conditions, then, single-unit responses to speech continued to be observed from fibers having low and high characteristic frequencies. Further exploration by Kiang and Moxon revealed that mixing even higher levels of low pass noise with the speech obscured changes in the firing rate of units having low characteristic frequencies, and the synchrony of firing was affected for units with high characteristic frequencies.

Applying this information to speech understanding in noise, Kiang and Moxon indicated that speech continues to be understood in a variety of conditions because of the "multiplicity of cues available." In the case of high-frequency hearing loss, however, there is loss of information from fibers having high characteristic frequencies not only for high-frequency speech components, but also for more intense low-frequency information. Only units with lower characteristic frequencies can carry the information; and moderate level low-frequency noise disrupts changes in their firing rates, too. Thus, normal ears can compensate for this loss of information from low-frequency units resulting from low-frequency background noise, because fibers with high characteristic frequencies could still carry the low-frequency information as well as the high-frequency information. However, high-frequency hearing loss with loss of units with high characteristic frequencies disrupts hearing not only of high-frequency speech components, but also low frequency speech components in low frequency noise backgrounds.

In a later publication Kiang (1980) showed neurograms (a display of neural activity for an entire array of nerve fibers) for "shoo cat" presented at different levels, interrupted 300 times per sec, in noise, center clipped, and peak clipped. As Kiang pointed out, there appears to be little relationship between the neurograms and the intelligibility of the speech stimulus. The neurogram for the high intensity "shoo cat" was altered considerably, but the speech was still intelligible. Interrupting the stimulus did not appreciably alter the neurogram, but the difference is clearly heard. Similarly, although "shoo cat" was still clearly intelligible in the noise, little if any synchrony of firing was seen in the neurogram. Furthermore, although center clipping markedly affects speech intelligibility considerably more than peak clipping, the neurograms were altered less for center clipped speech than for peak clipped speech. Kiang concluded that cues in neural firing patterns in terms of synchrony, subpopulations of fibers, and so on can be resolved ". . . by further research using presently available methods, but ultimate understanding requires more knowledge of how information contained in auditory nerve activity is processed by the central nervous system" (p. 835). Nevertheless, investigations of electrophysiologic responses to speech present exciting information to be pursued further.

ASSESSMENT OF CENTRAL AUDITORY NERVOUS SYSTEM FUNCTION

Kiang (1980) has noted the complexity of neural coding of speech signals in the auditory nerve and the lack of relation between observations of neurograms and the intelligibility of speech. This complexity is multiplied many times (figuratively and literally) in the central nervous system. As succinctly described by Lundborg et al. (1975), ≃30,000 fibers in the auditory nerve increase to ≃100,000 fibers at the level of the brainstem, to ≃400,000 auditory radiation fibers, and finally to more than 10,000,000 in the auditory cortex. Given this internal redundancy, and the external redundancy of multiple cues of speech signals, it is little wonder that difficult tasks must be developed to evaluate the central auditory nervous system.

Dichotic listening tasks provide unique opportunities to assess which speech cues are used most readily by the central auditory nervous system in identifying and differentiating various cues. For example, Speaks et al. (1981) presented voiced and voiceless plosive nonsense syllables dichotically to normal-hearing subjects and found that when competing against one another for identification, /pa/ and /ta/ were correctly identified significantly more often than /ba/ and /da/; /ka/ was heard correctly more often than /ta/, /ba/, /da/, and /ga/; /ga/ was identified correctly significantly more frequently than /pa/, /ba/, and /da/; /ba/ and /da/ were heard correctly least often. For eight of these 11 combinations in which a given nonsense syllable was heard correctly significantly more often than another, the dominant syllable was a voiceless plosive and seven of the eight involved a voiceless plosive over a voiced plosive. After reviewing various possible cues that might account for these observations, the authors concluded that greater peak intensity in the brief burst of frication noise at the moment of articulatory release for the dominant syllables could explain their findings. They cautioned, however, that other factors such as burst duration, voice, onset time, and aspiration energy also should be considered. They suggested that use of synthetic stimuli could help resolve such factors. Once again, it is apparent that use of computer generated stimuli in which various parameters of the signal can be varied individually and independently can provide information about auditory processing of speech sounds.

Use of synthetic stimuli in which the same formants, different formants, or portions of different formants are presented to the two ears allowed Cutting (1976) to describe six different fusions as products of central auditory nervous system function. If the first and second formants for /da/ are presented to both ears, sound localization occurs. If the formants of /ba/ are presented to one ear and formants for /ga/ are delivered to the other ear, psychoacoustic fusion takes place such that often the perception is neither /ba/ nor /ga/, but /da/. If the first formant of /da/ is presented to one ear and the second formant to the other ear, /da/ is heard because of spectral fusion by the central nervous system. When the first formant in its entirety and the steady state portion of the second formant for /da/ is delivered to one ear and only the second formant transition for /da/ is presented to the other ear, /da/ and a noise are heard for spectral/temporal fusion according to Cutting. Phonetic feature fusion occurs if formants for /ba/ are presented to one ear while formants for /ta/ arrive at the opposite ear and /da/ or /pa/ are heard. Presentation of three formants of /da/ to one side with three formants for /ra/ to the other results in the perception of /dra/ and, hence, phonologic fusion within the central auditory nervous system. Interestingly, investigation of other phonological fusions by Cutting and Day (1975) with formants for words such as bed, led, pay, lay, ray, red, go, low, row, paid, pail, and pair led them to conclude that their 68 normal listeners formed two distinct groups. For one group, fusion scores clustered around 39 percent with a range of 2 to 60 percent; for the other group the fusion scores clustered around 88 percent with a range of 70 to 100 percent. Certainly these observations on fusions in response to dichotic speech stimuli are intriguing and worthy of further investigation, not only to assess critical stimulus features for normal individuals, but also to assess performance of individuals having lesions in the central auditory nervous system.

Unfortunately, documenting the specific site of involvement in the central nervous system is problematic. Often it must be inferred from symptoms or radiologic studies. Even when a lesion is documented by radiologic studies or more precisely by surgical intervention, it must be remembered that a neoplasm or other type of lesion at one site can cause dysfunction from excess pressure or a compromise in blood supply at sites quite removed from the primary lesion. Nevertheless, much can be learned about central auditory processing of speech stimuli from dichotic listening studies with normal subjects and with patients having lesions of the central nervous system.

Also problematic in the assessment of function or dysfunction of the central auditory nervous system is the confounding influence of hearing loss. Speaks (1980) addressed this problem by stating, "Patients with central auditory deficits may have a coexisting peripheral impairment, unilateral or bilateral . . . The peripheral loss may exert a substantial effect on dichotic testing, thereby confounding the interpretation of central test findings . . . We cannot assume, in the absence of empirical evidence, that moving from difficult tests (e.g., CV nonsense syllables) to easy tests (e.g., digits or sentences) eliminates the contaminating influence of peripheral pathology on central tests" (p. 1858). In this light, the battery of five dichotic tests described by Niccum, Rubens, and Speaks (1981) merit consideration. They used digits: one, two, three, four, five, and six; high contrast words: pie, tree, cloud, book, door, and glove; vowel words: key, cow, car, bow, boy, and bear; consonant words: pan, fan, man, boat, coat, and goat; and nonsense CV syllables: /pa/, /ta/, /ka/, /ba/, /da/, and /ga/. The digits, and the high contrast, vowel, and consonant words can be depicted by pictures for presentation to individuals unable to respond in the oral mode. Presentation of these test materials to 16 aphasic patients revealed similar performance by these subjects for the digit, high contrast, and vowel word tests, and poorer performance for the consonant words presented dichotically. Sensitivity to dysfunction was better for the latter test. The dichotic consonant-vowel test materials proved too difficult for two of their patients and generally very difficult overall. It would seem to this writer, however, that these dichotic digit, high contrast, vowel, and consonant test materials merit investigation with hearing-impaired individuals who are otherwise "neurologically normal" in order to evaluate the influence of hearing loss on observed performance. As indicated by Speaks (1980), empirical evidence is needed to determine the presence or absence of the "contaminating influence of peripheral pathology on central tests" (p. 1858).

Recent technologic advances have allowed mapping activity of the human brain in awake subjects or patients in response to stimuli or when carrying out certain tasks by measuring metabolic activity in circumscribed regions of an intact human brain. As stated by Lassen, Ingvar, and Skinhøj (1978), ". . . during a test involving a specific type of cerebral function there is a local change in nerve cell activity and hence in the metabolic rate that gives rise to an increase in blood flow in a specific region" (p. 65). To measure this increase in blood flow, a radioactive isotope (xenon 133) dissolved in a saline solution is injected into one of the main arteries to the brain. Detectors placed near the head trace the movement of the radioactive isotope in the blood through the brain tissue of a single (either right or left) hemisphere. The signals from the detectors are processed by a computer and displayed on a television monitor. Different flow rates close to the surface of the cerebral cortex produce different colors on the television monitor. Using the technique, Lassen et al. (1978) observed that loud meaningless noises increased blood flow near the superior posterior portion of both temporal lobes. Flow in both areas was increased further upon hearing simple words such as "bang," "zoom," and "crack." More complex speech stimuli increased blood flow in the inferior posterior portion of the frontal lobe near Brocá's area.

Instead of injecting the radioactive material into a main artery of the brain which is an invasive technique restricted to use with patients who for diagnostic purposes must have cerebral arteriograms, it is now possible to inhale gases carrying a radioactive isotope (Stump and Williams, 1980). Hence, the inhalation technique for studying cerebral blood flow in specific regions of the cortex can be used with volunteer subjects including "normals." Another advantage of this method over the above-mentioned invasive technique is that data can be collected and analyzed from homologous areas of the brain tissue surface layers from both hemispheres simultaneously. Using the inhalation technique, Knopman et al. (1980) completed blood flow studies with normal subjects for a nonverbal and a verbal task. The nonverbal task was to discriminate between loud and soft noise bursts. In the verbal task the subjects were required to recognize a noun that meant something to eat in a list of other monosyllables. For both types of stimuli, statistically significant increases in blood flow were observed for the left hemisphere at a probe site just inferior to or straddling the Sylvian fissure posterior to the Rolandic fissure in the vicinity of Wernicke's area.

Another new method for studying functional brain activity in awake humans also based on measuring energy metabolism with a radioactive pharmaceutical is the recent application of positron emission tomography (PET) (Alavi et al., 1981; Toufexis, 1981). In the PET technique a radioactive tracer (^{18}F-2-deoxy-2-fluoro-D-glucose) is injected under local anesthesia via a radial artery catheter to awake volunteer subjects (including normals). This tracer is taken up by the brain at a rate proportional to that of glucose and its radioactive metabolic products remain trapped within the brain tissue for a sufficient period of time to be detected through the skull using position emission tomography. The PET technique can provide three-dimensional computer reconstructed images of areas of the brain that are activated by a specific sensory stimulus, thus permitting brain function to be mapped in awake humans. The PET technique has some important advantages over the regional cerebral blood flow methods, including substantially better resolution and computer reconstructed images in three rather than two dimensions. Greenberg et al. (1981) observed increased metabolic rate in the temporal lobe contralateral to the ear in which a factual story was heard. Attention to the verbal material was enhanced by informing the subjects that they would be questioned about the content of the story.

Such studies mark the beginning, no doubt, of work in mapping of metabolic activity in the cortex. Knopman et al. (1980) mentioned that they have begun to search for correlations between blood flow data and dichotic listening test results. Refinements of metabolic rate measurements in the future are likely to increase our understanding of processing of speech within the central nervous system. Cerebral blood flow studies and positron emission tomography investigations such as mentioned here suggest the start of a new and exciting era in the study of cerebral function including, of course, function of the central auditory nervous system.

SUMMARY

In this chapter, the author has attempted to review briefly some recent developments which, in his opinion, hold promise for improving speech audiometry. Study of features of speech stimuli critical to correct perception of speech sounds, other psychoacoustic phenomena and their relationship to speech understanding, use of computers for generating, storing, and analyzing speech stimuli, neural coding, and central auditory nervous system processing of speech were mentioned. Employing a variety of tests in evaluating the performance of the normal-hearing ear and the hearing-impaired ear of individuals having unilateral hearing losses is advocated.

REFERENCES

Alavi, A., M. Reivich, J. Greenberg, P. Hand, A. Rosenquist, W. Rintelmann, D. Christman, J. Fowler, A. Goldman, R. MacGregor, and A. Wolf. 1981. Mapping of functional activity in brain with ^{18}F-Fluoro-Deoxyglucose. Sem. Nucl. Med. 11:24–31.

American National Standards Institute. 1969. Methods for Calculation of the Articulation Index, ANSI-S3.5-1969. American National Standards Institute, New York.

Aniansson, G. 1974. Methods for assessing high frequency hearing loss in every-day listening situations. Acta Otolaryngol. (Suppl.) 320

Bilger, R. C., and M. D. Wang. 1976. Consonant confusions in patients with sensorineural hearing loss. J. Speech Hear. Res. 19:718–748.

Blumstein, S. E., and K. N. Stevens. 1980. Perceptual invariance and onset spectra for stop consonants in different vowel environments. J. Acoust. Soc. Am. 67:648–662.

Boothroyd, A. 1968. Developments in speech audiometry. Sound 2:3–10.

Cutting, J. E. 1976. Auditory and linguistic processes in speech perception: Influences from six fusions in dichotic listening. Psychol. Rev. 83:114–150.

Cutting, J. E., and R. S. Day. 1975. The perception of stop-liquid clusters in phonological fusion. J. Phonetics 3:99–113.

Dirks, D. D. Speech perception by the hearing impaired. In G. Studebaker and F. Bess (eds.) The Vanderbilt Hearing Aid Report. Monographs in Contemporary Audiology, Education Services Division, Instrumentation Associates, Inc., Upper Darby, Pa. In press.

Dirks, D. D., D. E. Morgan, and J. R. Dubno. 1982. A procedure for quantifying the effects of noise on speech recognition. J. Speech Hear. Disord. 47:114–123.

Dorman, D. E., M. Studdert-Kennedy, and L. J. Raphael. 1977. Stop consonant recognition: Release bursts and formant transitions as functionally equivalent, context dependent cues. Percept. Psychophysics 22:109–122.

Dreschler, W., and R. Plomp. 1980. Relation between psychophysical data

and speech perception for hearing impaired subjects. J. Acoust. Soc. Am. 68:1608–1615.
Dubno, J. R., and H. Levitt. 1981. Predicting consonant confusions from acoustic analysis. J. Acoust. Soc. Am. 69:249–262.
Dugal, R. L., L. D. Braida, and N. I. Durlach, 1978. Implications of previous research for the selection of frequency-gain characteristics. In G. A. Studebaker and I. Hochberg (eds.) Acoustical Factors Affecting Hearing Aid Performance, pp. 379–403. University Park Press, Baltimore.
Edgerton, B. J., and J. L. Danhauer. 1979. Clinical Implications of Speech Discrimination Testing Using Nonsense Stimuli. University Park Press, Baltimore.
Florentine, M., S. Buss, B. Scharf, and E. Zwicker. 1980. Frequency selectivity in normally-hearing and hearing-impaired observers. J. Speech Hear. Res. 23:646–669.
French, N. R., and J. R. Steinberg. 1947. Factors governing the intelligibility of speech. J. Acous. Soc. Am. 19:90–119.
Gengel, R. W. 1973. On the reliability of discrimination performance in persons with sensorineural hearing impairment using a closed set. J. Aud. Res. 13:97–100.
Gray, T. F., and C. E. Speaks. 1978. Ability of hearing impaired listeners to understand connected discourse. J. Am. Aud. Soc. 3:159–166.
Greenberg, J. H., M. Reivich, A. Alavi, P. Hand, A. Rosenquist, W. Rintelmann, A. Stein, R. Tusa, R. Dann, D. Christman, J. Fowler, R. MacGregor, and A. Wolf. 1981. Metabolic mapping of functional activity in human subjects with the [^{18}F] Fluorodeoxyglucose technique. Science 212:678–680.
Griffiths, J. D. 1967. Rhyming minimal contrasts: A simplified diagnostic articulation test. J. Acoust. Soc. Am. 42:235–241.
Hagerman, B. 1976. Reliability in the determination of speech discrimination. Scand. Audiol. 5:219–228.
Harris, J. D. 1980. On the use of a three-words-per-item format in tests for hearing of speech. J. Acoust. Soc. Am. 67:345–347.
Hecker, M. H. L., K. N. Stevens, and C. E. Williams. 1966. Measurements of reaction time for intelligibility tests. J. Acoust. Soc. Am. 39:1188–1189.
House, A. S., C. E. Williams, M. H. L. Hecker, and K. D. Kryter. 1965. Articulation testing methods. Consonantal differentiation in a closed-response set. J. Acoust. Soc. Am. 37:158–166.
Humes, L. E. Speech and temporal resolution by the hearing impaired. In G. Studebaker and F. Bess (eds.) The Vanderbilt Hearing Aid Report. Monographs in Contemporary Audiology, Education Services Division, Instrumentation Associates, Inc., Upper Darby, Pa. In press.
Irwin, R. J., L. K. Hinchcliff, and S. Kemp. 1981. Temporal acuity in normal and hearing impaired listeners. Audiology 20:234–243.
Kalikow, D. N., K. N. Stevens, and L. L. Elliott. 1977. Development of a test of speech intelligibility in noise using sentence materials with controlled word predictability. J. Acoust. Soc. Am. 61:1337–1351.
Kamm, C., E. C. Carterette, D. E. Morgan, and D. D. Dirks. 1980. Use of digitized speech materials in audiological research. J. Speech Hear. Res. 23:709–721.
Kiang, N. Y. S. 1980. Processing of speech by the auditory system. J. Acoust. Soc. Am. 68:830–835.

Kiang, N. Y. S., and E. C. Moxon. 1974. Tails of tuning curves of auditory nerve fibers. J. Acoust. Soc. Am. 55:620–630.

Knopman, D. S., A. B. Rubens, A. C. Klassen, M. W. Meyer, and N. Niccum. 1980. Regional cerebral blood flow patterns during verbal and nonverbal auditory aclivation. Brain Lang. 9:93–112.

Kruel, E. J., J. C. Nixon, K. D. Kryter, D. W. Bell, J. S. Lang, and E. D. Schubert. 1968. A proposed clinical test of speech discrimination. J. Speech Hear. Res. 11:536–552.

Kryter, K. D. 1962. Methods for calculation and use of the articulation index. J. Acoust. Soc. Am. 34:1689–1697.

LaCroix, P. G., and J. D. Harris. 1979. Effects of high-frequency cue reduction on the comprehension of distorted speech. J. Speech Hear. Disord. 44:236–246.

Lassen, M. A., D. H. Ingvar, and E. Skinhøj. 1978. Brain function and blood flow. Sci. Am. 239:62–71.

Levitt, H. 1971. Transformed up-down methods in psychoacoustics. J. Acoust. Soc. Am. 49:467–477.

Levitt. H., and L. R. Rabiner. 1967. Use of a sequential strategy in intelligibility testing. J. Acoust. Soc. Am. 42:609–612.

Levitt, H., and S. B. Resnick, 1978. Speech reception by the hearing impaired: Methods of testing and the development of new tests. Scand. Audiol. (Suppl.):107–130.

Lundborg, T., H. Rosenhamer, T. Murray, and N. Zwetnow. 1975. Information abundance of speech and speech testing in topical diagnosis within the C.N.S. Scand. Audiol. 4:9–17.

Markides, A. 1978. Whole-word scoring versus phoneme scoring in speech audiometry. Br. J. Audiol. 12:40–49.

Nabalek, A. K., and D. Mason. 1981. Effect of noise and reverberation on binaural and monaural word identification by subjects with various audiograms. J. Speech Hear. Res. 24:375–383.

Nelson, D. A., and R. C. Bilger. 1974. Pure-tone octave masking in listeners with sensorineural hearing loss. J. Speech Hear. Res. 17:252–269.

Niccum, N., A. B. Rubens, and C. Speaks. 1981. Effects of stimulus material on the dichotic listening performance of aphasic patients. J. Speech Hear. Res. 24:526–534.

Niemeyer, W. 1965. Speech audiometry with phonetically balanced sentences. Int. Audiol. 4:94–101.

Nixon, J. C. 1973. Investigation of the response for the modified rhyme hearing test. J. Speech Hear. Res. 16:658–666.

Olsen, W. O. 1981. The effects of noise and reverberation on speech intelligibility. In F. H. Bess, B. A. Freeman, and J. S. Sinclair (eds.), Amplification in Education, pp. 151–163. Alexander Graham Bell Association for the Deaf. Washington, D.C.

Owens, E. 1978. Consonant errors and remediation in sensorineural hearing loss. J. Speech Hear. Disord. 43:331–347.

Owens, E., M. Benedict, and E. D. Schubert. 1972. Consonant phonemic errors associated with pure-tone configurations and certain kinds of hearing impairments. J. Speech Hear. Res. 15:308–322.

Owens, E., and E. D. Schubert. 1977. Development of the California Consonant Test. J. Speech Hear. Res. 20:463–474.

Oyer, H. J., and M. Doudna. 1959. Structural analysis of word responses made by hard of hearing subjects on a discrimination test. Arch. Otolaryngol. 70:357–363.

Pederson, O. T., and G. A. Studebaker. 1972. A new minimal contrasts closed-response-set speech test. J. Aud. Res. 12:187–195.
Pratt, R. L. 1981. On the use of reaction time as a measure of intelligibility. Br. J. Audiol. 15:253–255.
Raffin, M. H. M., and D. Schafer. 1980. Application of a probability model based on the binomial distribution to speech-discrimination scores. J. Speech Hear. Res. 23:570–575.
Raffin, M. J. M., and A. R. Thornton. 1980. Confidence levels for differences between speech discrimination scores. J. Speech Hear. Res. 23:5–18.
Reed, C. 1975. Identification and discrimination of vowel-consonant syllables in listeners with sensori-neural hearing loss. J. Speech Hear. Res. 18:773–794.
Resnick, S. B., J. R. Dubno, S. Hoffnung, and H. Levitt. 1975. Phoneme errors on a nonsense syllable test. J. Acoust. Soc. Am. 58:S114.
Scharf, B. 1978. Comparison of normal and impaired hearing. II. Frequency analysis, speech perception. Scand. Audiol. (Suppl.):81–106.
Schultz, M. C., and E. D. Schubert. 1969. A multiple choice discrimination test (MCDT). Laryngoscope 79:382–399.
Sergeant, L., J. E. Atkinson, and P. G. LaCroix. 1979. The NSMRL tri-word test of intelligiblity (TTI). J. Acoust. Soc. Am. 65:218–222.
Sher, A. E., and E. Owens, 1974. Consonant confusions associated with hearing loss above 2000 Hz. J. Speech Hear. Res. 17:669–681.
Speaks, C. 1980. The evaluation of disorders of the central auditory system. In M. M. Paparella, and D. A. Shumrick (eds.), Otolaryngology. Volume II, The Ear. pp. 1846–1960. W. B. Saunders Company, Philadelphia.
Speaks, C. E., Carney, N. Niccum, and C. Johnson. 1981. Stimulus dominance in dichotic listening. J. Speech Hear. Res. 24:430–437.
Speaks, C., B. Parker, C. Harris, and P. Kuhl. 1972. Intelligiblity of connected discourse. J. Speech Hear. Res. 15:590–602.
Stevenson, P. W. 1975. Responses to speech audiometry and phonemic discrimination patterns in the elderly. Audiology 14:185–231.
Stump, D. A., and R. Williams. 1980. The noninvasive measurement of regional blood circulation. Brain Lang. 9:35–46.
Thornton, A. R., and M. J. M. Raffin. 1978. Binomial characteristics of speech discrimination scores. J. Speech Hear. Res. 21:507–518.
Toufexis, A. 1981. A brain marvel called PET. Time Sept. 14:74.
Tyler, R. S., E. J. Wood, M. Fernandes. 1982. Frequency resolution of hearing loss. Br. J. Audiol. 16:45–63.
Van Tassell, D. J., and E. S. A. Crump. 1981. Effects of stimulus level on perception of two acoustic cues in speech. J. Acoust. Soc. Am. 70:1527–1529.
Walden, B. E., D. M. Schwartz, A. A. Montgomery, and R. A. Prosek. 1981. A comparison of the effects of hearing impairment and acoustic filtering on consonant recognition. J. Speech Hear. Res. 24:32–43.
Wang, M. D., C. M. Reed, and R. C. Bilger, 1978. A comparison of the effects of filtering and sensorineural hearing loss on patterns of consonant confusions. J. Speech Hear. Res. 21:5–36.
Webster, J. C. 1972. Compendium of Speech Testing Material on Typical Noise Spectra for Use in Evaluating Communications Equipment. Technical Document 191. Human Factors Technology Division. Naval Electronics Laboratory Center, San Diego, California.

Author Index

Abbs, J. H., 47, 50
Achor, L. J., 264, 276, 283
Adams, K. M., 250, 276
Alavi, A., 391, 392, 393
Alencewicz, C. M., 204, 226
Alpiner, J. G., 189, 191, 214, 225, 358, 362, 363, 370
Altschuler, M. W., 214, 226
Anderson, C. M., 208-209, 228
Anianssen, G., 174, 191, 380, 392
Antablin, J. K., 105, 126, 138, 201
Antonelli, A., 233, 235, 236, 249, 276-277
Applebaum, E. L., 250, 262
Asp, G. J., 369-370
Aspinall, K. B., 166, 191
Atherly, G. R. C., 175, 198
Atkinson, C. J., 163, 197
Atkinson, J. E., 378, 395

Bailey, H. A. T., 159, 198, 316, 318
Ball, K., 148, 156, 194
Bamford, J. M., 147, 154, 192
Barber, C. G., 366, 374
Barford, J., 347, 350
Barney, H. L., 35, 45, 52
Barry, S. J., 171, 191
Beasley, D. S., 42, 51, 133, 161, 164, 170, 197, 199, 232, 237, 238, 252, 256-259, 276, 278, 280, 282
Beattie, R. C., 85, 122, 133, 135, 161, 165, 169, 191-193, 211, 226, 335, 338, 339, 344, 350
Beck, E. L., 333, 351
Beck, L. B., 333, 350
Becker, M., 321, 351
Bell, D. N., 7, 10, 99, 100, 124, 136, 160, 161, 196, 357, 372, 378, 381, 394
Bench, J., 147, 154, 192
Benedict, M., 139, 198, 358, 373, 376, 394
Benitez, J. T., 235, 280
Benson, R. W., 7, 10, 19, 24, 104, 105, 124, 132, 148, 195, 354, 372
Berg, F. S., 363, 365, 369
Berger, K. N., 361, 371
Berger, K. W., 204, 207, 214, 218, 220, 225, 226, 361, 371
Bergman, M., 235, 237, 238, 276, 277
Berlin, C. I., 233, 241, 247, 248, 259, 264, 277
Berlin, H. L., 277, 259, 280, 281
Berry, C., 369, 370
Berry, J. 369, 370
Bess, F. H., 8, 9, 42, 50, 51, 127, 128, 134, 157, 165, 168, 169, 171, 175, 183, 185, 192, 193, 195, 200, 237, 238, 280, 335, 338, 344, 352
Bettsworth, A., 112, 123, 185, 186, 193
Bickford, B. J., 333, 352
Bilger, R. C., 89, 122, 169, 200, 338, 344, 352, 356, 362, 371, 376, 377, 383, 392, 394, 395
Billger, J. M., 252, 255, 283
Binnie, C. A., 366, 371
Birk-Nielsen, H., 175, 194
Blegvad, B., 204, 220, 228
Blesser, B., 368, 371
Block, M. G., 74, 75, 78
Blosser, D., 166, 196, 204, 220, 323, 351
Blumstein, S. E., 47, 50, 379, 392
Bocca, E., 232, 235, 236, 242, 249, 277
Bode, D. L., 162, 192

Author Index

Boothroyd, A., 133, 192, 354, 371, 378, 392
Borden, G. L., 50
Bosatra, A., 204, 226
Bouwmeester, I., 183, 193
Bower, D. R., 112, 123, 185, 186, 193, 210, 211, 214, 227, 305–307, 318
Bowling, L. S., 95, 100, 102, 103, 122
Bowman, W. D., 113, 124
Bradley, W. A., 171, 195
Braisa, L. D., 380, 393
Brandy, W. T., 7, 10, 160, 192
Bratt, G. W., 175, 192, 238, 276
Breakey, M. R., 74, 75, 77, 119, 122
Broadbent, D. E., 246, 277
Brooks, R., 156, 192
Browning, K. M., 133, 201
Brunt, M., 241, 244, 245, 256, 277
Bryant, W. S., 90, 122
Bucheit, W., 239, 279
Buchwald, J. S., 263, 277
Bucy, P. C., 249, 283
Buining, E., 316, 319
Burchfield, S. A., 133, 161, 164, 170, 199
Burgi, E. J., 163, 197
Burke, K. S., 164, 192, 200
Burkhard, M. D., 216, 228, 335, 350
Burney, P. A., 321, 350
Buss, S., 383, 393
Byrke, D. 218, 224, 226

Cager, D. W., 211, 226
Calearo, C., 232, 233, 235–237, 242, 249, 277
Caley, K. E., 133, 201
Campanelli, P. A., 164, 192
Campbell, G. A., 128, 192
Campbell, R. A., 162, 192
Carhart, R., 8, 10, 41, 52, 104, 111, 122–124, 132, 148, 161, 162, 166, 168, 175, 187, 188, 192, 193, 201, 204, 226, 237, 239, 241, 243, 249 250, 262, 263, 279, 281–283, 305–307, 318, 319, 321–328, 331, 338–340, 348–350, 354, 363, 371
Carney, A. E., 44, 50, 388, 395

Carr, R. R., 116, 123
Carter, C. W., 18, 24
Carterette, E. C., 379, 393
Carver, W. F., 161, 193, 224, 226
Cassinari, V., 232, 235, 277
Causey, G. D., 174, 194
Cervellera, G., 236, 237, 262
Chaiklin, J. B., 85, 104, 113, 123, 126, 163, 198
Chermak, G., 321, 350
Cherow-Skalka, E., 146, 158, 194
Cherry, C., 99, 123
Cherry, E. C., 249, 277
Christen, R., 218, 224, 226
Christman, D., 391–393
Church, G., 238, 278
Clack, T. D., 141, 183, 193, 195
Clark, J. G., 256, 281
Clark, T., 369, 371
Clefft, I., 192
Clemis, J. D., 161, 193, 224, 226, 262, 277
Clevenger, J. P., 161, 193
Cohen, R. L., 184, 193
Coles, R. R. A., 313, 318
Collins, M. J., 188, 197
Colten, S., 183, 198
Conn, M., 100–102, 123
Connors, S., 148, 156, 194
Cooley, J. W., 29, 50
Cooper, F. S., 44–47, 49–52 47, 49
Cooper, J. C., 170, 193
Corbit, J. D., 47, 49, 50
Costello, J. M., 363, 371
Costello, M. R., 253, 277, 278
Cox, B. P., 95, 100, 102, 103, 123
Cox, R. M., 216, 217, 223, 226, 334–337, 346, 350, 352
Cramer, K. D., 89, 123
Creston, J., 164, 200
Crowley, A. L., 339, 340, 342, 347, 351
Crump, E. S. A., 379, 395
Cullen, J. K., Jr., 241, 247, 250, 259, 260, 277, 280, 283
Curry, E. T., 95, 100, 102, 103, 123, 163, 197
Cutts, B. P., 170, 193
Cutting, J. E., 388, 389, 392

Author Index

Dadson, R. S., 206, 228
Dalsgaard, S. C., 335, 350
Daly, D. D., 246, 282
Damianopoulous, E., 316, 319
Dancer, J., 100–102, 123
Danaher, E. M., 183, 193, 333, 350
Danhauer, J. L., 129, 170, 193, 356, 371, 378, 393
Dann, R., 391, 393
Davis, H., 7, 10, 16–19, 21–24, 44, 52, 74, 75, 77, 85, 93, 104, 105, 112, 119, 122, 124, 126, 128, 132, 140, 148, 173, 193, 195, 200, 211, 226, 354, 355, 371, 372
Dawson, G. J., 260, 281
Day, R. S., 389, 392
Dayal, V. S., 239, 278
deBoer, E. J., 183, 193
Decker, R. L., 84, 100, 113, 125
De Filippo, C. L., 367, 371
Delattre, P. C., 45, 46, 50, 51, 52
Delk, J. H., 111, 125
Dempsey, C., 252, 278
Denenberg, L. J., 214, 226
deQuiros, J., 232, 236, 278
Derlacki, E. L., 262, 277
Dermody, P., 259, 260
Dewey, G., 17, 24, 130, 132, 193
DiGiovanni, D., 317, 318
Dirks, D. D., 8, 10, 63, 74, 75, 104, 106–108, 112, 113, 117, 119, 123, 125, 126, 141, 142, 145, 175, 185, 186, 193, 203–215, 218–222, 226, 227, 243, 279, 305–307, 316, 318, 327, 350, 356, 371, 379, 380, 382, 392, 393
Disarno, N. J., 163, 193
Dixon, R. F., 104, 123
Dobie, R. A., 264, 277
Doerfler, L. G., 19, 24, 55, 77
Dorman, D. E., 379, 392
Dorman, M. F., 47, 50
Doudna, M., 358, 377, 394
Downs, M. P., 110, 125
Dreschler, W., 383, 392
Dubno, J. R., 129, 130, 188, 197, 199, 333, 351, 356, 371, 378, 379, 382, 392, 393, 395
Dudley, B., 103, 126
Duffy, J. R., 141, 194

Dugal, R. L., 380, 393
Dumbleton, C., 145, 199
Dunn, H. K., 31, 51
Durlach, N. I., 380, 393
Durrant, J. D., 232, 278

Eagles, E. L., 55, 77
Edgerton, B. J., 85, 100, 122, 129, 133, 135, 161, 165, 169, 191, 192, 193, 211, 226, 335, 338, 339, 344, 350, 356, 371, 378, 393
Edman, T. R., 44, 52
Eilers, R. E., 48, 50, 158, 193
Eimas, P. D., 47–50, 52
Eisenberg, R. B., 110, 123
Eisenbrey, A. B., 235, 280
Egan, J. P., 17, 18, 24, 130, 131, 166, 169, 182, 193, 354, 371
Egolf, D. P., 216, 226
Eldert, E., 7, 10, 19, 24, 104, 105, 124, 132, 148, 195, 354, 372
Elkins, E., 174, 193, 194
Elliott, L. L., 142, 147–149, 156, 194, 196, 362, 372, 381, 393
Elman, J. L., 48, 51
Elpern, B. S., 95, 100, 102, 103, 164, 194, 224, 226
Enfield, M. L., 256, 279
Epstein, A., 355, 371
Erber, N. P., 89, 123, 147, 150, 151, 152, 172, 194, 204, 226, 369, 371
Erdman, S. A., 356, 366, 374
Everitt, W., 236, 237, 278
Ewertson, H. W., 175, 194

Fairbanks, G., 136, 166, 175, 194, 195, 236, 237, 278, 357, 371
Faist, L. H., 369, 374
Falconer, G. A., 16, 24
Fant, C. G. M., 31, 33, 35, 37, 49, 51
Farrell, D. R., 333, 352
Favor, C., 369, 374
Feldmann, H., 89, 91, 123
Fernandes, M., 384, 395
Feth, L. L., 216, 226
Finitzo-Hieber, T., 146, 158, 194
Finney, D. J., 106–107
Fisher, L. B., 188, 194

Flaherty-Rintelmann, A., 258, 276
Flake, C., 145, 200
Fleischer-Gallagher, A. M., 260, 283
Fletcher, H., 11-14, 24, 85, 89, 90, 91, 93, 110, 113, 123, 128, 194
Fletcher, S. G., 40, 51
Florentine, M., 383, 393
Flottorp, G., 207, 221, 229
Flower, R. M., 112, 113, 124
Flowers, A., 253, 278
Font, J., 104, 123
Forbis, N. K., 7, 8, 10, 132, 134, 159, 164, 198, 286, 295, 311, 318
Forman, B., 237, 276
Fowler, E. P. 111, 124
Fowler, J., 391-393
Francis, S. L., 369, 374
Frankmann, J. P., 363, 373
Freeman, B. A., 238, 258, 259, 276, 278
Freeman, J., 333, 351
Freeman, L., 129, 130, 199
French, N. R., 18, 24, 40, 41, 51, 112, 124, 182, 194, 333, 350, 380, 393
Fristoe, M., 146, 194

Gabrielsson, A., 333, 350
Gaddis, S., 171, 191
Gardner, W. H., 113, 125
Gatling, L. W., 219, 228
Gengel, R. W., 160, 169, 194, 377, 393
Gerber, S. E., 41, 51, 188, 194
Gerlin, I. J., 146, 158, 194
Gerstman, L. J., 45, 46, 50, 51, 52
Geschwind, N., 246, 283
Gibler, A., 157, 192
Gilman, S., 216, 226
Gilroy, J., 234-236, 242, 244, 245, 248, 249-251, 254, 278, 280
Giolas, T. G., 141, 175, 194, 355, 362, 367, 371
Gladstone, V. S., 159, 194
Glantz, J., 316, 319
Glasscock, M. E., 175, 192, 199
Glorig, A., 111, 125, 166, 175, 195
Goetzinger, C. P., 156, 164, 166, 171, 192, 194, 196, 354,372
Goldman, A., 391, 392

Goldman, R., 146, 194
Goldstein, D. P., 332-334, 347, 350, 352
Goldstein, R., 232, 278
Goodglass, H., 246, 278, 282, 283
Goodman, A., 232, 278
Graham, J. T., 111, 124
Gravel, J. S., 134, 195
Gray, T. F., 335, 350, 381, 382, 393
Green, D. M., 1, 10, 80-82, 112, 124
Green, E. J., 365, 372
Greenberg, J., 391-393
Greetis, E. S., 305-307, 318
Griffiths, J. D., 136, 195, 357, 372, 378, 393
Grimm, D., 161, 201
Gruber, J., 89, 124
Grubb, P., 164, 166, 195
Guerkink, N. A., 252, 261, 281

Haenel, J. L., 133, 201
Hagberg, E. N., 204, 214, 226
Hagerman, B., 168, 195, 376, 393
Hahlbrock, K., 171, 195
Haines, H. L., 111, 124, 141, 195, 361, 372
Halle, M., 38, 49, 51
Hammer, L. C., 239, 278
Hampton, D. B., 367, 374
Hand, P., 391-393
Harbert, F., 183, 195, 317, 319
Harriman, E., 367, 374
Harris, J. D., 111, 124, 141, 195, 355, 361, 372, 377, 378, 381, 382, 393-395
Harris, K. S., 50
Harris, R. W., 333, 334, 347, 350
Harris, W. D., 367, 374
Hart, C. W., 239, 243, 250, 262, 281
Haskins, H. A., 145, 146, 195
Haspiel, G., 146, 200
Hass, W., 153, 201
Hattler, K. W. 166, 198
Hawkins, C. P., 259, 260, 278
Hawkins, D. B., 205, 216, 217, 226
Hawkins, J. E., 15, 16, 24, 85, 91-92, 104-105, 113, 124, 196, 306, 318
Hawkins, R. R., 159, 198
Hawley, M. E., 90, 124

Author Index

Hayashi, R., 233, 249, 278, 281
Hayes, D., 162, 187, 188, 196, 240, 279
Haynes, D., 327-331, 339, 344, 351
Hecker, M. H. L., 136, 195, 357, 372, 378, 385, 393
Hedgecock, L. D., 347, 350
Heilman, K. M., 239, 278
Heinz, J. M., 45, 51
Hennebert, D., 249, 278
High, W. S., 166, 175, 195
Hill, W., 220, 228
Hinchcliff, L. K., 384, 393
Hinchcliffe, R., 204, 226
Hipskind, N. M., 214, 227
Hirsh, I. J., 7, 10, 19, 22, 24, 85, 92, 93, 104, 105, 113, 124, 132, 140, 148, 169, 190, 195, 200, 250, 278, 338, 344, 352, 354, 355, 361, 369, 371, 373
Hixon, T. J., 37, 52
Hochberg, I., 220, 227
Hochberg, J., 47, 51
Hodgson, W. R., 164, 196, 223, 227, 232, 235, 278
Hoel, R., 183, 200
Hoffnung, S., 129, 130, 199, 333, 335-337, 346, 351, 352, 378, 395
Holland, A. L., 363, 372
Holmes, D. W., 214, 227, 228
Hood, J. D., 7, 10, 160, 176, 181, 195, 204, 207, 210-212, 227, 312, 318
Hood, R. B., 325, 350
Hoople, G., 171, 195
Horton, K., 369, 372
House, A. S., 35, 40, 43, 44, 52, 136, 195, 357, 372, 378, 393
Howard, M. T., 332, 333, 335, 346, 351
Howie, D. G., 129, 130, 199, 333, 351
Huang, C. M., 263, 277
Hudgins, C. V., 15, 16, 24, 91, 92, 104-105, 144, 195, 211, 226
Hughes, G. W., 38, 51
Hughes, L. F., 259, 277, 281
Hughson, W., 89, 91, 111, 124, 321, 350
Humes, L. E., 169, 185, 192, 195, 383, 393

Huntington, D. A., 174, 199
Hutcherson, R. W., 141, 142, 195

Illmer, R., 252, 255, 279
Ingham, J., 316, 318
Ingvar, D. H., 390, 394
Irons, F., 368, 374
Irwin, R. J., 384, 393
Isard, S., 367, 372

Jackson, P. L., 366, 371
Jakobson, R., 49, 51
Jacquat, W. S., 156, 196
Jaeger, R., 236, 237, 278
Jannetta, P. J., 247, 248, 277
Jeffers, J., 332, 350
Jerger, J., 8, 10, 84, 100, 104, 112, 124, 126, 133, 140, 143, 147, 162, 169, 174, 175, 177, 183-188, 191, 195, 196, 204, 227, 234, 235, 240-243, 245, 278, 279, 283, 310, 318, 327-331, 339, 344, 351, 361, 374
Jerger, S., 84, 104, 112, 124, 140, 155, 162, 174, 175, 184-186, 196, 204, 227, 234, 235, 240, 241, 243, 245, 263, 279
Jerome, J. J., 339, 340, 342, 347, 351
Jetty, A. J., 133, 161, 164, 170, 199
Jirsa, R. E., 164, 196
Johnson, C., 305, 306, 318, 388, 395
Johnson, D. W., 256, 279
Johnson, E. W., 119, 124, 175, 196
Johnson, J. I., 204, 217-221, 228
Johnson, R. M., 74, 75, 78, 112, 126
Johnston, K. L., 258, 280
Jokinen, K., 249, 282
Jones, C. I., 366, 374
Jones, J. H., 90, 91, 124, 321, 351
Jones, K. O., 148, 156, 196
Jones, P. L., 259, 260, 278
Josey, A. F., 175, 185, 192, 199
Jusczyk, P., 48, 50

Kalikow, D. N., 142, 196, 362, 372, 381, 393
Kamm, C., 112, 123, 185, 186, 193, 204, 209-214, 218-222, 226, 227, 379, 393

Author Index

Kärber, G., 107, 124
Karlin, J. E., 15, 16, 24, 91, 92, 104, 105, 124
Kasden, S., 171, 196, 199
Katz, D., 147–149, 156, 194, 196
Katz, J., 241, 244, 245, 252, 255, 279
Katinsky, S., 239, 279
Keating, L. W., 361, 371
Keith, R. W., 169, 184, 193, 196, 252, 280
Kelsey, P. A., 141, 195
Kemps, S., 384, 393
Kiang, N. Y. S., 112, 124, 386, 387, 393
Kille, E., 148, 156, 194
Killion, M. C., 74, 75, 77, 329, 351
Kimura, D., 233, 245–247, 280
King, R., 232, 278
King, W. P., 164, 192
Kirkpatrick, L. L., 247, 280
Kiukaanniemi, H., 182, 183, 196
Klassen, A. C., 391, 393
Kline, D. G., 247, 248, 277
Klodd, D. A., 165, 193, 335, 338, 344, 350
Knopman, D. S., 391, 393
Knox, A. W., 159, 197
Knudsen, V. O., 90, 91, 124, 321, 351
Koen, M., 368, 373
Koenig, W., 18, 24, 31, 51
Konkle, D. F., 1, 42, 51, 55, 134, 195, 232, 237, 238, 261, 280, 283
Kopra, L. L., 166, 196, 204, 220, 227, 323, 351
Korsan-Bengtsen, M., 235, 238, 280
Koval, A., 147, 154, 192
Krogh, H. J., 204, 220, 228
Kruel, E. J., 7, 10, 99, 100, 124, 136, 160, 161, 196, 357, 372, 378, 381, 394
Kryter, K. D., 7, 10, 112, 124, 136, 160, 161, 195, 196, 357, 372, 378, 380, 381, 393, 394
Kuhl, P. K., 48, 51, 381, 382, 395
Kupperman, G. L., 160, 194
Kurdziel, S., 169, 198, 234, 237–240 243, 250, 262, 280–282

Lacroix, P. G., 355, 361, 372, 378, 394, 395

Lacy, L. Y. 31, 51
Ladefoged, P., 33, 51
Lamb, S. H., 175, 194, 362, 367, 371
Lambert, W. E., 367, 373
Landes, B., 149, 198
Lane, C., 316, 319
Lang, J. S., 7, 10, 136, 160, 161, 196, 357, 372, 378, 381, 394
Langhofer, 356, 371
LaRiviere, C., 367, 374
Larson, G. W., 156, 196
Larson, L. L., 358, 372
Larson, V. D., 165, 169, 200, 335, 338, 344, 352
Lasky, E. Z., 162, 192
Lassen, M. A., 390, 394
Lazzaroni, A., 232, 236, 237, 277
Leatherwood, R. W., 333, 350
Lee, F., 238, 280
Lehiste, I., 132, 138, 197
Leiser, R. P., 251, 280
Leppler, J. G., 170, 193
Lerman, J. W., 146, 149, 197, 256, 282
Leshowitz, B., 183, 197
Leventhal, G., 367, 372
Levin, S., 148, 156, 194
Levitt, A., 114, 125
Levitt, H., 10, 38–40, 51, 116, 125, 128, 129, 131, 148, 162, 163, 188, 197, 209, 210, 227, 356, 372, 378, 379, 382, 393, 394, 395
LeWarre, R. M., 356, 371
Lewis, S., 196
Libby, E. R., 329, 351
Liberman, A. M., 44–47, 49–52, 247, 282
Lichtwitz, L., 90, 125
Licklider, J. C. R., 40, 42, 51, 85, 125, 250, 280
Liden, G., 113, 125, 182–184, 197, 308, 318
Lieberman, P., 367, 372
Linden, A., 233, 249, 380
Lindner, W. A., 82, 125
Lindstrom, R., 183, 197
Ling, D., 147, 157, 197
Lipke, D. W., 97, 126
Lorge, L., 132, 138, 143, 144, 200
Lovrinic, J. H., 163, 197, 232, 239, 279

Author Index

Lowe-Bell, S., 247, 248, 259, 277
Lowe, S. S., 233, 241, 247, 248, 259, 277, 280
Lowry, J. F., 218, 220, 226
Lozar, J., 333, 352
Lundborg, T. H., 238, 280, 388, 394
Lybarger, S. F., 216, 227
Lynn, G. E., 165, 197, 231, 234–238, 242, 244, 245, 248–254, 278, 280, 282

McCandless, G., 204, 207, 212, 225, 227
McConnell, F., 338, 339, 351
McDonald, D., 338, 339, 351
McDonald, V. B., 339, 340, 342, 347, 351
McGinnis, M. S., 163, 193
McLaughlin, R. M., 149, 197
McLennan, R. O., Jr., 159, 197
McNamee, J., 156, 197
McPherson, L. T., 323, 352
MacMillan, N. A., 85, 125
MacGregor, R., 391–393
Madory, R. D., 188, 197, 339, 351
Maki, J. E., 164, 197, 238, 256, 257, 258
Malmquist, C., 169, 196, 316, 318, 339, 351
Mangabeira-Albernaz, P., 316, 318
Manning, W. H., 164, 197, 258, 280
Mansur, R., 145, 197
Margolis, R. H., 79, 214, 227, 228
Markides, A., 164, 197, 378, 394
Markle, D., 204, 227
Marquis, R. J., 211, 226
Martin, E. S., 183, 197, 198, 333, 351
Martin, F. N., 1, 7, 8, 10, 132, 134, 159, 163, 164, 198, 220, 227, 256, 281, 286, 287, 298, 311, 316–318,
Martin, M. C., 221, 227
Mason, D., 376, 394
Matkin, N. D., 8, 10, 89, 109, 125, 128, 133, 144, 158, 162, 164, 168, 169, 172, 173–175, 354, 372
Matzker, J., 232, 233, 242, 248, 249, 265, 281
Matthews, J., 363, 372
Melnick, W., 55, 62, 63, 169, 170, 200
Mermelstein, P. 45, 52

Merrell, H. B., 163, 197
Meyer, M. W., 391, 393
Mickey, R., 204, 209, 212, 213, 220–222, 227
Migliavacca, F., 233, 235, 277
Mikus, B., 238, 282
Miller, D. L., 204, 207, 212
Miller, G. A., 40, 42, 44, 51, 52, 85, 125, 169, 198, 356, 358, 365–367, 372
Miller, G. W., 175, 192
Miller, J. D., 48, 51, 232, 261, 283
Miller, L. S., 169, 194
Milner, B., 246, 281
Miltenberger, G. E., 260, 281
Minifie, F. D., 37, 52
Mirabile, P. J., 259, 281
Montgomery, A. A., 333, 337, 344, 346, 347, 351, 352, 356, 366, 371, 374, 377, 379, 395
Moore, J. M., 158, 193, 198, 201, 367, 372
Morgan, D. E., 63, 77, 104, 106, 141, 142, 195, 203, 205–211, 214, 215, 227, 327, 350, 379, 382, 392, 393
Morales-Garcia, C., 239, 281
Morimoto, M., 233, 249, 278, 281
Morton, J., 368, 372
Mosher, N. A., 133, 161, 164, 170, 199
Moxon, E. C., 112, 124, 386, 393
Munson, W., 113, 123
Murray, T., 238, 280, 388, 394
Musiek, F. E., 235, 239, 244, 245, 246, 247, 250, 252, 261, 262, 281
Mussell, S. A., 331, 351
Myatt, B., 149, 198
Myers, C. K., 111, 124, 361, 372

Nabalek, A. K., 376, 394
Nelson, D. A., 163, 198, 383, 394
Neutzel, J. M., 362, 371
Newby, H. A., 104, 112, 125, 174, 199
Niccum, N., 391, 393, 395
Nicely, P., 356, 358, 365, 366, 372
Nichols, R. H., 211, 226
Nickel, B., 246, 283
Nielson, K., 156, 198

Author Index

Niemeyer, W., 174, 198, 381, 394
Nigro, G. N., 48, 50
Nixon, J. C., 7, 10, 99, 100, 124, 136, 160, 161, 196, 357, 372, 377, 378, 381, 394
Nixon, R. F., 174, 199
Noble, W. G., 175, 198
Noffsinger, D., 169, 198, 234, 238, 239, 240, 243, 250, 251, 260, 262, 263, 277, 278, 280–282
Norman, D. A., 40, 52
Norris, J., 316, 318
Northern, J. L., 110, 125, 166, 198
Novak, R. E., 116, 125

Ochs, M. G., 134, 195
O'Conner, J. D., 45, 52
Oelschlaeger, M. L., 257, 282
Ohde, R. N., 48, 52
Ohta, R., 233, 249, 278, 281
Olsen, W., O., 8, 10, 74, 75, 89, 104, 105, 109, 119, 125, 126, 128, 133, 144, 162, 164, 168, 169, 172–175, 184, 198, 201, 238–241, 243, 250, 243, 250, 251, 262, 263, 280–282, 354, 372, 375, 378, 394
Olson, A. E., 214, 227
O'Neill, J. J., 363, 373
Orchik, D. J., 188, 198, 238, 256–258, 277, 282, 346, 351
Ormson, K., 257, 282
Osberger, M. J., 183, 193, 333, 350
Owens, E., 89, 125, 138, 139, 175, 189, 194, 198, 200, 353, 355, 358–362, 367, 371, 373, 376–378, 394, 395
Owens, S. L., 369, 374
Oyer, H. J., 358, 363, 373, 377, 394

Pack, G., 244, 245, 279
Palva, A., 249, 282
Pappas, J., 316, 318
Parker, B., 381, 382, 395
Parker, C., 335, 337, 347, 351
Parker, W., 112, 125
Pascoe, D. P., 133, 188, 198
Pederson, O. J., 182, 199

Pederson, O. T., 137, 199, 357, 373, 378, 394
Penley, E. D., 133, 161, 164, 170, 199
Pennington, C. D., 159, 163, 198, 220, 227, 286, 318
Penrod, J. P., 7, 10, 160, 199
Pestalozza, G., 169, 199
Peterson, B., 156, 196
Peterson, C. E., 211, 226
Peterson, G. E., 35, 45, 52, 132, 138, 197
Peterson, J. L., 104, 124, 183, 196
Phillips, D., 169, 199
Pickett, J. M., 183, 193, 197, 198, 333, 350, 351, 367, 373
Pinheiro, M. L., 235, 239, 244, 247, 254, 255, 261, 262, 281, 282
Pisoni, D. B., 47, 52
Plakke, B., 256, 257
Plomp, R., 383, 392
Pollack, D., 369, 373
Pollack, I., 84, 100, 125, 169, 182, 199, 218, 219, 227, 367, 373
Pollack, M. C., 223, 228
Poole, J., 7, 10, 160, 176, 181, 195, 204, 207, 210–211, 212, 227, 239, 240, 281
Popelka, G., 214, 227, 228
Porter, R. J., 247, 259, 281, 282
Porter, L. S., 111, 123
Posner, J., 224, 228
Pratt, R. L., 385, 394
Preide, V. M., 313, 317–319
Preslar, M. J., 55, 78
Pronovost, W., 145, 199
Prosek, R. A., 333, 344, 346, 351, 352, 355, 366, 374, 377, 379, 395
Proud, G. O., 171, 194
Punch, J. L., 332, 333, 335, 337, 344, 346, 347, 350–352

Quaranta, A., 236, 237, 262, 282
Quiggle, R. R., 111, 112

Rabiner, L. R., 116, 125, 382, 394
Rabinowitz, W. P., 362, 371
Radley, J. P. A., 38, 51
Raffin, M. J. M., 166–168, 171,

Raffin—*continued,* 199, 201, 338, 343, 345, 349, 352, 376, 395
Raica, A. N., 260, 381
Rampp, D. R., 260, 283
Randolph, K. J., 361, 372
Rane, R. L., 204, 214, 226
Raphael, L. J., 47, 50, 379, 392
Redell, R. C., 147, 152, 201
Reed, C., 365, 373, 376, 377, 385, 395
Rees, N. S., 252, 275
Reeves, A. G., 244, 245, 247, 248, 250, 262, 281
Reid, L., 323, 352
Reivich, M., 391-393
Resnick, S., 10, 128-131, 148, 160, 164, 188, 197, 199, 249, 283, 321, 333, 351, 378, 394, 395
Reynolds, E. G., 7, 10, 19, 24, 93, 104, 105, 124, 148, 195, 354, 372
Rintelmann, W. F., 1, 113, 125, 133, 150, 156, 161, 164, 170, 172, 199, 231, 232, 237, 238, 252, 257, 261, 276, 277, 280, 282, 283, 309, 318, 391-393
Ritter, R., 207, 214, 228
Rittmanic, P. A., 183, 199
Robinson, D. W., 206, 228
Robinson, M., 171, 196, 199
Roddy, N., 188, 198, 346, 351
Rodel, M. A. T., 369, 373
Roe, T. G., 161, 199
Roeser, R. J., 246, 282
Rose, D. E., 165, 199, 361, 371
Rosenberg, S., 367, 368, 373
Rosenhamer, H., 238, 280, 388, 394
Rosenquist, A., 391-393
Ross, D. A., 211, 226
Ross, M., 146, 149, 174, 197, 199, 214, 223, 224, 228, 256, 282
Rowe, M. J., 264, 282
Ryan, J. T., 247, 280
Rubens, A. B., 389, 391, 393, 394
Rubenstein, H., 84, 100, 125
Rubin, M., 220, 228
Rupp, R. R., 169, 199
Rzcezkowski, C., 362, 371

Sachs, E., Jr., 244-246, 262, 281
Sachs, R. M., 216, 228, 335, 350

Sahgal, V., 239, 243, 250, 262, 281
Sambataro, C., 169, 199
Sanders, D. A., 357, 363, 364, 359, 373
Sanders, J. W., 113, 125, 175, 199, 286, 287, 293, 298, 317, 318
Sanders, T. R. B., 57, 78
Sanderson-Leepa, M. E., 150, 156, 172, 199, 257, 282
Sawusch, J. R., 48, 52
Schafter, D., 376, 395
Scharf, B., 214, 228, 383, 393, 395
Scharf, D. J., 48, 52
Scherr, C. K., 366, 374
Schmitz, H., 208, 228
Schoeny, Z. G., 250, 262, 282
Schubert, E. D., 7, 10, 89, 125, 135, 136, 138, 139, 160, 161, 175, 194, 196, 198, 200, 354, 357-359, 361, 362, 364, 367, 371-373, 376-378, 381, 394, 395
Schuchman, G. I., 323, 353
Schuknecht, H. F., 183, 200
Schulhoff, C., 246, 282
Schultz, M. C., 89, 125, 354, 358, 373, 378, 395
Schultz, M. D., 135, 200
Schumaier, D. R., 133, 161, 164, 170, 199
Schwartz, D. M., 41, 52, 139, 165, 169, 170, 195, 200, 238, 282, 321, 333, 335, 337, 338, 341-344, 346-348, 351, 352, 355, 366, 373, 374, 377, 379, 395
Schwimmer, S., 237, 277
Scott, B. L., 45, 52, 367, 371
Sedge, R. K., 323, 352
Sergeant, L., 378, 395
Sever, J., 169, 170, 200
Shankweiler, D. P., 44, 46, 49, 51, 52, 233, 247, 282, 283
Shapiro, I., 204, 216, 221, 223, 228
Shapiro, M. T., 169, 170, 200
Shaw, C. K., 164, 197
Shaw, E. A. G., 74, 78, 206, 228
Shepard, D. E., 369, 374
Sher, A. E., 355, 373, 376, 377, 395
Sherman, R. E., 256, 279
Sherrick, G., 316, 318
Shore, I., 169, 200, 338, 344, 352

Shutts, R. E., 164, 192, 200
Siegenthaler, B. M., 146, 159, 194, 200
Silber, E. F., 338, 339, 351
Silverman, S. R., 7, 10, 11, 17-19, 22-24, 85, 93, 104, 105, 124, 126, 128, 132, 140, 148, 173, 190, 193, 195, 200, 207, 208, 211, 212, 228, 354, 361, 372, 373
Sims, D. G., 367, 373
Siqueland, P., 48, 50
Sivian, L. J., 73, 78
Sjören, H., 333, 350
Skinhoj, E., 390, 394
Skinner, M. W., 188, 200
Skinner, P. H., 223, 227, 264, 283
Slosberg, R. M., 129, 130, 199, 333, 351
Small, V., 253, 278
Smiarowski, R. A., 323, 352
Smith, B., 249, 283
Smith, M. J., 205, 226
Snow, J., 232, 261, 283
Snyder, J. M., 113, 125, 308, 309, 318
Sortini, A., 145, 200
Sparks, R., 246, 283
Speaks, C. E., 143, 153, 169, 196, 200, 234, 240, 242, 279, 283, 310, 319, 328, 335, 339, 350, 351, 361, 374, 381, 382, 388, 389, 390, 393-395
Spearman, C., 107, 125
Spencer, R., 317, 319
Sperry, R., 246, 281
Spitzer, J. B., 243, 245, 283
Stach, B., 165, 200
Starr, A., 264, 276, 283
Stein, A., 391, 393
Steinberg, J. C., 11, 24, 90, 91, 112, 123, 124, 128, 182, 194, 333, 350
Steinberg, J. L., 40, 41, 51
Steinberg, J. R., 380, 393
Stephens, S. D., 204, 208, 209, 220, 228
Stevens, K. N., 35, 40, 43-45, 47-52, 142, 196, 362, 372, 379, 381, 385, 392, 393
Stevens, S. S., 15, 16, 24, 85, 91, 92, 104, 105, 113, 124, 207, 211, 221, 226, 229, 306, 318
Stevenson, P. W., 378, 395

Steward, J. L., 55, 78
Stewart, K., 19, 24
Stinson, M., 368, 374
Stowe, A. N., 367, 374
Strange, W., 44, 52
Stream, R. W., 74, 75, 77, 107, 108, 113, 118, 119, 123, 125, 126
Studdert-Kennedy, M., 43, 44, 46, 47, 49, 51, 233, 283, 379, 392
Studebaker, G. A., 137, 148, 156, 196, 199, 286, 287, 292, 293, 298, 307, 309, 312-317, 319, 334-337, 346, 350, 352, 357, 373, 374, 378, 394
Stump, D. A., 390, 395
Summerfield, A. B., 111, 125
Summers, R., 55, 78
Surr, R. K., 41, 52, 139, 170, 200, 355, 373
Sussman, H. M., 47, 50
Suter, A. H., 174, 200
Svihovec, D. V., 85, 100, 133, 135, 161, 192
Swets, J. A., 80-82, 124, 126
Swisher, L. P., 239, 277
Swoboda, P., 103, 126

Talbott, C. B. 358, 373
Talis, H. P., 169, 196
Tarantino, L., 239, 278
Tartter, V. C., 47, 52
Taylor, L., 246, 281
Taylor, P. C., 251, 280
Taylor, W., 249, 277
Telleen, C. C., 367, 373
Thiagarajan, S., 365, 374
Thomas, W. G., 55, 78
Thompson, C. L., 241, 247, 250, 259, 277, 280
Thompson, E. A., 89, 91, 111, 124
Thompson, G., 158, 183, 200
Thorndike, E. L., 132, 138, 143, 144, 200
Thornton, A. R., 166-168, 171, 199, 201, 338, 343, 345, 349, 352, 376, 395
Thurlow, W. R., 17, 19, 24, 85, 126, 173, 200
Tillman, T. W., 8, 10, 41, 52, 74, 78, 84, 100, 104, 105, 119, 124, 126,

Tillman—*continued*, 132, 133, 148, 161, 183, 196, 201, 237, 249, 283, 305–307, 318, 354, 374
Tobey, E. A., 260, 283
Tobias, J. V., 166, 169, 201, 368, 374
Townsend, T. H., 25, 42, 50, 55, 183, 192
Toufexis, A., 391, 395
Trammell, J., 234, 279, 369, 374
Tree, D. R., 216, 226
Treisman, M., 316, 319, 367, 374
Tukey, J. W., 29, 50
Tusa, R., 391, 393
Tyler, R. S., 384, 395

Ullrich, K., 161, 201
Urbantschitsch, V., 11, 24

VanTassell, D. J., 379, 395
Ventry, I. M., 100–102, 104, 113, 123, 126, 204, 217–221, 228, 243, 245, 283
Verbrugge, R. R., 44, 52
Vermeulen, V., 169, 170, 200
Victoreen, J. A., 223, 228
Viehweg, R., 112, 113, 124
Viemeister, N. F., 44, 50
Vigorito, J., 48, 50
Voiers, W. D., 358, 374
Voroba, B., 114, 125

Waldron, D. L., 166, 196
Walden, B. E., 321, 323, 333, 341–344, 346, 349, 351, 352, 355, 356, 366, 374, 377, 379
Wait, D., 369, 374
Wallenfels, H. G., 207, 228
Walsh, T. E., 17–19, 24, 85, 126, 173, 200
Wang, M. D., 89, 122, 356, 371, 376, 377, 392, 395
Wark, D. J., 223, 226
Wathen-Dunn, W., 97, 26
Watson, L. A., 204, 228, 324, 352
Weber, S., 147, 152, 201
Webster, J. C., 376, 395
Wedenberg, E., 369, 374
Wegal, P., 316, 319
Wepman, J., 153, 201
White, E. B., 153, 201
White, E. J., 254, 256, 261, 283

White, R. E. C., 188, 197, 335, 336, 337, 346, 352
White, S. D., 73, 78
Widin, G. P., 44, 50
Wiener, F. M., 182, 193
Wilber, L. A., 1, 10, 41, 52, 55, 62, 78, 132, 201
Wilder, B. J., 239, 278
Wiley, T., 214, 228
Willeford, J., 241, 244, 252–256, 283
Wilner, H. I., 235, 280
Williams, C., 112, 124, 136, 195, 357, 372, 378, 385, 390, 393, 395
Williams, D., 257, 282
Williams, F., 37, 52
Wilson, D. H., 235, 239, 244, 245, 247, 248, 250, 262, 281
Wilson, I. M., 192
Wilson, M. D., 147, 153, 154, 156, 201
Wilson, R. H., 63, 74, 75, 77, 79, 104–108, 113, 117–119, 123, 126, 133, 138, 158, 201, 205, 206, 208, 209, 227, 305–307, 318, 319
Wilson, W. R., 158, 193, 198
Winitz, H., 367, 374
Witlen, R. P., 369, 374
Witt, L. H., 147, 150, 172, 194
Witter, H. L., 332, 352
Wolf, A., 391–393
Wood, C. C., 48, 49, 53
Wood, E. J., 384, 395
Woodcock, R., 146, 194
Woodford, C. M., 214, 227, 228
Woods, R. W., 219, 220, 228
Woodward, M. F., 366, 374
Worthington, D. W., 355, 366, 374

Yanovitz, A., 333, 352
Young, I. M., 183, 195, 317, 319
Young, L., 103, 126, 305, 306, 318

Zaner, A., 204, 227
Zerlin, S., 334, 335, 344, 352
Zwetnow, N., 238, 280, 388, 394
Zwicker, A., 207, 221, 229
Zwicker, E., 383, 393
Zwislocki, J. J., 216, 229, 293, 316, 319, 335, 352

Subject Index

Abbreviated speech recognition tests, 164–168
Accelerated speech, 236–237
Acoustic analyses, of test stimuli and results, 379–380
Acoustic patterns, decoding, 45–49
Acoustic reflex threshold
  loudness discomfort level and, 212–214
  measurement, 263
Adaptation paradigm, 49
Adaptive procedure, preselected performance level determined by, 382
Adaptive testing, for speech recognition assessment, 162–163
Adequate masking, 300
AI, *see* Articulation index
Alternating speech test, 254, 255
American National Standards Institute (ANSI), 57, 58, 59, 62–76, 292
American National Standard Specification for Audiometers, 62, 98
Amplitude cross sections, 96, 97, 98
Amplitude spectrum, 29
"Analysis by Synthesis," 49
Anechoic chamber, 71–72
ANSI, *see* American National Standards Institute
ANT, *see* Auditory Numbers Test
Antiphasic condition, 115–116
Aperiodic sound, 26–27
Approximants, 37
Armed Forces National Research Committee on Hearing and Bioacoustics (CHABA), 22, 140, 188, 361–362, 367
ART, *see* Acoustic reflex threshold
Articulation functions, 234

Articulation index, 380
Articulation testing, 12–13, 14
Attenuation steps, size of, 104
Attenuator linearity, of a speech audiometer, 67–68
Audio cassette tape recordings, 70
Audiometer, 55–56
  calibration, 61–76
  development of, 90–91
  pure tone, 59–61
  speech, 59–61, 63–64
  standards for, 56–59
Auditory brainstem response (ABR), 263–264
Auditory modalities, in phoneme recognition, 365–366
Auditory numbers test (ANT), 147, 151–152
Auditory perceptual problems, in children, 251–261
Auditory skills curriculum, 370
Auditory Skills Instructional Planning System, 369
Auditory training, 11, 363–364
  for children, 364–370
Aural rehabilitation, 131, 189
  continuous speech and, 368
  equipment innovation for, 368–369
  for children, 369–370
  phoneme recognition and, 364–365
  sentences and, 367
    context in, 367–368
  speech recognition and, 190, 353
    phoneme recognition and, 355–356
    phoneme recognition within words, 357–359
    self-report scales and, 362–363
    sentence test and, 359–362
    word recognition and, 354–355
  tracking, 367

Subject Index

Azimuth position, recognition threshold for spondaic words and, 118–119
  see also Loudspeaker, location of

Binaural tests
  for central auditory nervous system disorders, 233, 241–251
  filtered speech, 242, 248–249
  fusion, 242, 254, 255
Binomial characteristics, of speech recognition tests, 166–168
BKB-PR, see Picture-related BKB sentence list for children
BKB sentence test (BKB-ST), 147, 154, 155
Blood flow, in functional brain activity, 390–391
Bone conduction, speech recognition by, 171
Bone conduction pure tone audiometer, 309, 310
Bone conduction speech audiometry, 295, 307
  masking and, 311
Brainstem evoked response (BSER), 263–264
Brainstem lesions, patients with, 274–275
Broadband noise, 169, 303
BSER, see Brainstem evoked response

Calibration, 56
  of audiometer, 61–76
California consonant test (CCT), 138–140, 189, 359, 360, 378
CANS, see Central auditory nervous system (CANS)
Carrier phrase, in speech recognition, 159
Categorical perception, 43–44
CCT, see California consonant test
Central auditory nervous system (CANS)
  assessment of function, 387–392
  disorders, 231–234, 275–276, 389
    auditory perceptual problems in children, 251–261

  binaural tests for, 233, 241–251
  cases illustrating, 264–275
  monaural tests for, 233, 234–241
  nonspeech measures for, 261–264
Central Institute for the Deaf (CID), 15, 19, 131–132, 140–142
  Everyday Sentence Test, 22
  sentence lists, 238
    revised, 238
  W-1 test, 83, 102
  W-2 test, 93, 105
  W-22 test, 22, 132, 135, 148, 156, 188, 354, 355, 358
    error analysis of, 378
    split-half reliability for the, 164–165
    10-word speech recognition test from, 165
Central masking, 316–317
Cerebral function, 390–392
CHABA, see Armed Forces National Research Committee on Hearing and Bio-Acoustics
Children
  auditory perceptual problems in, 251–261
  auditory training for, 369–370
  speech recognition assessment among, 144–159
Children's Perception of Speech (CHIPS), 147
CID, see Central Institute for the Deaf
Closed nonsense syllable test, error analysis of, 378
Closed response speech test, error analysis of, 378
Closed set, 190
Closed-set response, 163
Closed-set response monosyllabic test, 135–140, 378
Cochlea, disorders of the, 176–177, 184–187
Committee on Hearing and Bio-Acoustics, Armed Forces National Research (CHABA), 22, 140, 188, 361–362, 367
Competing message (speech), 239
  connected speech as, 5
  speech recognition assessment using, 168–171

Subject Index

Competing sentence test, 241, 244, 253–254
Computer generated stimuli, for auditory processing, 388
Conditioned orienting response (COR), 110
Conditioned techniques, 110
Conductive hearing loss, 176, 180–181
Connected speech, 5–6
Consonants, 36–38
  duration of, 40
  frequency of, 39–40
  recognition, 358–359
  speech perception and, 45
Consonant-vowel syllable test, 241, 247–248, 259–260
Context, in facilitating sentence understanding, 367–368
Continuous noise, in speech recognition assessment, 169–171
Continuous speech, 38
  in aural rehabilitation, 368
Contralateral masking, 286–287
  clinical applications of, 302–317
  functions, 295–302
  rationale for, 287–295
Contralateral paradigm, 288, 289
Coupler, 64, 65
Crest factor, 96–97
Criteria for Permissible Ambient Noise During Audiometric Testing, 76
Cross hearing, 285–286
  see also Contralateral masking
"Cross masking," 295
CVs, *see* Consonant-vowel syllable test

Detection threshold, 15, 82–86, 111
Diagnosis, speech recognition and, 175–187, 190
Dichotic listening tasks, 388
Digitized speech, for aural rehabilitation, 369
Digits, auditory test employing, 245–247
Diotic listening condition, *see* Binaural tests
DIP, *see* Discrimination by Identification of Pictures

Discomfort, *see* Loudness discomfort level
Discrimination, 17, 18–19, 89, 363
  of phonemes, 365
Discrimination by Identification of Pictures (DIP), 146
Distortion
  intensity and, 42
  speech audiometer and, 68

Earphone
  audiometer output directed to, 64–70
  measurements, 70
  reference sound pressure level for, 67
Effective gain, of a hearing aid, 323
Effective masking level (EML), 296–297
  contralateral masking and, 312–316
  for masker, 304–307
Efficiency in noise, of a hearing aid, 324, 326–327
Electropsysiologic responses, to speech, 386–387
EML, *see* Effective masking level
Error analyses, responses to test materials, 376–378
Everyday speech sentences, 361–362, 367

Familiarity, with spondees, 100–102
Far ear, 117–118
Feature detectors, in speech perception, 47–48
Fenestration operation, 18–19
Filtered speech
  low-pass, 41, 254
  tasks, 235–236
"Filtering effect," 183
Filters, spectrum obtained by, 29–30, 31
First-order sentential approximations, 238
Five Sound Test, 147, 157–158
Flowers-Costello test of central auditory abilities, 253
Formula approach, for appropriate masking levels, 313–316

Subject Index

4C test, 14
Free field, 71, 73
Frequency, speech perception and, 40–41
Frequency pattern perception test, *see* Pitch pattern perception test
Frequency resolution, 383–384
Frequency response, 65
   for speech audiometers, 65–66
Fricatives, 37
Fusions, in response to dichotic speech stimuli, 388–389

Gap detection experiments, temporal resolution by, 384–385
GFW, *see* Goldman-Fristoe-Woodstock Test of Auditory Discrimination
Goldman-Fristoe-Woodstock Test of Auditory Discrimination (GFW), 146
Griffiths' rhyming minimal contrasts test lists, error analysis of, 378

Half list testing, 164–168
Handicap scales, speech recognition assessment and, 190
Head shadow effect, 118
Hearing aid evaluation, 348–350
   Carhart method, 186–187, 322–327
   Jerger and Hayes method, 327–331
   loudness discomfort level for, 204
   most comfortable loudness level for, 204, 217, 223–225
   noise background and, 171
   nonsense syllable test for, 129–130, 131, 356
   objective strategies for, 322–331
   reliability of method of, 337–348
   saturation sound pressure level for, 214–217
   speech recognition measures for, 187–189, 190
   subjective strategies for, 331–337
   reliability of, 346–348
Hearing-aid-processed speech, intelligibility and, 334–337, 346–348

Hearing loss
   central auditory nervous system and, 389, 390
   loudness discomfort level and, 211–212
   most comfortable loudness level and, 221–223
   shape of, 182–183
   speech recognition and, 181–183
Hearing performance inventory (HPI), 362–363
HF lists, *see* High frequency lists
High frequency lists (HF), 133–135, 188
Homogeneity
   for intelligibility, 5
   spondees and, 100–104
Homophasic condition, 115
HPI, *see* Hearing performance inventory

Identification tests
   of phonemes, 365
   variability in performance, 376
IEC Artificial Ear, of the Wide Band Type for the Calibration of Earphones Used in Audiometry, An, 70
Infants, feature detectors in, 48
Inhalation technique, for functional brain activity, 390–391
Instructions, loudness discomfort level reliability and, 207–208
Intelligibility, 89
   hearing-aid-processed speech and, 334–337, 346–348
   homogeneity for, 5
   intensity and, 41–42
   neurograms and, 387
   spondees and, 100–102
   threshold of, 15–17
Intelligibility functions, 234
Intelligibility test, 12–13, 14
Intensity, speech perception and, 41–42
Intensity level, of speech recognition tests, 161
   for children, 172

Interaural attenuation
  definition of, 310
  masking and, 291-295
  value, 308-309
International Kindergarten
  Vocabulary list, 145
Intracranial tumors, word recognition
  ability and, 112-113
Invariance, in speech signal, 46-47
Ipsilateral masking functions, 296, 307
Ipsilateral masking paradigm, 296, 298
Ipsilateral paradigm, 288, 289
"Isophonemic" word lists, 133
  error analysis of, 378

Kent State University (KSU) test, 361

LDL, *see* Loudness discomfort level
Learning disabled, auditory perceptual problems and, 251-261
Liquid glides, 356
Listener responses
  recording, 8
  types of, 6-7
Listening check, of the audiometer, 63
Live voice techniques
  monitored, 160, 161
  for speech testing, 7-8
Long-time spectral average, 39
Loudness discomfort level (LDL), 203-205
  clinical use of, 212-217
  hearing loss and, 211-212
  of a hearing aid, 323
  reliability, 207-210
  for speech, 210-211
  validity of, 205-207
  see also Most comfortable loudness level
Loudness level, for speech recognition materials, 161-162
Loudspeaker, 71
  location of and spondee recognition threshold, 116-119
  see also Sound field speech audiometry
Low cut-off frequency, for hearing aid evaluation, 333
Low-pass filtered speech, 41, 254

MAF, *see* Minimal audible field
MAP, *see* Minimal audible pressure
Masked threshold, 383
Maskee, 288
Masker, 288
Masking, 168-169, 286
  central, 316-317
  definition of, 288-291
  functions, 295-302
  levels, 312-316
  speech audiometer and, 68-69, 71
  speech recognition and, 183-184
  speech recognition threshold and, 113
  when to do, 307-312
  see also Contralateral masking
Masking dilemma, 302
Masking level difference (MLD), 113-116
  pure tone task and, 262-263
  for speech, 250-251
Maximum masking level, 301, 302
MCDT, *see* Multiple choice discrimination test
MCL, *see* Most Comfortable loudness level
Metabolic activity, in the cortex, 391-392
Microprocessors, for aural rehabilitation, 368-369
Minimal audible field (MAF), 73-75
Minimal audible pressure (MAP), 73-75
Minimal brain dysfunction, auditory perceptual problems, 251-261
Minimum audible field, 119
Minimum audible pressure, 119
Minimum masking level, 297-298, 300-301, 302
MLD, *see* Masking level differences
Modified rhyme hearing test (MRHT), 136-137, 161, 165
Modified rhyme test (MRT), 136, 238, 357, 378

Subject Index

Monaural tests, for central auditory nervous system disorders, 233–241
Monitored live voice, in speech recognition test, 160, 161
Monosyllabic words
  for hearing assessment, 3
  speech recognition by, 190
    in children, 144–145, 149–152
    closed-set response, 135–140
    open-set response and, 130–135
Most comfortable loudness (MCL) level, 137, 161, 203–205
  clinical use of, 223–225
  hearing loss and, 221–223
  reliability, 218–220
  stimulus effects and, 220–221
  validity, 217–218
MRHT, see Modified rhyme hearing test
MRT, see Modified rhyme test
Multiple choice discrimination test (MCDT), 135–136
  error analysis of, 378
Multiple-choice test
  for speech recognition, 135–137, 138–139, 145
  for word recognition, 358–359
Myatt and Landes test, 149

Nasality, 357, 364
Nasals, 37, 45
National Bureau of Standards, coupler and, 64, 65
National Research Council Committee on Hearing and Bioacoustics, Armed Forces (CHABA), 22, 140, 188, 361–362, 367
Near ear, 117–118
Neural coding, of speech, 386–387
Noise
  audiometer and, 68
  in an audiometric test room, 76
  in contralateral masking, 303–304
  prose presented with, 381–382
  speech recognition and, 174, 184
  speech recognition assessment using, 168–171
  speech understanding in, 386–387

Nonsense syllables
  identification of, 379
  in phoneme recognition, 355–356
  speech recognition assessment and, 128–130, 190
Nonsense syllable test (NST), 3, 129–130, 131, 133, 148, 157, 333
Nonspeech measures, for central auditory nervous system disorders, 261–264
Northwestern University
  auditory test #2, 241, 243
  auditory test #4, 132
  auditory test #6 (NU #6), 132–133, 137, 140, 148, 150, 153, 156, 160, 161, 180, 188, 237, 238, 257, 309, 354, 355
  error analysis of, 378
  hearing aid evaluation, 338–339
  split-half reliability for, 164–165
  10-word speech recognition test from, 165
  auditory test #20 (NU #20), 241, 243–244
  children's perception of speech test (NU-CHIPS), 149–150
NST, see Nonsense syllable test

Oklahoma University Closed Response Test (OUCRT), 148
Open-ended set of test materials, errors from an, 377
Open-response design, for speech recognition assessment, 144–145
Open set, 190
Open-set monosyllabic lists, 130–135
OUCRT, see Oklahoma University Closed Response Test
Overmasking, 300

Paired-comparison subjective approach, for hearing aid evaluation, 331–332
PAL, see Psycho-Acoustic Laboratory
PAL PB-50, 130–132, 135, 144, 145, 325

Pascoe high frequency (PHF), 133–135
PBF, *see* Phonetically balanced familiar lists
PB-50, PAL, 130–132, 135, 144, 145, 325
PB-500, 156
PBK-50, *see* Phonetically balanced kindergarten list
PB Max, 18, 22–23, 160
Pediatric speech intelligibility test, 147, 155–156
Perception, *see* Speech perception
Perception of Words and Word Patterns, 147
Performance-intensity (PI) function, 184–185, 187, 234–235, 310
  in speech recognition assessment, 161–162
Periodic sound, 27, 28, 29, 30
PET, *see* Position emission tomography
PHF, *see* Pascoe high frequency word list
Phonemes, 40
  intensities of, 38, 39
  recognition
    in aural recognition, 364–366
    for aural rehabilitation, 355–359, 364–365
Phonemic balance, 166
Phonetically balanced familiar lists (PBF), 144
Phonetically balanced kindergarten list (PBK-50), 145, 146, 150, 257, 258
Phonetically balanced monosyllables, 184–187
Phonetically balanced (PB) word lists, 234
  PAL PB 50, 130–132, 135, 144, 145, 325
Phonetic balance, 17–18
Phonetic feature fusion, 389
PI, *see* Performance-intensity function
Picture identification task (PIT), 138
Picture-pointing speech recognition task, 145, 149–150
Picture-related BKB sentence lists for children (BKB-PR), 154

PIT, *see* Picture identification task
Pitch pattern test, 255, 261
Position emission tomography (PET), 391
Presentation mode, 109
  for speech recognition assessment, 159–163
  for subjects difficult to test, 109–110
Programmed instruction
  in auditory rehabilitation, 370
  for aural rehabilitation, 368–369
  for phoneme recognition, 361–365
  for sentence materials, 367
Prose, in a noise background, 381–382
Psycho-Acoustic Laboratories (PAL), 15, 16, 17, 21, 91–93, 128–129, 130–132
  auditory test No. 9, 16, 91–92, 93, 105
  auditory test No. 12, 92
  auditory test No. 14, 92
  PAL-8 sentences, 361
  PAL-PB, 130–132, 135, 144, 145, 325
Psychometric function, 79–82
Psychophysical method, loudness discomfort level reliability and, 208–210
Psychophysical tuning curves, 383–384
PTA, *see* Pure tone audiometry
Pure tone audiometer, 59–61
Pure tone audiometry (PTA), 1, 308
  bone conduction, 309, 310
  techniques, 2
Pure tone masking level difference task, 262–263
Pure tone stimuli, for conditioned techniques, 110
Pure tone thresholds, 111, 383–384
  speech recognition threshold and, 121

QUAH, *see* Quantification of the auditory handicap
Quality judgments, hearing aid evaluation by, 332–334

Subject Index

Quantification of the auditory handicap (QUAH), 174
Questionnaires, for quantification of a hearing handicap, 175

Radioactive material, brain activity studied with, 390
Rapidly alternating speech perception test (RASP), 242, 249–250, 255
RASP, see Rapidly alternating speech perception test
Reaction time, for responses to speech stimuli, 385–386
Recognition, 89
Recognition thresholds, 82–86, 111
Recorded materials, on speech recognition test, 160, 161
Reference sound pressure level, 73
  of a speech audiometer, 66–67
Response mode, 105, 109–110
  subjects difficult to test and, 109–110
Responses, see Listener responses
Resynthesis task, 242
Retrocochlear lesions, assessment of, 239
Reverberation, speech understanding and, 376
Revised CID sentence lists, 238
Rhyme test, 357
Rhyming minimal contrasts, error analysis of, 378
RI, see Rollover index
"Rollover effect," 185, 234–235
Rollover index (RI), 185–186

SAI, see Social adequacy index
Saturation sound pressure level (SSPL), 204
  loudness discomfort level and, 214–217
SE, see Single elimination tournament strategy
Segmentation, speech signal and, 46
Self-report scales, in aural rehabilitation, 362–363
Sensorineural hearing loss, 176
Sentence recognition score, 89

Sentences
  in aural rehabilitation, 359, 361–362, 367–368
  everyday speech, 361–362, 367
  for hearing assessment, 5, 188
  loudness discomfort level for, 211
  speech recognition assessment by, 140–144, 190
    in adults, 140–144
    in children, 152–157
  see also Synthetic sentence(s)
Sentential approximation, see Synthetic sentences
Sequential testing, see Adaptive testing
SERT, see Sound effects recognition test
Shadowing techniques, see Threshold shift
Sibilance, 356
Signal-to-noise (S/N) ratio, 381, 382
  for hearing aids, 324
Single elimination (SE) tournament strategy, 335–337
S/N ratio, see Signal-to-noise ratio
Social adequacy of hearing
  assessment of, 19–22
  social adequacy index for, 173–174, 354–355
  speech recognition and, 190
Social adequacy index (SAI), 173–174, 354–355
Social efficiency, speech-recognition tests estimating, 173–175
Sonorance, 364
Sonorants, 356, 357
Sound, analysis of, 27–33
Sound effects recognition test (SERT), 146, 158–159
Sound field speech audiometry, 71–73, 116–119
  calibration guidelines for, 73–76
Spearman-Kärber method, 107–109
Spectrograms, 31–33, 46
  speech, 96, 97
Spectrum, 29–31
  average, 39
  level, 80
  of vowels, 34, 36
Speech, neural transmission of, 386–387

Subject Index 415

Speech audiometer, 59-61, 63-64
  see also Audiometer
Speech awareness threshold, 88
  see also Speech detection threshold
Speech detection threshold, 87
Speech discrimination, see Speech recognition
"Speech frequencies," 112
Speech mode, 43-45
Speech-in-noise tasks, 239-240
Speech perception, 40-42
  models of perception, 49-50
  problems in children, 251-261
  processing, 42-48
Speech perception in noise (SPIN) test, 141, 142, 148, 156-157, 362
Speech reception threshold, 88, 89
  historical perspective, 91
Speech recognition, 127
  assessment, 163-164
  materials
    for adults, 128-144
    for children, 144-159
  procedural strategies in, 159-173
  score, 89
  tests
    binomial characteristics of, 166-168
    clinical utilization of, 173-191
  see also Aural rehabilitation
Speech recognition threshold, 109
  derivation, 107-109
  determinants of, 111-119
  estimation of the, 106-107
  evaluation, 119-122
  presentation mode in, 103-105
  protocol, 105-106
  pure tone thresholds and, 111-113
  response mode, 105
  sound field in, 116-119
Speech signals, analyzing, 33-40
Speech sounds
  composition of, 26-27
  frequency content of, 38-39
Speech spectrograms, 96, 97
Speech spectrum noise, in contralateral masking, 304-305
Speech stimuli, 2-3
  loudness discomfort level for, 210-211

  mechanism assessment and perspective of, 89-93
  most comfortable loudness level and, 220-221
  physical characteristics of, 97-105
  types of, 306
SPIN, see Speech perception in noise test
Spondaic words, see Spondees
Spondee Recognition Test, 147
Spondees
  auditory thresholds established by, 91-95
  effective masking level obtained with, 304-306
  familiarity with, 100-102
  for hearing assessment, 4-5
  homogeneity, 100-104
  information content, 99, 100
  intelligibility, 100-102
  loudness discomfort level for, 211
  masking level difference for, 113-116
  physical characteristics of, 97-105
  presentation mode, 103-105
  redundancy, 99, 100
  response modes with, 105
  speech recognition assessment in children, 150-151
SSI, see Synthetic sentence identification (SSI) test
SSIC, see Synthetic sentence identification for children test
SSI-CCM, see Synthetic sentence identification-contralateral competing message test
SSI-ICM, see Synthetic sentence identification-ipsilateral competing message task
SSPL, see Saturation sound pressure level
Staggered spondaic word (SSW) test, 241, 244-245, 255, 256
Standardization, audiometers and, 56-59
Stops, 37-38
  recognition, 45-46
Suprathreshold speech audiometric measures, masking and, 309-310, 311
Swinging speech test, 249

Syllables, 44–45
　consonant-vowel syllable test, 241, 247–248
　for hearing assessment, 3
　recognition score, 89
Synthetic sentence identification for children (SSIC) test, 147, 153–154
Synthetic sentence identification-contralateral competing message (SSI-CCM) test, 241, 242–243
Synthetic sentence identification-ipsilateral competing message (SSI-ICM) task, 240–241
Synthetic sentence identification (SSI) test, 141, 143–144, 156, 188, 240, 310, 328
　hearing aid evaluation and, 338–339
Synthetic sentences, 258
Synthetic stimuli, for central auditory nervous system function, 388–389

TAC, *see* Test of auditory comprehension
Tangible reinforcement operant conditioning assessment (TROCA), 110
Temporal resolution, 384–385
Test of auditory comprehension (TAC), 369
Third-order sentential approximations, 238
Threshold, 15–17
　definition, 79, 80
　detection experiment and, 82
　of discomfort or tolerance, *see* Loudness discomfort level
　estimating the, 105–109
　historical perspective, 89–93
　masked, 383
　measurement, 93–110, 308–309
　psychometric function and, 79–82
　pure tone, 111–113, 383–384
　recognition experiment and, 82
　of social adequacy, 173–174
　speech detection, 82–88
　speech reception, 88, 89
　speech recognition, 82–87
　unmasked, 383
　see also Speech recognition threshold
Threshold of audibility, 88
　see also Speech detection threshold
Threshold difference, 81–82
Threshold shift, for appropriate masking level, 312–313
Time-compressed speech tests, 236–239, 257–258
Tolerance limit, of a hearing aid, 323–324
Tracking, an aural rehabilitation, 367
Transverse interhemispheric auditory tracts, lesions involving the, 273–274
True sensory threshold, 80
Two-choice response tests, 358

Uncomfortable loudness level, *see* Loudness discomfort level
Undermasking, 300
Undistorted speech tests, for central auditory nervous system disorders, 234–235
University of Oklahoma closed response speech test (UOCRST), 137–138, 156
UOCRST, *see* University of Oklahoma closed response speech test
Up-down transformed response testing, *see* Adaptive testing

Verbal-recall response mode, 105
Visually reinforced infant speech discrimination (VRISD), 158
Visual modalities, in phoneme recognition, 365–366
Visual reinforcement audiometry (VRA), 110
Voice onset time (VOT), 47, 48, 49
Voicing, 356
Voicing differences, 364
Volume measurements of Electrical Speech and Program Waves, 69
Volume unit (VU) meter, 60, 61, 98–99

deflection, 98–99
speech audiometer, 69–70
VOT, *see* Voice onset time
Vowels
 frequency and, 39–40
 production of, 33–36
 recognition of, 358–359
 speech perception and, 45
VRISD, *see* Visually reinforced infant speech discrimination
VU, *see* Volume unit meter

Waveform, 27–29
Willeford test battery, 254–255, 256

WIPI, *see* Word intelligibility by picture identification test
Word discrimination in quiet, of a hearing aid, 324–325
Word intelligibility by picture identification (WIPI), 146, 147, 149, 150, 152, 153, 256–258
Word recognition tests
 for aural rehabilitation, 354–355
 for hearing aid evaluation, 338–339
 variability in performance, 376
World War II, speech audiometry and, 11, 14–18, 91–93, 131